1998
YEAR BOOK OF
HAND SURGERY®

Statement of Purpose

The YEAR BOOK Service

The YEAR BOOK series was devised in 1901 by practicing health professionals who observed that the literature of medicine and related disciplines had become so voluminous that no one individual could read and place in perspective every potential advance in a major specialty. In the final decade of the 20th century, this recognition is more acutely true than it was in 1901.

More than merely a series of books, YEAR BOOK volumes are the tangible results of a unique service designed to accomplish the following:

- to *survey* a wide range of journals of proven value
- to *select* from those journals papers representing significant advances and statements of important clinical principles
- to provide *abstracts* of those articles that are readable, convenient summaries of their key points
- to provide *commentary* about those articles to place them in perspective.

These publications grow out of a unique process that calls on the talents of outstanding authorities in clinical and fundamental disciplines, trained literature specialists, and professional writers, all supported by the resources of Mosby, the world's preeminent publisher for the health professions.

The Literature Base

Mosby and its editors survey more than 1,000 journals published worldwide, covering the full range of the health professions. On an annual basis, the publisher examines usage patterns and polls its expert authorities to add new journals to the literature base and to delete journals that are no longer useful as potential YEAR BOOK sources.

The Literature Survey

The publisher's team of literature specialists, all of whom are trained and experienced health professionals, examines every original, peer-reviewed article in each journal issue. More than 250,000 articles per year are scanned systematically, including title, text, illustrations, tables, and references. Each scan is compared, article by article, to the search strategies that the publisher has developed in consultation with the 270 outside experts who form the pool of YEAR BOOK editors. A given article may be reviewed by any number of editors, from one to a dozen or more, regardless of the discipline for which the paper was originally published. In turn, each editor who receives the article reviews it to determine whether the article should be included in the YEAR BOOK. This decision is based on the article's inherent quality, its probable usefulness to readers of that YEAR BOOK, and the editor's goal to represent a balanced picture of a given field in each volume of the YEAR BOOK. In addition, the editor indicates when to include figures and tables from the article to help the YEAR BOOK reader better understand the information.

Of the quarter million articles scanned each year, only 5% are selected for detailed analysis within the YEAR BOOK series, thereby assuring readers of the high value of every selection.

The Abstract

The publisher's abstracting staff is headed by a seasoned medical professional and includes individuals with training in the life sciences, medicine, and other areas, plus extensive experience in writing for the health professions and related industries. Each selected article is assigned to a specific writer on this abstracting staff. The abstracter, guided in many cases by notations supplied by the expert editor, writes a structured, condensed summary designed so that the reader can rapidly acquire the essential information contained in the article.

The Commentary

The YEAR BOOK editorial boards, sometimes assisted by guest commentators, write comments that place each article in perspective for the reader. This provides the reader with the equivalent of a personal consultation with a leading international authority—an opportunity to better understand the value of the article and to benefit from the authority's thought processes in assessing the article.

Additional Editorial Features

The editorial boards of each YEAR BOOK organize the abstracts and comments to provide a logical and satisfying sequence of information. To enhance the organization, editors also provide introductions to sections or individual chapters, comments linking a number of abstracts, citations to additional literature, and other features.

The published YEAR BOOK contains enhanced bibliographic citations for each selected article, including extended listings of multiple authors and identification of author affiliations. Each YEAR BOOK contains a Table of Contents specific to that year's volume. From year to year, the Table of Contents for a given YEAR BOOK will vary depending on developments within the field.

Every YEAR BOOK contains a list of the journals from which papers have been selected. This list represents a subset of the more than 1,000 journals surveyed by the publisher and occasionally reflects a particularly pertinent article from a journal that is not surveyed on a routine basis.

Finally, each volume contains a comprehensive subject index and an index to authors of each selected paper.

The 1998 Year Book Series

Year Book of Allergy, Asthma, and Clinical Immunology: Drs. Rosenwasser, Borish, Gelfand, Leung, Nelson, and Szefler

Year Book of Anesthesiology and Pain Management®: Drs. Tinker, Abram, Chestnut, Roizen, Rothenberg, and Wood

Year Book of Cardiology®: Drs. Schlant, Collins, Gersh, Graham, Kaplan, and Waldo

Year Book of Chiropractic®: Dr. Lawrence

Year Book of Critical Care Medicine®: Drs. Parrillo, Balk, Calvin, Franklin, and Shapiro

Year Book of Dentistry®: Drs. Meskin, Berry, Jeffcoat, Leinfelder, Roser, Summitt, and Zakariasen

Year Book of Dermatologic Surgery®: Drs. Greenway, Papadopoulos, Whitaker, and Barrett

Year Book of Dermatology®: Dr. Thiers

Year Book of Diagnostic Radiology®: Drs. Osborn, Groskin, Dalinka, Maynard, Pentecost, Rebner, Ros, Smirniotopoulos, and Young

Year Book of Drug Therapy®: Drs. Lasagna and Weintraub

Year Book of Emergency Medicine®: Drs. Wagner, Dronen, Davidson, King, Niemann, and Roberts

Year Book of Endocrinology®: Drs. Bagdade, Braverman, Horton, Kannan, Landsberg, Molitch, Morley, Nathan, Odell, Poehlman, Rogol, and Ryan

Year Book of Family Practice®: Drs. Berg, Bowman, Davidson, Dexter, and Scherger

Year Book of Gastroenterology®: Drs. Aliperti and Fleshman

Year Book of Geriatrics and Gerontology®: Drs. Beck, Burton, Ostwald, Rabins, Reuben, Roth, Shapiro, and Whitehouse

Year Book of Hand Surgery®: Drs. Amadio and Hentz

Year Book of Hematology®: Drs. Spivak, Bell, Ness, Quesenberry, Wiernik, and Horowitz

Year Book of Infectious Diseases: Drs. Keusch, Barza, Bennish, Poutsiaka, Skolnik, and Snydman

Year Book of Medicine®: Drs. Klahr, Cline, McCallum, Frishman, Utiger, Malawista, Mandell, and Jett

Year Book of Neonatal and Perinatal Medicine®: Drs. Fanaroff, Maisels, and Stevenson

Year Book of Nephrology, Hypertension, and Mineral Metabolism: Drs. Schwab, Bennett, Emmett, Hostetter, Kuman, and Toto

Year Book of Neurology and Neurosurgery®: Drs. Bradley and Gibbs

Year Book of Nuclear Medicine®: Drs. Gottschalk, Blaufox, Neumann, Strauss, and Zubal

Year Book of Obstetrics, Gynecology, and Women's Health: Drs. Mishell, Herbst, and Kirschbaum

Year Book of Occupational and Environmental Medicine®: Drs. Emmett, Frank, Gochfeld, and Hessl

Year Book of Oncology®: Drs. Ozols, Eisenberg, Glatstein, Loehrer, Tallman, and Wiersma

Year Book of Ophthalmology®: Drs. Wilson, Augsburger, Cohen, Eagle, Grossman, Laibson, Maguire, Nelson, Penne, Rapuano, Sergott, Spaeth, Tipperman, Ms. Gosfield, and Ms. Salmon

Year Book of Orthopedics®: Drs. Morrey, Beauchamp, Currier, Tolo, Trigg, Swiontkowski

Year Book of Otolaryngology–Head and Neck Surgery®: Drs. Paparella and Holt

Year Book of Pathology and Laboratory Medicine: Drs. Raab, Cohen, Olson, Sirgi, and Stanley

Year Book of Pediatrics®: Dr. Stockman

Year Book of Plastic, Reconstructive, and Aesthetic Surgery®: Drs. Miller, Bartlett, Garner, McKinney, Ruberg, Salisbury, and Smith

Year Book of Psychiatry and Applied Mental Health®: Drs. Talbott, Ballanger, Frances, Lydiard, Meltzer, Schowalter, and Tasman

Year Book of Pulmonary Disease®: Drs. Jett, Maurer, Ryu, Strollo, and Wenzel

Year Book of Rheumatology®: Drs. Panush, Hadler, LeRoy, Liang, Reichlin, Simon, and Weinblatt

Year Book of Sports Medicine®: Drs. Shephard, Drinkwater, Eichner, Torg, Alexander, and Mr. George

Year Book of Surgery®: Drs. Copeland, Bland, Deitch, Eberlein, Howard, Luce, Seeger, Souba, and Sugarbaker

Year Book of Thoracic and Cardiovascular Surgery®: Drs. Ginsberg, Wechsler, and Williams

Year Book of Urology®: Drs. Andriole and Coplen

Year Book of Vascular Surgery®: Dr. Porter

1998
The Year Book of HAND SURGERY®

Editors
Peter C. Amadio, M.D.
Vincent R. Hentz, M.D.

Editors Emeritus
Robert A. Chase, M.D.
James H. Dobyns, M.D.

International Assistant Editors
Massimo Ceruso, M.D.
Guy Foucher, M.D.
Seiichi Ishii, M.D.
Priv.-Doz. Dr. Med. C.L. Jantea
Caroline LeClercq, M.D.
Alberto Lluch, M.D., Ph.D.
Yasuo Ueba, M.D.

Mosby

St. Louis Baltimore Boston Carlsbad Naples New York Philadelphia Portland London
Madrid Mexico City Singapore Sydney Tokyo Toronto Wiesbaden

Mosby
Dedicated to Publishing Excellence

A Times Mirror
Company

Publisher: Theresa Van Schaik
Developmental Editor: Jaime Chatman
Manuscript Editor: Stephanie M. Geels
Production Assistant: Laura Bayless
Manager, Literature Services: Idelle L. Winer
Illustrations and Permissions Coordinator: Chidi C. Ukabam

1998 EDITION

Printed in the United States of America
Composition by Reed Technology and Information Services, Inc.
Printing/binding by Maple-Vail

Editorial Office:
Mosby, Inc.
11830 Westline Industrial Drive
St. Louis, MO 63146

International Standard Serial Number: 0739–5949
International Standard Book Number: 0–8151–0163–5

Editors

Peter C. Amadio, M.D.

Professor of Orthopedic Surgery, Mayo Medical School; Consultant, Department of Orthopedics and Surgery of the Hand, Mayo Clinic, Rochester, Minnesota

Vincent R. Hentz, M.D.

Professor of Surgery and Chief, Division of Hand Surgery, Stanford University School of Medicine, Stanford, California

Editors Emeritus

Robert A. Chase, M.D.

Emile Holman Professor of Surgery and Anatomy, Emeritus, Stanford University School of Medicine, Stanford, California

James H. Dobyns, M.D.

Emeritus Professor of Orthopedic Surgery, Mayo Foundation, Rochester, Minnesota; Clinical Professor, University of Texas Health Science Center, San Antonio, Texas

International Assistant Editors

Massimo Ceruso, M.D.

Hand Surgery and Reconstructive Microsurgery Department, Azienda Ospedaliera Careggi—Università degli Studi di Firenze, Centro Traumatologico Ortopedico, Firenze, Italia

Guy Foucher, M.D.

Chirurgien, Strasbourg, France

Seiichi Ishii, M.D.

Professor of Orthopedic Surgery, Sapporo Medical University, Sapporo, Japan

Priv.-Doz. Dr. Med. C.L. Jantea

Upper Limb Service, Orthopaedic Department, Heinrich-Heine-University Dusseldorf, Dusseldorf, Germany

Caroline LeClercq, M.D.

Ancien Chef de Clinique, Assistante des Hospitaux de Paris, Institut de la Main, Paris, France

Alberto Lluch, M.D., Ph.D.

Assistant Professor of Orthopedic Surgery, University of Barcelona, Institut Kaplan for Surgery of the Hand and Upper Extremity, Barcelona, Spain

Yasuo Ueba, M.D.

Professor, Division of Occupational Therapy, College of Medical Technology, Kyoto University, Kyoto, Japan

Contributing Editors

Marie A. Badalamente, Ph.D.
State University of New York, Stonybrook, New York

Robert D. Beckenbaugh, M.D.
Professor of Orthopedic Surgery, Mayo Medical School; Consultant, Department of Orthopedics and Surgery of the Hand, Mayo Clinic, Rochester, Minnesota

Keith Bengtson, M.D.
Consultant in the Department of Physical Medicine and Rehabilitation, Mayo Medical Center, Rochester, Minnesota

Richard A. Berger, M.D., Ph.D.
Associate Professor of Orthopedic Surgery and Anatomy, Mayo Medical School; Consultant, Departments of Orthopedics, Surgery of the Hand, and Anatomy, Mayo Clinic, Rochester, Minnesota

Gabrielle Bergman, M.D.
Assistant Professor of Radiology, Stanford University Hospital, Stanford, California

Thomas H. Berquist, M.D.
Professor of Radiology, Mayo Medical School; Chair, Department of Diagnostic Radiology, Mayo Clinic, Jacksonville, Florida

Charles Burgar, M.D.
Assistant Professor of Functional Restoration, Stanford University Hospital, Stanford, California

R. Cadossi, M.D.
Department of Hematology, University of Bologna, Bologna, Italy

Michele Chammas, M.D., Ph.D.
LaPeyronie University Hospital, Division of Orthopedic and Hand Surgery, Montpellier, France

Kerri Colbert, O.T.R., C.H.T.
Division of Hand Surgery, Stanford Health Services, Stanford, California

William P. Cooney, III, M.D.
Professor of Surgery, Mayo Medical School; Chair, Division of Hand Surgery, Department of Orthopedic Surgery, Mayo Clinic, Rochester, Minnesota

Jasper R. Daube, M.D.
Professor of Neurology, Mayo Clinic; St. Mary's Hospital, Rochester, Minnesota

Paul Dell, M.D.
Professor and Chief of Hand and Microsurgery, University of Florida, Gainesville, Florida

Edward Diao, M.D.
Assistant Professor, Department of Orthopedic Surgery, University of California at San Francisco, San Francisco, California

William Engber, M.D.
Associate Professor of Orthopedic Surgery, University of Wisconsin, Madison, Wisconsin

Roslyn B. Evans, O.T.R./L., C.H.T.
Indian River Hand Rehabilitation, Inc., Vero Beach, Florida

Joseph M. Failla, M.D.
Senior Staff, Department of Orthopedic Surgery; Head of Section of Hand Surgery, Henry Ford Hospital, Detroit, Michigan

Earl Fleelger, M.D.
Director, Hand Program, Albert Einstein Medical Center, Philadelphia, Pennsylvania

Alan A. Freeland, M.D.
Professor of Orthopedic Surgery, Director of Hand Surgery Service, University of Mississippi Medical Center, Jackson, Mississippi

Carolyn Gordon, O.T.R., C.H.T.
Division of Hand Surgery, Stanford Health Services, Stanford, California

John W. Hallett, Jr., M.D.
Professor of Surgery, Mayo Medical School, Mayo Clinic, Rochester, Minnesota

Michelle A. James, M.D.
Associate Clinical Professor of Orthopaedic Surgery, University of California Davis Medical Center; Chief Hand Surgeon and Medical Director of Rehabilitation, Shriner's Hospital for Children, Sacramento, California

Craig H. Johnson, M.D.
Senior Associate Consultant, Division of Plastic and Reconstructive Surgery, Department of Surgery and Division of Hand Surgery, Department of Orthopedic Surgery, Mayo Clinic, Rochester, Minnesota

Jesse B. Jupiter, M.D.
Associate Professor of Orthopedic Surgery; Director, Orthopedic Hand Service, Massachusetts General Hospital, Boston, Massachusetts

Morton L. Kasdan, M.D.
Clinical Professor of Plastic and Reconstructive Surgery, University of Louisville, Louisville, Kentucky

Julia A. Katarincic, M.D.
Instructor in Orthopedics, Mayo Medical Center, Rochester, Minnesota

Michael Keith, M.D.
Professor of Orthopedic Surgery, Case Western Reserve University, Cleveland, Ohio

L. Andrew Koman, M.D.
Professor, Surgical Sciences, Department of Orthopaedic Surgery, Bowman Gray School of Medicine, Wake Forest University, Winston-Salem, North Carolina

Prem Lalwani, O.T.R., C.H.T.
Division of Hand Surgery, Stanford Health Services, Stanford, California

Lewis B. Lane, M.D.
Associate Clinical Professor of Orthopedic Surgery, Albert Einstein College of Medicine; Chief, Hand Surgery, Long Island Jewish Medical Center, New Hyde Park, New York; Chief, Department of Orthopedics, North Shore University Hospital, Manhasset, New York

Maurice LeBlanc, M.S.M.E., C.P.
Chief, Applied Technology, Rehabilitation R&D Center, VA Palo Alto Health Care System, Palo Alto, California

William L. Lineaweaver, M.D.
Associate Professor of Functional Restoration–Hand Surgery, Stanford University School of Medicine, Stanford, California

Ronald L. Linscheid, M.D.
Professor of Orthopedic Surgery, Mayo Medical School; Consultant Emeritus, Department of Orthopedics and Surgery of the Hand, Mayo Clinic, Rochester, Minnesota

Susan E. Mackinnon, M.D.
Professor of Surgery, Chief Division of Plastic and Reconstructive Surgery, Washington University School of Medicine, St. Louis, Missouri

John M. Markley, Jr., M.D.
Clinical Assistant Professor, University of Michigan, Department of Surgery, Section of Plastic Surgery, University Hospital; Primary Active Staff, St. Joseph Mercy Hospital, Ann Arbor, Michigan

N. Bradley Meland, M.D.
Associate Professor of Plastic Surgery, Mayo Medical School; Head, Section of Hand Surgery, Mayo Clinic, Scottsdale, Arizona

Peter A. Nathan, M.D.
Portland Hand Surgery and Rehabilitation Center, Portland, Oregon

Edward R. North, M.D.
Washington Hand Surgery, Kirkland, Washington

Shawn W. O'Driscoll, M.D.
Associate Professor of Orthopedic Surgery, Mayo Medical School; Consultant, Department of Orthopedics, Mayo Clinic, Rochester, Minnesota

A. Lee Osterman, M.D.
Professor of Orthopedic and Hand Surgery, Thomas Jefferson University Hospital, Philadelphia Hand Center, Philadelphia, Pennsylvania

Clayton A. Peimer, M.D.
Professor, Department of Orthopedics, State University of New York at Buffalo School of Medicine; Chief of Hand Surgery, Department of Orthopedics, Millard Fillmore Hospital, Buffalo, New York

Vincent D. Pellegrini, Jr., M.D.
Department of Orthopedics and Rehabilitation, The Pennsylvania State University/The Milton S. Hershey Medical Center, Hershey, Pennsylvania

Leonard K. Ruby, M.D.
Professor of Orthopedic Surgery, Tufts University School of Medicine, Boston, Massachusetts

Jaiyoung Ryu, M.D.
Associate Professor of Orthopedic Surgery, University of West Virginia, Morgantown, West Virginia

Saleh M. Shenaq, M.D.
Professor and Chief, Professor of Surgery, Director, Plastic Surgery and Microsurgery Research Laboratory, Division of Plastic Surgery; Professor of Neurosurgery, Department of Neurosurgery and Vice-Chairman, Research, Department of Surgery, Baylor College of Medicine; Chief of

Plastic Surgery Section, Chief of Surgery, The Institute for Rehabilitation and Research, Houston, Texas

Barry P. Simmons, M.D.
Associate Professor, Harvard Medical School; Chief, Hand and Upper Extremity Surgical Service, Brigham and Women's Hospital, Boston, Massachusetts

Anthony A. Smith, M.D.
Associate Professor, Mayo Medical School; Senior Associate Consultant, Section of Hand Surgery, Mayo Clinic Scottsdale, Scottsdale, Arizona

Anthony A. Stans, M.D.
Instructor of Orthopedic Surgery, Mayo Graduate School of Medicine; Senior Associate Consultant, Mayo Clinic, Rochester, Minnesota

Peter J. Stern, M.D.
Professor and Chairman, Department of Orthopedic Surgery, University of Cincinnati College of Medicine, Cincinnati, Ohio

Robert M. Szabo, M.D., M.P.H.
Professor of Hand, Microvascular, and Orthopedic Surgery, University of California, Davis, California

Julio Taleisnik, M.D.
Clinical Professor of Surgery (Orthopedics), University of California, Irvine, California

Francisco J. Valero-Cuevas, Ph.D.
Research Associate and Lecturer, Mechanical Engineering Department, Stanford University, Stanford, California

Steven F. Viegas, M.D.
Professor and Chief, Division of Hand Surgery, Department of Orthopaedic Surgery and Rehabilitation; Professor of Anatomy and Neuroscience, The University of Texas Medical Branch, Galveston, Texas

Peter Wu, M.D.
Assistant Professor of Physical Medicine and Rehabilitation, Stanford Health System, Stanford, California

Felix M. Zajac, Ph.D.
Director, Rehabilitation R&D Center, VA Palo Alto Health Care System; Professor, Departments of Medical Engineering and Functional Restoration, Stanford University, Stanford, California

Table of Contents

Journals Represented

Mosby and its editors survey more than 1,000 journals for its abstract and commentary publications. From these journals, the editors select the articles to be abstracted. Journals represented in this YEAR BOOK are listed below.

Acta Neurochirurgica
Acta Orthopaedica Scandinavica
Acta Radiologica
American Journal of Industrial Medicine
American Journal of Occupational Therapy
American Journal of Orthopedics
American Journal of Roentgenology
Annales de Chirurgie Plastique et Esthetique
Annales de Chirurgie de la Main
Annals of Plastic Surgery
Annals of Rheumatic Diseases
Archives of Environmental Health
Archives of Physical Medicine and Rehabilitation
Archives of Surgery
Arthroscopy
British Journal of Plastic Surgery
Canadian Association of Radiologists Journal
Canadian Journal of Neurological Sciences
Clinical Anatomy
Clinical Biomechanics
Clinical Orthopaedics and Related Research
European Journal of Plastic Surgery
Giornale Italiano di Ortopedia e Traumatologia
Handchirurgie, Mikrochirurgie, Plastische Chirurgie
Injury
International Journal of Sports Medicine
Journal of Biomechanics
Journal of Bone and Joint Surgery (American Volume)
Journal of Bone and Joint Surgery (British Volume)
Journal of Clinical Rheumatology
Journal of Hand Surgery (American)
Journal of Hand Surgery (British)
Journal of Hand Therapy
Journal of Neurology, Neurosurgery and Psychiatry
Journal of Occupational and Environmental Medicine
Journal of Orthopaedic Trauma
Journal of Pediatric Orthopedics
Journal of Reconstructive Microsurgery
Journal of Rheumatology
Journal of Vascular Surgery
La Main
Microsurgery
Minerva Ortopedica E Traumatologica
Modern Pathology
Occupational and Environmental Medicine
Pain
Pediatric Dermatology

Physical Therapy
Plastic and Reconstructive Surgery
Radiology
Revista Espanola de Cirugia de la Mano
Revue de Chirurgie Orthopedique
Revista di Chirurgia e Riabilitazione della Mano e dell'Arto
Scandinavian Journal of Rheumatology
The 1996 Jefferson Orthopaedic Journal

Standard Abbreviations

The following terms are abbreviated in this edition: acquired immunodeficiency syndrome (AIDS), cardiopulmonary resuscitation (CPR), central nervous system (CNS), cerebrospinal fluid (CSF), computed tomography (CT), deoxyribonucleic acid (DNA), electrocardiography (ECG), health maintenance organization (HMO), human immunodeficiency virus (HIV), intensive care unit (ICU), intramuscular (IM), intravenous (IV), magnetic resonance (MR) imaging (MRI), and ribonucleic acid (RNA).

Note

The Year Book of Hand Surgery® is a literature survey service providing abstracts of articles published in the professional literature. Every effort is made to assure the accuracy of the information presented in these pages. Neither the editors nor the publisher of the Year Book of Hand Surgery® can be responsible for errors in the original materials. The editors' comments are their own opinions. Mention of specific products within this publication does not constitute endorsement.

To facilitate the use of the Year Book of Hand Surgery® as a reference tool, all illustrations and tables included in this publication are now identified as they appear in the original article. This change is meant to help the reader recognize that any illustration or table appearing in the Year Book of Hand Surgery® may be only one of many in the original article. For this reason, figure and table numbers will often appear to be out of sequence within the Year Book of Hand Surgery®.

Introduction

The production of this 1998 edition of the YEAR BOOK OF HAND SURGERY was associated with a number of changes brought about by the consolidation of activities of Mosby–Year Book, Inc. These changes included moving the editorial office from Chicago to St. Louis; as a consequence, we said goodbye to our former developmental editor, Catherine Flanagan, and hello to our new publisher, Terry Van Schaik, and to assistant developmental editors Brenda Orf and Jaime Chatman. We thank them for making the transition relatively painless.

As always, we have depended on the expertise and energy of our contributing editors and international editors, Drs. Foucher, Ishii, Jantea, LeClercq, Lluch, and Ueba, to make this anthology more valuable. To this group of international editors, we welcome Dr. Massimo Ceruso of Florence who has taken over for Dr. Antonio Landi as the international editor for Italy.

Thanks go to our families for their acceptance of additional time away, and to our secretaries and staff at Stanford and Mayo.

Finally, we continually seek suggestions from our readers on how to improve the YEAR BOOK. Your comments, happy or harsh, are always welcome.

Vincent R. Hentz, M.D.

Peter C. Amadio, M.D.

1 Anatomy and Biomechanics

The Cutaneous Innervation of the Palm: An Anatomic Study of the Ulnar and Median Nerves

Martin CH, Seiler JG III, Lesesne JS (Emory Univ, Atlanta, Ga)

J Hand Surg (Am) 21A:634–638, 1996 1–1

Background.—Persistent tenderness has been associated with the traditional incisions used in open carpal tunnel release. Some authorities have suggested that such scars are the result of an injury to cutaneous nerves and possible neuroma formation. However, no specific information on the origin of these nerves is available. Also, the radial extent of the ulnar-based palmar cutaneous innervation has not been defined. The anatomy of the median and ulnar nerve contributions to the cutaneous innervation of the palm was reported, with specific reference to a longitudinal palmar incision in the axis of the ring finger.

Methods and Findings.—Twenty-five fresh-frozen cadaveric hands were dissected. The palmar cutaneous branch of the median nerve was observed in all. In 1 hand, the palmar cutaneous branch of the median nerve was isolated as it crossed the incision. In another 2 specimens, the terminal branches of the nerve were identified at the incision margin. A classic palmar cutaneous branch of the ulnar nerve was discovered at a mean of 4.9 cm proximal to the pisiform in 4 hands. In another 10 hands, a nerve of Henle arose a mean of 14 cm proximal to the pisiform, traveling with the ulnar neurovascular bundle to the wrist flexion crease. In 24 hands, 1 or more transverse palmar cutaneous branches originating a mean of 3 mm distal to the pisiform in Guyon's canal were observed; their origin and destination varied greatly. An incision in the ring finger axis in 16 of these hands would have probably affected at least 1 branch of the ulnar-based cutaneous innervation to the palm. Cutaneous branches of the ulnar nerve would likely cross the line of dissection often during an open carpal tunnel release.

Conclusion.—These findings suggest that there is no true "internervous plane" in the palm for an approach to the carpal canal. Careful dissection in the palm is necessary to preserve crossing cutaneous nerves when open carpal tunnel release is performed through a longitudinal palmar incision.

▶ I can think of no area of the body where an incision could be made in a true internervous plane. This has been shown by many investigators and has been emphasized again recently by studies such as that by DaSilva.[1] The authors quite correctly confirm the regularly recommended care in preserving identifiable cutaneous nerve branches crossing the incision made for open carpal tunnel release. Nerves emerging from the ulnar cutaneous branches are documented in this study.

R.A. Chase, M.D.

Reference

1. DaSilva MF, Moore DC, Weiss A-PC, et al: Anatomy of the palmar cutaneous branch of the median nerve: Clinical significance. *J Hand Surg (Am)* 21A:639–643, 1996.

Correlative MR-Anatomic Study of the Median Nerve

Ikeda K, Haughton VM, Ho K-C, et al (Med College of Wisconsin, Milwaukee)

AJR 167:1233–1236, 1996 1–2

Introduction.—Few reports have described the normal median nerve, and specifically the fascicles within the collagenous epineurium. Magnetic resonance imaging of the fine structure of the median nerve could be useful in assessing its suitability for anastomosis, in evaluating nerve trauma in patients with carpal tunnel syndrome, and in evaluating median nerve tumors. The MRI appearance and anatomy of the median nerve were correlated.

Methods.—Three cadaver wrist specimens containing the carpal tunnel were imaged with an experimental 3-T scanner. The specimens were then sectioned, stained, and examined on the gross and microscopic levels with cryomicrotomy and microscopy.

Results.—The MRI scans showed the median nerve, tendons, and connective tissues within the carpal tunnel. The median nerve could be identified by its anatomical relationships to other structures. An average of 16 fascicles were seen in the proximal and distal parts of the nerve (Fig 3). By comparison, histologic section revealed an average of 19 fascicles. On MRI, the nerve fascicles appeared as small, irregular structures of higher signal intensity than the nerve sheath. The epineurium and perineurium have a lower signal intensity, similar to that of the tendons.

Conclusion.—High-resolution MRI techniques can show the internal structure of the median nerve. Such techniques could be clinically useful in the investigation of neuritis, tumor, degeneration, or fatty proliferation of

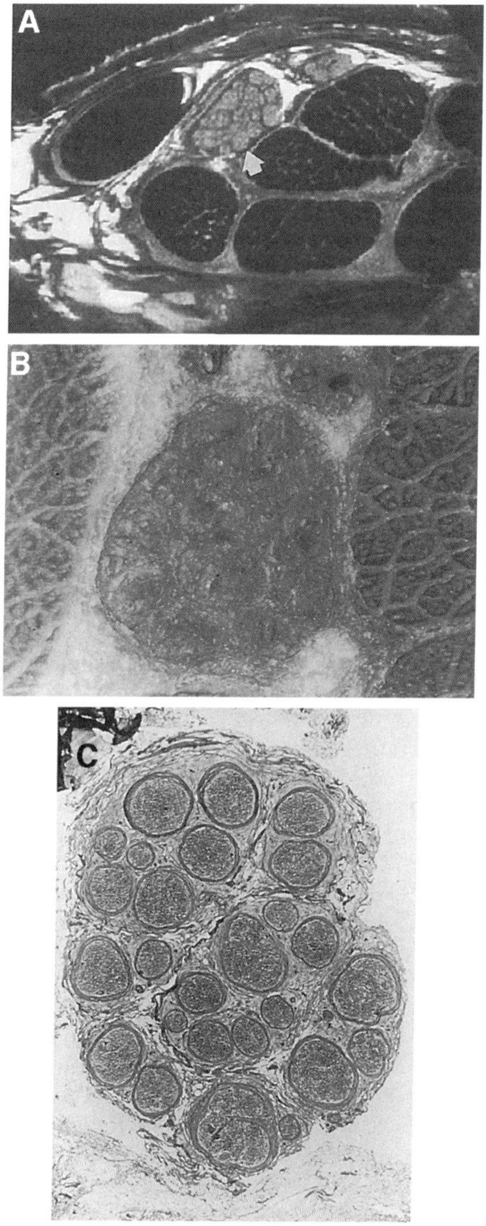

FIGURE 3.—Magnetic resonance imaging, cryomicrotomy, and histology of proximal median nerve. **A**, in MR image (TR/TE, 500/28; 12 excitations), fascicles and sheath are distinguished in median nerve (*arrow*). **B**, in corresponding magnification of cryomicrotome section, nerve has roughly elliptical shape. **C**, in histologic section, multiple fascicles bounded by nerve sheath are better seen. More fascicles are distinguished in **C** than in **A**; Bodian stain. (Courtesy of Ikeda K, Haughton VM, Ho K-C, et al: Correlative MR-anatomic study of the median nerve. *AJR* 167:1233–1236, 1996.)

the median nerve. They could help to evaluate the nerve before biopsy, or perhaps could one day replace biopsy.

▶ As MRI technology evolves, it will become a formidable tool in assisting in the diagnosis of and the location of nerve pathology. The photographs in the article are quite amazing in clarity and detail.

V.R. Hentz, M.D.

Excursion and Strain of the Median Nerve

Wright TW, Glowczewskie F, Wheeler D, et al (Univ of Florida, Gainesville)

J Bone Joint Surg (Am) 78A:1897–1903, 1996 1–3

Objective.—The effect of motion and strain on the median nerve with respect to movement and position of the shoulder, wrist, elbow, and fingers has not been studied. The relationship between excursion and strain of the median nerve with movement, and the potential mechanism for the production of peripheral neuropathy were investigated using cadaveric upper extremities.

Methods.—The excursion of the median nerve was measured in 5 fresh-frozen transthoracic cadaver specimens at various angles of flexion and extension. Strain was measured in triplicate using a Microstrain DVRT displacement gauge to record percent elongation, and a strip-chart recorder to register instantaneous strain. Magnitudes of the differences between wrist and elbow excursion measurements and strain measurements and their directions were analyzed statistically.

Results.—The mean total excursion of the median nerve at the wrist was 19.6 mm with the wrist flexed at 65 degrees vs. extended to 60 degrees; 9.7 mm for hyperextended fingers vs. fully flexed fingers; 23.8 mm for the shoulder adducted to 30 degrees, elbow flexed to 90 degrees, wrist extended to 60 degrees, fingers hyperextended to 35 degrees, and the forearm pronated to 60 degrees; and 9.1 mm at the elbow when the shoulder was adducted to 110 degrees vs. 30 degrees. Abduction of the shoulder to 30 degrees caused the greatest amount of distal excursion, and abduction to 110 degrees caused the greatest amount of proximal excursion, a total of 30.1 mm. Strain as a result of nerve wrinkling occurred consistently when the wrist was flexed. Mean total changes in strain at the wrist, depending on joint motion, were 7.5% for the shoulder, 3.7% for the elbow, 9.6% for the wrist, and 19.0% for the fingers. At the elbow, mean total changes in strain with joint motion were 13.3% for the shoulder, 14.8% for the wrist, and 10.3% for the fingers. Movement of the wrist and finger joints produced significant median nerve excursion at the wrist. Shoulder and elbow movement resulted in significant excursion at the elbow. Analysis of the relation between excursion and strain at the wrist and elbow demonstrated that composite positioning of the joints significantly increased tension and excursion in the nerve. Any interference with normal nerve glide can result in mechanical damage to the nerve.

Conclusions.—Position and movement of joints have a significant effect on the excursion and strain on the median nerve. Physical limitation of excursion of the nerve can cause damage. These findings may shed some light on the pathophysiology of peripheral neuropathy.

► This excellent anatomical study underlines the importance of nerve gliding, and demonstrates the marked effect of movement of even remote joints on nerve gliding. Both wrist and shoulder movement induce gliding at the elbow, for example. The significant impact of shoulder movement on nerve gliding might help explain the etiology of thoracic outlet syndrome; if gliding is blocked for some reason, then shoulder movement might induce unacceptable nerve stretching. One might have wished therefore that the authors had repeated their experiment after simulation of nerve fixation by scar or fracture. Perhaps that will be the subject of a future work.

P.C. Amadio, M.D.

Guyon's Canal Revisited: An Anatomic Study of the Carpal Ulnar Neurovascular Space

Cobb TK, Carmichael SW, Cooney WP (Mayo Clinic and Found, Rochester, Minn)

J Hand Surg (Am) 21A:861–869, 1996 1–4

Background.—During dissection of the carpal tunnel, the floor of Guyon's canal appeared to be involved intimately with the ulnar part of the roof of the carpal tunnel, which is inconsistent with the commonly held belief that the hook of hamate acts as the radial border of this space. The radial boundary of the canal was found to extend radially to the hook of hamate, as Guyon originally described. The anatomical boundaries of the ulnar neurovascular space were described.

Methods and Findings.—Twenty-five fresh-frozen and thawed unembalmed specimens were dissected. Gross dissections, transverse and sagittal sections, and histologic assessment were done. The roof of Guyon's canal did not connect to the hamate bone but extended radially to the hook of hamate, attaching to the flexor retinaculum. This structure permits the ulnar artery and sensory component of the ulnar nerve to course radially to the hook of hamate, where they lie on the flexor retinaculum. Three segments were identified on the roof and radial border. A proximal segment begins near the pisiform and extends distally to the level of the hook of hamate but does not attach to it directly; a central segment contains only adipose tissue; and a distal fascial layer includes the palmaris brevis muscle. The floor of the space is composed of the muscles of the hypothenar eminence, their fibers of origin, and the flexor retinaculum (Fig 9).

Conclusions.—Although Guyon accurately described the proximal part of the carpal ulnar neurovascular space, his description has been misinterpreted. The hook of hamate apparently is not the radial boundary of the

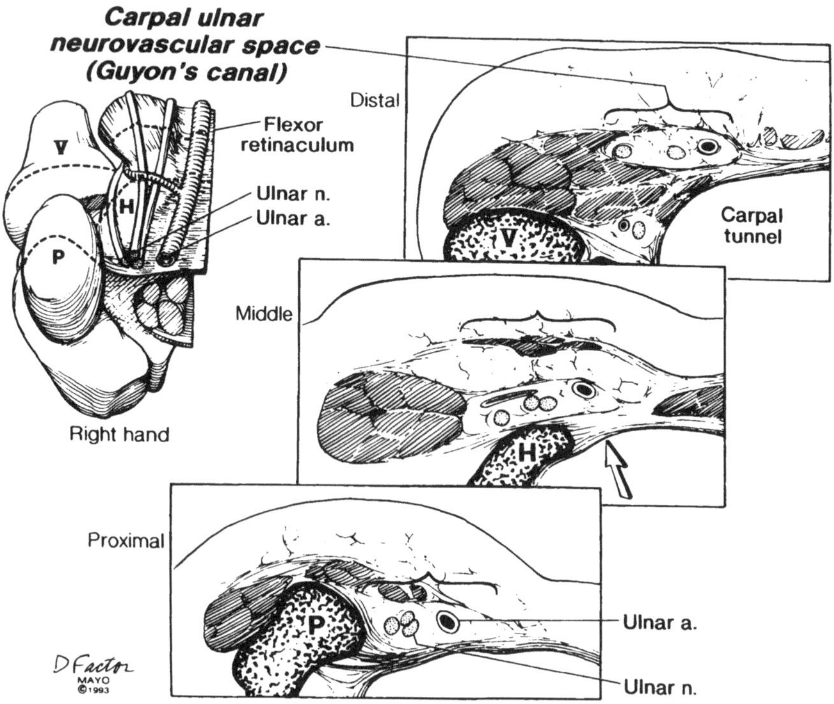

FIGURE 9.—Carpal ulnar neurovascular space. **A**, space viewed from proximal to distal. **B**, transverse sections at level of pisiform (*P*), hook of hamate (*H*), and fifth metacarpal (*V*). *Arrow* shows approximate location of endoscopic release of the flexor retinaculum (transverse carpal ligament). Note the potential vulnerability of ulnar artery. This specimen does not have a segmented carpal ulnar neurovascular space roof. *Abbreviations: A*, artery; *n*, nerve. (Courtesy of the Mayo Foundation. From Cobb TK, Carmichael SW, Cooney WP: Guyon's canal revisited: An anatomic study of the carpal ulnar neurovascular space. *J Hand Surg [Am]* 21A:861–869, 1996.)

canal. An understanding of the anatomical relationships in the carpal ulnar neurovascular space is necessary to avoid complications during carpal tunnel surgery.

▶ This study reinforces our knowledge of the variations in the radial border of the carpal ulnar neurovascular space (Loge de Guyon). Having seen instances of iatrogenic injury to the ulnar neurovascular structures in carpal tunnel release, I applaud this study as a reminder to hand surgeons that such injury may occur in *either* open or endoscopic carpal tunnel release. Review of this study, along with many others, is critical for anyone considering an endoscopic approach to *ulnar* tunnel release.

I have mixed feelings about renaming this space. Beneath my anatomical hat, I applaud the descriptive name; beneath my historian hat, I would be sad to see the noble name of "Loge de Guyon" disappear.

R.A. Chase, M.D.

Anatomic Study of the Ulnar Nerve and Related Vascular Anatomy at Guyon's Canal: A Practical Classification System

Lindsey JT, Watumull D (Metairie, La; Univ of Texas, Garland)

J Hand Surg (Am) 21A:626–633, 1996 1–5

Background.—The current literature regarding the anatomy of the nerves and related vascular anatomy in Guyon's canal is contradictory and inaccurate. Furthermore, descriptions of this region rarely include the hypothenar branching patterns. The various anatomical patterns of the ulnar nerve and artery at Guyon's canal were reported.

Methods and Findings.—Thirty-one fresh upper extremities from adult cadavers were microdissected. Two patterns of division of the ulnar nerve trunk were evident. In pattern A, present in 25 specimens, the ulnar nerve bifurcated into a main sensory trunk and a motor branch. In pattern B, observed in 6 specimens, the ulnar nerve trifurcated into 2 common digital sensory branches and a motor branch. There were also 3 patterns of hypothenar muscle innervation and 2 of vascular supply to the hypothenar musculature. Hypothenar innervation patterns were type 1 (single branch) in 10 specimens, type 2 (2 branches) in 14, and type 3 (3 or more branches) in 7. Seventeen specimens were found to have a major vascular arcade passing from the ulnar artery to the hypothenar musculature palmar to the entire ulnar nerve; 6 had the arcade passing palmar to the motor part of the nerve only; and 8 had no axial arterial supply. None of the specimens had a deep branch of the ulnar artery coursing with the deep motor branch of the ulnar nerve and contributing to a deep palmar arterial arcade (Table 1).

Conclusion.—This study did not verify the classically held belief that a deep branch of the ulnar artery accompanies the motor branch of the ulnar nerve, contributing to the ulnar arterial supply to the deep palmar arterial arch. This concept should be critically re-examined.

▶ This paper describes important observations of details of the structural relationships in Guyon's canal regarding the ulnar artery and ulnar nerve and their branches. Of particular importance to surgeons is that in approximately one third of the cases in this series, there was a single motor nerve branch to the hypothenar muscles. Therefore, innervation of the opponens and flexor digiti minimi muscles depends on motor nerves passing through the abductor digiti minimi. Thus, careful proximal dissection of the abductor digiti minimi muscle for a Huber transfer is critical for avoiding iatrogenic paralysis of the muscles that are promoted in importance with the donor loss by transfer of the abductor digiti minimi. I find it hard to believe that no arterial branch of the ulnar artery accompanies the deep motor branch of the ulnar nerve and hope to see further injection/dissection studies to prove this point.

R.A. Chase, M.D.

TABLE 1.—Innervation Patterns of the Hypothenar Muscles With Reference to the Proximal Aspect of the Pisiform Bone

	Type		
	1	*2*	*3*
No. of Specimens	10	14	7
No. of Branches	1	2	3 or more
Patterns	A: Within Guyon's canal (80%; average, 16 mm; range, 11–25 mm) B: Distal to canal (10%; 30 mm distal to pisiform) C: Proximal to canal (10%; 25 mm proximal to pisiform)	A: Branches within canal (68%; average, 18 mm; range, 0–32 mm) B: Distal to canal (32%; average, 30 mm; range, 27–46 mm)	A: All branches within canal (76%; average, 20 mm; range, 3–30 mm) B: Distal to canal (24%; average, 31 mm; range, 30–40 mm)

(Courtesy of Lindsey JT, Watumull D: Anatomic study of the ulnar nerve and related vascular anatomy at Guyon's canal: A practical classification system. *J Hand Surg [Am]* 21A: 626–633, 1996.)

The Internal Topography of the Axillary Nerve: An Anatomic and Histologic Study as it Relates to Microsurgery

Aszmann OC, Dellon AL (Univ of Maryland, Baltimore; Johns Hopkins Univ, Baltimore, Md)

J Reconstr Microsurg 12:359–363, 1996 1–6

Objective.—In nerve reconstruction, the main thing the surgeon can do to influence recovery is to promote correct fascicular alignment. As the use of interfascicular nerve grafting and repair increases, several studies have examined the internal topography of the peripheral nerves as it applies to microsurgery. The topography of the individual fascicle groups of the axillary nerve was studied throughout its course, from the posterior cord to its passage through the quadrangular space.

Methods.—The internal topography of the axillary nerve was studied using ×3.5 loupe magnification in 40 cadaver brachial plexuses. Another 10 axillary nerves were excised *in toto* for histologic serial sections to determine fascicular arrangement.

Results.—The axillary nerve was almost always completely separated from the thoracodorsal nerve at its origin. The axillary nerve was monofascicular through most of its course. However, at a mean of 35 mm proximal to the quadrangular space, it divided into inferomedial and superolateral branches. The motor fascicular group for the deltoid muscle was always located most superiorly, at the level of the quandrangular space. This motor portion of the nerve represented a distinct entity, localized up to 45 mm proximal to the quadrangular space.

Conclusions.—The motor fascicular portion of the axillary nerve is consistently located near the level of the quadrangular space. This has important implications for surgical reconstruction of the axillary nerve. The surgeon should be careful to identify, match, and align the motor fascicle correctly, to avoid wasteful axonal regeneration into the functionally unrelated fascicles running to the teres minor and the lateral shoulder skin.

► This useful article outlines the fascicular anatomy of the axillary nerve, and emphasizes that the motor branch to the deltoid remains in the superolateral quadrant throughout nearly the entire course of the nerve. This knowledge should help surgeons who wish to graft the nerve for deltoid function.

P.C. Amadio, M.D.

Biomechanical Changes of Cadaveric Finger Flexion: The Effect of Wrist Position and of the Transverse Carpal Ligament and Palmar and Forearm Fasciae

Kang H-J, Lee S-G, Phillips CS, et al (Seoul, Korea; Univ of Chicago)
J Hand Surg (Am) 21A:963–968, 1996 1–7

Background.—Carpal tunnel syndrome is the most common nerve entrapment syndrome. It is usually treated by division of the transverse carpal ligament (TCL), including the palmar fascia and the distal forearm fascia. Long-term complications of this surgical decompression include decreased grip strength and bowstringing of the flexor tendons. It has been proposed that the TCL is an important retinacular pulley for the digital flexors. The effects of wrist positioning and TCL sectioning on the biomechanics of finger flexion were investigated in cadaveric hands.

Methods.—The profundus tendon of the index, long, and ring fingers of 6 cadaveric hands were individually pulled 3 times each with the wrist in neutral, 30-degree extension, and 30-degree flexion. The movements were repeated after TCL transection. Changes in excursion, load, and work of the flexor tendons were recorded.

Results.—Wrist extension improved excursion efficiency, whereas wrist flexion reduced excursion efficiency by 16% after TCL transection. The reduction in load efficiency and work efficiency was also greatest in the flexed position. There was a significant decrease in excursion efficiency of the flexor tendons with the wrist in the flexed position.

Conclusions.—These biomechanical measurements in cadaveric hands demonstrate that the TCL is an important retinacular pulley for the digital flexor tendons. The acute weakness that can result after TCL release can be modified by holding the wrist in a mild extension position to minimize anterior displacement of flexor tendons and increase the efficiency of tendon excursion during postoperative exercise.

▶ This well-constructed cadaveric study examines the influence of wrist position and division of the TCL and palmar fascia on the biomechanics of the finger flexion. The hypothesis that the TCL is an important retinacular pulley for the digital flexors is clearly stated and appears to be validated by the results. Although it is intuitive that digital flexor strength is diminished by wrist flexion, this paper provides a scientific argument for the decreased grip strength that may be seen clinically after division of the TCL. Furthermore, it provides support for postoperative therapy protocols that place the wrist in a neutral or extended position. Despite their findings, clinical experience has not demonstrated adverse effects when the wrist is not immobilized after carpal tunnel decompression.[1]

P.J. Stern, M.D.

Reference

1. Cook AC, Szabo RM, Birkholz SW, et al: Early mobilization following carpal tunnel release: A prospective randomized study. *J Hand Surg (Br)* 20B:228–230, 1995.

The Vascularization of the Common Synovial Sheath and the Tendons of the Flexor Muscles of the Carpal Tunnel [French]

Zbrodowski A, Gajisin S, Bednarkiewicz M (Centre Médical Universitaire, Geneva; Hôpital Cantonal Universitaire, Geneva)

Ann Chir Main 15:248–256, 1996 1–8

Background.—Surgical reconstruction of the hand must take into consideration its vascular anatomy as well as its physiology. This study examined the superficial and deep flexor tendons in the wrist, the common synovial sheath, the vascularization of these structures, and their relationships within the carpal tunnel.

Methods.—The upper extremities of 200 fresh human cadavers were prepared by injecting colored latex or an aqueous solution of India ink with gelatin into the brachial artery. The flexor retinaculum ligament was cut along its median line, the tendon sheath was opened along its palmar surface, and the flexor tendons were cut at the level of the digital sheath. The mesotendons were cut away and vascular relationships were examined by a stereomicroscope.

Findings.—The vascularization of the superficial and deep flexor tendons is quite variable (Fig 4). Before entering the carpal tunnel, flexor tendons receive blood most commonly from radial and ulnar arterioles that branch at the level of the tendon. Within the carpal tunnel (Fig 8), 4 different blood supplies can be found: (1) Branches of the radial and ulnar

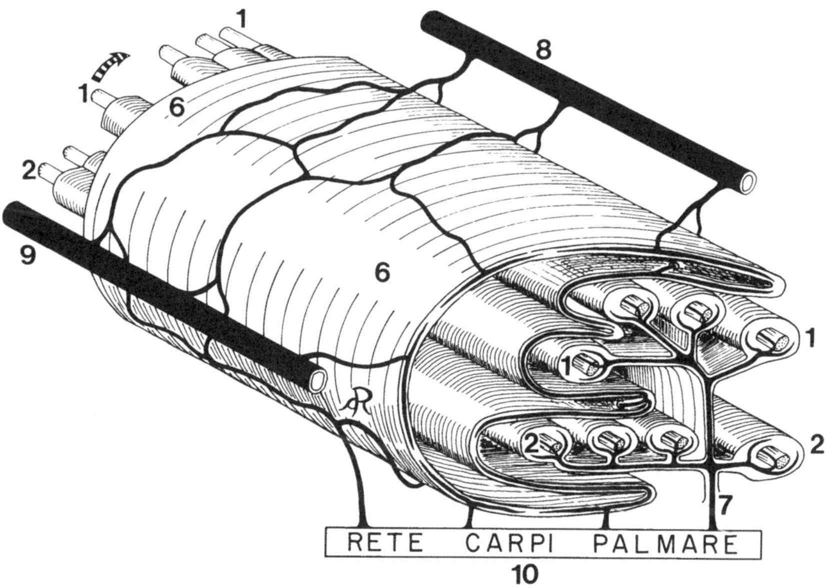

FIGURE 4.—Schematic drawing illustrating the vascularization of the carpal sheath and flexor tendons. (Courtesy of Zbrodowski A, Gajisin S, Bednarkiewicz M: The vascularization of the common synovial sheath and the tendons of the flexor muscles of the carpal tunnel [French]. *Ann Chir Main* 15:248–256, 1996.)

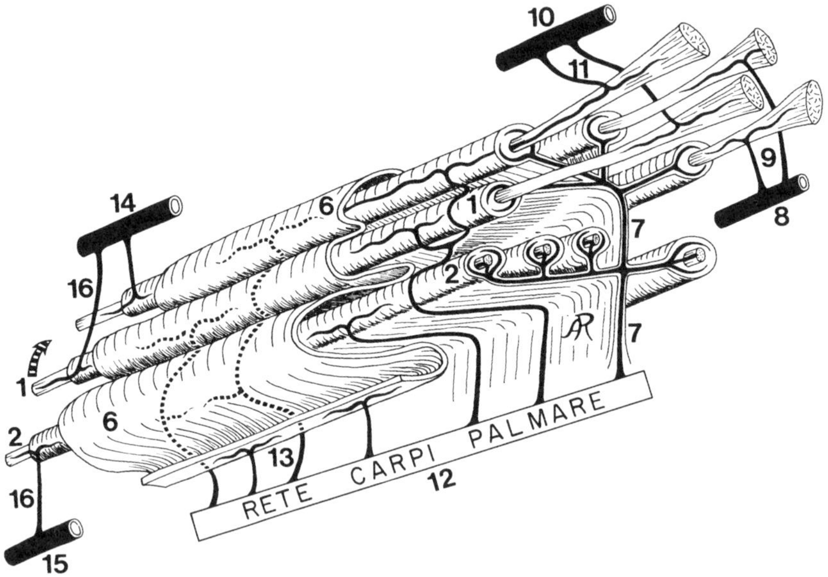

FIGURE 8.—Schematic drawing of the vascularization of the content of the carpal tunnel. (Courtesy of Zbrodowski A, Gajisin S, Bednarkiewicz M: The vascularization of the common synovial sheath and the tendons of the flexor muscles of the carpal tunnel [French]. *Ann Chir Main* 15:248–256, 1996.)

arteries; (2) Branches of the artery that supplies the median nerve; (3) Branches from the superficial arterial arch; and (4) Carpal "mesotendinal" arteries (carpal arteries in the base of the mesotendon). Once in the palm, the flexor tendons are vascularized by arterial branches of the arcus palmaris profundus and by palmar metacarpal arteries. Rich networks of arteries, veins, and nerves are seen throughout the course of the tendons.

The mesotendon of the common synovial sheath gives some attachment to the tendons, while also providing passage for blood vessels and nerves.

Conclusions.—The deep and superficial flexor tendons of the hand have a varied and rich vascular supply. The neurovascular bundles of the mesotendon contribute to the flexor tendon blood supply, as do the ulnar and radial arteries. Overall, however, the most important vascular supply for tendons seems to be the deep networks that provide (directly or via branches) a blood supply along the length of the tendon.

▶ This report contains beautiful, detailed illustrations of the blood supply of the flexor tendons and tenosynovium in the region of the carpal canal. Especially nice is Figure 4, which shows the vessels to the synovial sheath and Figure 8, which shows vessels to the individual tendons. (Both are included in this abstract.) The complicated arrangement of the visceral and parietal layers is nicely shown. What an incredible effort to study 200 cadaver extremities in this way!

The authors showed that flexor tendons and their tenosynovia are nourished by vessels from different sources. The flexor tendons receive direct vessels from the radial and ulnar arteries that form ascending and descending branches from branches off a median artery, when present, from transverse palmar carpal arteries off the ulnar and radial arteries that course at the distal border of the pronator quadratus to anastomose as the palmar carpal network of arteries, and distally in the palm from branches off the palmar arches. The mesotendon is described and compared to bowel mesentery, with a described function of allowing the tendon blood supply to have excursion with tendon motion. The greatest length of the mesotendon is from the carpal canal floor to the superficial flexor tendon, measuring 64 mm, and certainly consistent with tendon excursion.

Under the common synovial sheath, there is a zone of little vessel penetration into the palmar surface of the tendons. The size of the neurovascular bundles into the tendons was measured, with vessels ranging from 0.4–0.6 mm. The tenosynovium is nourished by direct vessels from the radial and ulnar arteries, which appear to have rich anastomoses.

I can see a great deal of clinical significance for these data:

1. When performing a flexor tenosynovectomy in a rheumatoid patient, it may be possible to find the tenosynovial vessel off the radial and ulnar arteries and to cauterize them first to limit hematoma formation.
2. The small size of the tendon vessels and their intrafascicular branches may have a role in the development of trigger finger. With shear between individual tendon fascicles, there may be microdamage to the intrafascicular tissue, with a fibrous reparative process resulting. I have seen fibrous tissue formed between tendon fascicles in trigger finger tendon biopsy samples and these small vessels may be the source of the tissue.
3. One could imagine that these small intratendinous and intrasynovial vessels are affected in diabetes mellitus. Perhaps this could explain development of trigger finger and carpal tunnel syndrome associated with diabetes, and could be the basis of thickening of these tissues.
4. No mention was made of communication between digital flexor tenosynovial sheaths, but this is obviously important in the spread proximally of flexor tenosynovitis.

J.M. Failla, M.D.

Variations of the Flexor Digitorum Superficialis Tendon of the Little Finger

Gonzalez MH, Whittum J, Kogan M, et al (Univ of Illinois, Chicago)
J Hand Surg (Br) 22B:277–280, 1997 1–9

Objective.—Understanding the various anomalies of the flexor digitorum superficialis tendon (FDS) of the little finger is important when repairing lacerations. Because most observations regarding the fifth flexor tendon have been anecdotal, an investigation of the anatomy of the FDS to the little finger was conducted.

Methods.—Seventy unpaired cadaveric hands were dissected, and anomalies of the FDS of the little finger were photographed. Widths of the radial and ulnar insertions, and widths at the A-1 pulley with the finger, distance from the end of the tendon to the metacarpophalangeal (MCP) joint, length of the proximal phalanx, and width of the radial slip were measured.

Results.—The average radial and ulnar slip widths were 1.9 and 2.0 mm, respectively, with a correlation coefficient suggesting equal lengths. The average diameter of the little finger and ring finger slip widths were 3 and 5.4 mm, respectively, with a correlation coefficient suggesting proportional sizes. The average length from the decussation of the FDS to the MCP joint was 16.2 mm, and the mean length of the fifth proximal phalanx was 44.7 mm. Here the correlation coefficient suggested that the point of decussation is independent of the size of the fifth phalanx. Nine hands (13%) had anatomical variations of the FDS.

Conclusion.—Variation in the FDS of the little finger are common. A thorough knowledge of little finger anatomy is necessary when performing repairs to the tendon or harvesting the tendon for tendon transfer.

▶ It is commonly stated that the FDS of the little finger is often absent or anomalous, but there is little in the literature that describes the frequency of these findings. This paper suggests that anomalies of the FDS of the littler finger may be less common than generally supposed; only 9 of 70 hands had any anomaly, and in only one was the FDS absent. Dysfunction of the FDS in a little finger that has been injured should not automatically be assumed to be caused by anomaly or congenital absence.

P.C. Amadio, M.D.

Anatomy of the Extensor Tendons to the Index Finger

Gonzalez MH, Weinzweig N, Kay T, et al (Univ of Illinois, Chicago; Cook County Hosp, Chicago)

J Hand Surg (Am) 21A:988–991, 1996 1–10

Background.—Knowledge of the anatomical relationship of the extensors to the index finger is important in tendon repair and extensor indicis proprius (EIP) transfer. The position and variations of the extensors to the index finger were studied anatomically.

Methods and Findings.—Seventy-two cadaver hands, including 30 fresh-frozen and 42 embalmed specimens, were dissected. In 58 hands, classic descriptions were confirmed: a single slip of the extensor digitorum communis (EDC) and of the EIP ran to the index finger, and the EIP was ulnar to the EDC at the level of the metacarpal head. A double slip of the EIP was noted in 10 hands. A double slip of the EDC running to the index finger was observed in 2 hands. In another 2 hands, a single slip of the EIP was either volar or radial to the EDC at the level of the metacarpal head. Nineteen percent of the hands had anatomical variants of the EIP and EDC tendons at the level of the metacarpal head. Also, 2 hands had aberrant tendons (Fig 4).

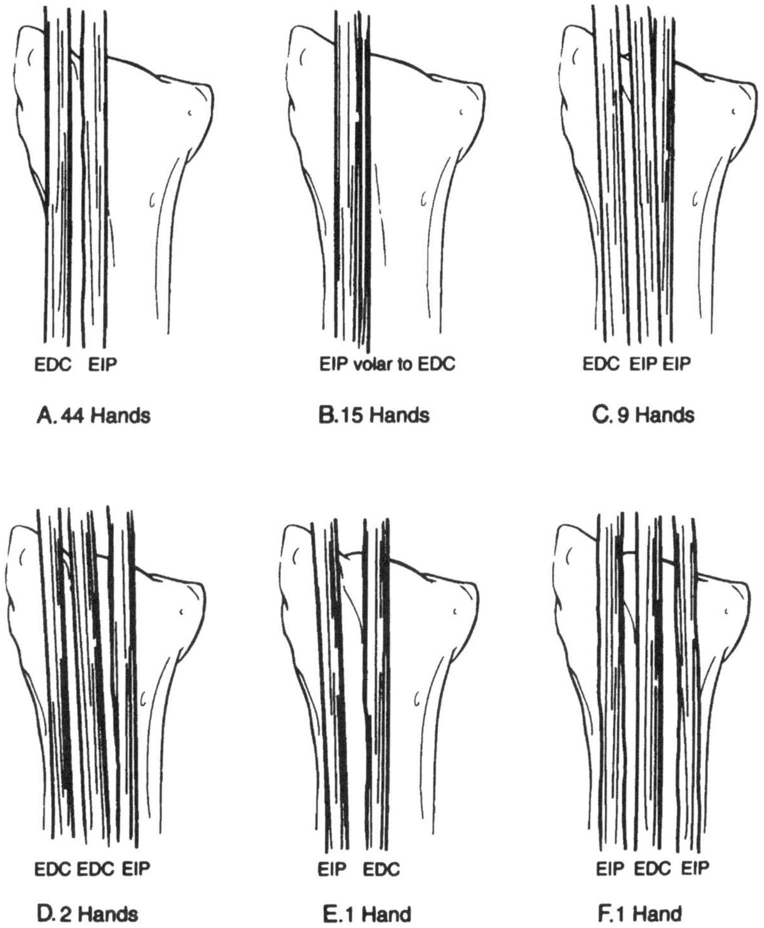

FIGURE 4.—Accessory slip of extensor indicis proprius (*EIP*) tendon. *Abbreviation: EDC,* extensor digitorum communis. (Courtesy of Gonzalez MH, Weinzweig N, Kay T, et al: Anatomy of the extensor tendons to the index finger. *J Hand Surg [Am]* 21A:988–991, 1996.)

Conclusions.—Surgeons performing tendon transfers using the EIP muscle must be aware of anatomical variants. Only 81% of the hands studied were found to have a single tendon slip of EIP lying ulnar to a single slip of EDC.

▶ Hand surgeons need to be aware of all sorts of variations from classic anatomical descriptions. The nomenclature used in this paper is at variance with modern anatomical nomenclature using Paris Nomia Anatomica. The words communis and proprius have been dropped, and thus the terms extensor indicis and extensor digitorum are proper. Nonetheless, this study reinforces the need to be alert to such variations when performing extensor indicis transfers, as any surgeon knows who has attempted to reflect a tendon out from a proximal incision when the distal section is incomplete. This happens most frequently with the other independent finger extensor, extensor digiti minimi, which regularly has 2 tendons of insertion, a fact sometimes not known to an experienced surgeon.

R.A. Chase, M.D.

The Extensor Tendons of the Fifth Digit: Anatomy and Classification [French]

Rupnik J, Leclercq C (Institut de la Main, Paris)

La Main 2:3–9, 1997 1–11

Introduction.—The extensor apparatus of the little finger depends upon two sources: the extensor digiti minimi (EDM) and the extensor digitorum (ED). Several variations in number, size, and topography of these tendons have been described. Our purpose has been to classify these variations, with a special focus of the use of extensor digiti minimi as a source of tendon transfer.

Material.—Thirty cadaver upper-limbs have been used (15 of which were fresh and 15 embalmed) for dissection of the tendons of extensor digitorum to the little finger (ED-5) and EDM from its origin on the muscle belly to the extensor hood.

Results.—EDM was always present, with two tendons in 80% cases. When three tendons were present, the most radial ran towards the fourth finger and fused with ED-4 at the extensor hood level. ED-5 and the junctura tendinum were missing in 2 cases (6%). When the ED-5 was present (94%), it separated from ED-4 distally most of the time (distal metacarpal) and proximally in 2 cases (proximal metacarpal).

Discussion.—Several previous studies have dealt with anatomical variations of the extensor tendons to the little finger. Although their description is identical to ours regarding EDM, some figures differ somewhat regarding the presence of ED-5: 44% (Schenck, 1964) and 70% (Gonzales, 1995; El Badawi, 1995) versus 94% in our series. One possible explanation may be the difficulty in differentiating splitting tendons from junctura in some cases. However their figures are in concordance with ours regarding the percentage of cases with no ED-5 and no junctura between ED-4 and EDM (1% to 6%). In these cases, one must not use EDM as a source of transfer or graft; this will result in a complete extension lag at the metacarpophalangeal joint level. Based on the presence and topography of ED-5, with percentages of each type met in 518 dissections (our series added to the above mentioned) we have established a classification of extensor tendons to the little finger (Table 1). When harvesting EDM, one must be aware of the possible absence of ED-5 and always look for it before raising EDM.

TABLE 1.—Anatomy of ED-5 in 6 Series

	Authors' series 30	SCHENCK 57	MESTDAGH 150	GODWIN 50	EL BADAWI 181	GONZALES 50	TOTAL (%) 518
Type A	26 (86%)	10 (17%)	134 (89%)	58 (96%)	73 (40%)	12 (24%)	59%
distal metacarpal							
Type B	2 (6%)	3 (5%)	9 (6%)	1 (2%)	54 (30%)	23 (46%)	18%
proximal metacarpal							
Type C absent	2 (6%)	32 (56%)	2 (1%)	1 (2%)	54 (30%)	15 (30%)	20%
junctura	0	30	?	1	54	12	19%
no junctura	2	2	?	0	0	3	1%
unknown		12	5				3%

(Courtesy of Rupnik J, Leclercq C: The extensor tendons of the fifth digit: Anatomy and classification [French]. *La Main* 2:3–9, 1997.)

This may lead to an extensive approach up to the proximal metacarpal level.

► The EDM is used as a tendon transfer and as a source for tendon grafts. The authors remind us that the common digital extensor contribution to the fifth finger is reliably absent in enough individuals so that the anatomy of extensor mechanism to the ED-5 at the level of the distal metacarpal must be explored and analyzed if one chooses the EDM as a graft or transfer resource. What hand surgeons may not appreciate is that the anatomy of this mechanism should be evaluated more proximally than is commonly done, even to the level of the proximal metacarpal.

V.R. Hentz, M.D.

The Abductores Pollicis Muscles: Clinical Considerations Based on Electromyographical and Anatomical Studies

Brandsma JW, Oudenaarde EV, Oostendorp R (Natl Inst of Allied Health Professions, Amersfoort, The Netherlands; Univ of Nijmegen, The Netherlands; Free Univ of Brussels, Belgium)

J Hand Ther 9:218–222, 1996 1–12

Introduction.—The multiple insertions of the abductor pollicis longus (APL) muscle are related to its distinct deep and superficial divisions. The deep division acts mainly as a dorsal flexor of the hand, whereas the superficial division is a prime mover of the first carpometacarpal joint. The abductor pollicis brevis (APB) is also a prime mover of the first carpometacarpal joint; the functions of the APL and APB appear to be closely related. Given its importance in the function of the thumb and hand, it is important to understand the function of the APL. Clinically relevant information on the APL and APB from anatomical and electrophysiologic studies was reviewed.

Clinical Considerations.—Knowledge of the abductores pollicis muscles is potentially relevant in many different clinical situations. Both the deep and superficial divisions of the APL are innervated by the radial nerve. The function of the APL cannot be sufficiently isolated for voluntary muscle testing, so strength tests for wrist dorsiflexion and finger extension are done. The median nerve innervates the APB; strength of palmar abduction of the thumb is more likely to be evaluated than the APB itself. The APL and APB together have been considered responsible for true palmar abduction of the thumb. The authors' studies have shown that electromyographic activity of the APB is greatest with the hand in palmar flexion—this is explained by the connection between the APB and the deep division of the APL. This connection may also explain the inability of patients with low and median ulnar palsies to perform palmar abduction of the thumb. Activation of the deep division of the APL is greatest with dorsal flexion of the hand, regardless of forearm position. In patients with suspected median or radial nerve impairment or both, it may be best to test thumb abduction with the hand and forearm in different positions.

Patients with radial nerve paralysis or APL tendon rupture would be expected to have limited palmar abduction, opposition, and radial abduction of the thumb. It is important to restore the paralyzed APL, which must be strong to hold out the first metacarpal joint against the force of the strong adductor. The consequences of failure to reactivate the APL after radial palsy are unclear. The APL may be used to restore abduction of the thumb or index finger. In patients with ulnar or median nerve paralysis, the APL should probably not be used unless there is no alternative. The use of the APL to restore index finger abduction ignores that the muscle's multiple insertions represent distinct divisions. Use of the APL has been reported in other common reconstructive situations as well, including carpal instability, thumb osteoarthritis, and tendovaginitis of the first extensor compartment. The possible consequences of APL dysfunction in these cases are unknown.

Discussion.—The abductores pollicis muscles play an important role in the function of the hand and thumb. For accurate clinical assessment and reconstructive surgery, it is essential to understand the function of the APL. More study is needed to determine the best hand and forearm position for strength testing of the APB and APL. When the APL is used for reconstructive surgery, it is important to accurately state which divisions or tendons of the muscle are used.

▶ Further observations on the structure and function relations of the APB and APL are important for surgeons who plan to use all or a part of the APL in tendon transfers. Muscle tendon units consisting of 2 muscle bellies in series is not unusual. The cited example of the flexor carpi ulnaris and abductor digiti minimi is but one. More relevant to the subject of the article are fibers of the palmaris longus coursing to the APB, because it must be considered in thumb abduction functions. Simultaneous electromyographic study of the palmaris longus together with 2 normal thumb abductors would be of interest.

R.A. Chase, M.D.

Pronator Quadratus Revisited

Stuart PR (Freeman Hosp, Newcastle-upon-Tyne, England)

J Hand Surg (Br) 21B:714–722, 1996 1–13

Background.—The anatomy and function of the pronator quadratus muscle have not been thoroughly described. The gross and microscopic anatomy of the pronator quadratus was reported, as well as the findings of in vivo studies.

Methods.—Six preserved specimens were dissected to confirm previous findings, which were then elaborated on in a study of the anatomical and architectural features of pronator quadratus in 40 fresh-frozen specimens. Gross cross-sectional anatomy was investigated in serial sections of 2 fresh-frozen cadaver specimens. Comparative anatomy was studied in fresh upper limb specimens from several primate species. The relationship of the muscle to the distal radioulnar joint capsule was studied in detail

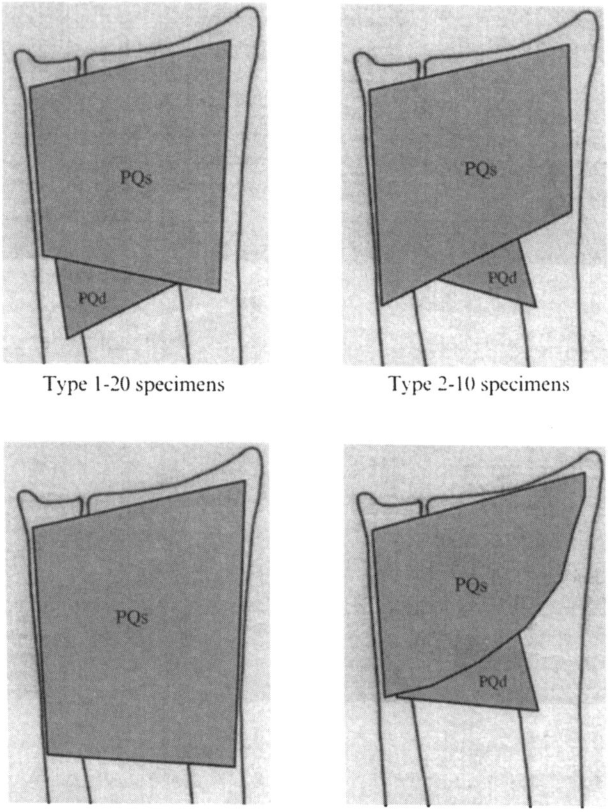

FIGURE 4.—Gross anatomical arrangement of pronator quadratus (*PQ*). *Abbreviations: PQs*, superficial head of PQ; *PQd*, deep head of PQ. (Courtesy of Stuart PR: Pronator quadratus revisited. *J Hand Surg [Br]* 21B:714–722, 1996.)

using sagittal, coronal, and transverse histologic sections of the distal radius and ulna. Microscopic studies were performed on fresh postmortem specimens from a young donor to determine muscle fiber type distribution within pronator quadratus. In vivo assessments were performed using MRI and electromyography.

Findings.—Two independent heads to the pronator quadratus muscle were found consistently. The origin of the superficial head was a short tendon on the dorsoulnar border of the ulna. It inserts into a broad flat facet on the volar surface of the radius. The origin of the deep head is similar, although with a slightly less distinct tendon and from a slightly more volar position on the ulna. The deep head insertion is to the whole of the ulnar border of the distal radial shaft extending dorsally to the interosseous membrane, filling the axilla of the distal radioulnar joint. The in vivo studies clearly showed the pronator quadratus to be the main pronator of the forearm. Pronator teres fired only in maximal pronation and resisted pronation. The deep head of the pronator quadratus consistently fired during supination and grip maneuvers, supporting the hypothesis that the deep head plays an important role in preventing radioulnar joint diastasis during forearm rotation and grip.

Conclusions.—Inspection of the gross anatomy has demonstrated the consistent division of pronator quadratus muscle into 2 distinct heads. Morphological patterns were also defined (Fig 4), and the architecture characterized. The superficial head is the primary mover in forearm pronation, with the deep head serving as a dynamic stabilizer of the distal radioulnar joint.

► This elegant and exhaustive study of the pronator quadratus establishes several important points. Not only does it confirm the consistent presence of 2 heads but it shows the separate functional roles of each. Like the fleshy, short intrinsic muscles of the hand, the pronator quadratus serves a capital role, in fact, the primary role, in pronation of the forearm. Its other more subtle but important function is as a dynamic stablizer and capsuled manager for the distal radioulnar joint, much as the articularis genus tends the knee joint capsule.

R.A. Chase, M.D.

Biomechanics of the Intact and Surgically Repaired Proximal Interphalangeal Joint Collateral Ligaments

Dzwierzynski WW, Pintar F, Matloub HS, et al (Med College of Wisconsin, Milwaukee)

J Hand Surg (Am) 21A:679–683, 1996 1–14

Background.—Injuries to the collateral ligament of the proximal interphalangeal (PIP) joints are a common occurrence, especially in the workplace and during sports activities. Treatments range from splinting to open repair with ligament reconstruction. Although all repair techniques provide stability in most patients, all are associated with loss of joint motion. The biomechanical strength and failure modes of intact and surgically repaired PIP collateral ligaments were evaluated.

Methods and Findings.—Eighty-five fresh cadaver fingers were evaluated, including 38 intact ligaments. Native ligament strength was found to be 162.5 newtons. The 47 ligament repair preparations included suture repair, pull-out wire repair, and repair using a Mitek suture anchor (Mitek Surgical Products Inc., Norwood, Mass). The native ligament strengths in each of these groups were 27.8 newtons, 35.9 newtons, and 38.4 newtons, respectively. The intact ligaments had a significantly greater breaking strength than that of any repaired ligaments. In all repairs, the ligaments failed at the repair site. Ligaments undergoing pull-out wire and Mitek anchor repairs were significantly stronger than those undergoing the suture technique.

Conclusions.—These repair techniques do not provide the stability of the intact PIP lateral collateral ligament. Thus, providing some protection against axial stress in the early postoperative period may be appropriate.

▶ The authors studied a biomechanical character (axial distraction force) of intact PIP joint collateral ligament and of the same after 3 different types of repair after rupture. An inevitable flaw of the study was that there was no healing process in cadaver specimens. All repaired ligaments failed at the site of the repair as expected, and the tested repair techniques could not provide the stability to start early motion, also as expected. Therefore, the authors conclude that it may be prudent to provide some protection against axial stress in the early postoperative period. And this may cause limitation of the joint motion. I personally believe that Dr. Moberg was right when he stated that immobilization in the position of function, while leaving the collateral ligament as slack as possible, was the best method for bringing the ends of the ruptured hand ligament together to restore normal alignment in total ligament ruptures of the hand.[1] Of course, there is an exception, such as the thumb metaphalangeal ulnar collateral ligament rupture with Stener lesion.

J. Ryu, M.D.

Reference

1. Moberg E: Fractures and ligamentous injuries of the thumb and fingers. *Surg Clin North Am* 40:297, 1960.

Kinematics of the Trapeziometacarpal Joint: A Biomechanical Analysis Comparing Tendon Interposition Arthroplasty and Total-Joint Arthroplasty

Imaeda T, Cooney WP, Niebur GL, et al (Mayo Clinic and Found, Rochester, Minn)

J Hand Surg (Am) 21A:544–553, 1996 1–15

Background.—Osteoarthritis commonly involves the trapeziometacarpal joint. The kinematics of the trapeziometacarpal joint after ligament reconstruction with tendon interposition (LRTI) arthroplasty and total-joint arthroplasty were studied.

Methods.—Fifteen cadaver hands were examined. Normal joints were compared with simulated total-joint arthroplasties of the ball and socket and fibrous suspension arthroplasties of LRTI.

Findings.—The pivot point after LRTI significantly shifted palmarly and ulnarly in reference to the trapezial coordinate system, compared with normal trapeziometacarpal joint motion. After total-joint arthroplasty, the pivot point shifted slightly palmarly and radially. In a comparison of rotation axes during thumb flexion-extension and abduction-adduction motion, the center of flexion-extension shifted palmarly and the center of abduction-adduction shifted ulnarly after LRTI. After total-joint arthroplasty, the center of rotation for flexion-extension shifted distally and palmarly. The shift for that of abduction-adduction was palmar and proximal. Passive circumduction was greater after LRTI arthroplasty compared with the normal joint, but was less after total-joint arthroplasty.

Conclusions.—These kinematic changes suggest a suspensory ligament function of reconstruction with LRTI arthroplasty. Total-joint arthroplasty, by contrast, results in axes of rotation that reflect the joint replacement instead of those of the normal joint.

► In a complicated biomechanical analysis, the authors demonstrate that neither the popular LRTI procedure nor a total-joint replacement using a fixed ball-and-socket articulation come close to re-creating the flexion-extension and abduction-adduction axes of the normal human trapeziometacarpal joint. Their findings are consistent with intuitive reasoning because of the concave-convex topography of the trapeziometacarpal articulation; the dorsovolar concave metacarpal contour suggests a flexion-extension axis proximal to the joint within the trapezium, whereas the convex radio-ulnar contour suggests an abduction-adduction axis distal to the joint line within the base of the thumb metacarpal. Both the LRTI and the fixed articulation total-joint replacement contain a single axis for both planes of motion, determined by the volar-ulnar pivot position of the ligament reconstruction on the metacarpal cortex for the LRTI compared with the distally displaced ball-and-socket articulation of the total-joint replacement. If the design engineer and arthroplasty surgeon continue to aspire to the ideal of re-creating normal kinematics of the trapeziometacarpal joint, only a resurfacing arthroplasty with reciprocal concave and convex contours will provide an acceptable solution.

V.D. Pellegrini, Jr., M.D.

Passive Axial Rotation of the Metacarpophalangeal Joint

Krishnan J, Chipchase L (Repatriation Gen Hosp, Daw Park, Australia)

J Hand Surg (Br) 22B:270–273, 1997 1–16

Background.—The metacarpophalangeal (MCP) joint is a complex hinge joint with 2 degrees of freedom: flexion/extension and radial/ulnar deviation. Axial rotation occurs at this joint but is not under conscious control. This is called essential axial rotation. Essential axial rotation assists in the dexterousness of the hand (Fig 2). The range of passive axial rotation in the MCP joints of normal, healthy volunteers was described.

Methods.—The study group consisted of 45 men and 55 women. Age, gender, and hand dominance were recorded for each participant, An Isotrak electromagnetic tracking system was used to evaluate MCP joint rotation. With the wrist maintained at 30 degrees extension and each MCP joint at 0 degrees extension, the joint was first supinated and then pronated. One examiner conducted all tests. Intra-examiner reliability was confirmed with 10 volunteers on 2 separate days.

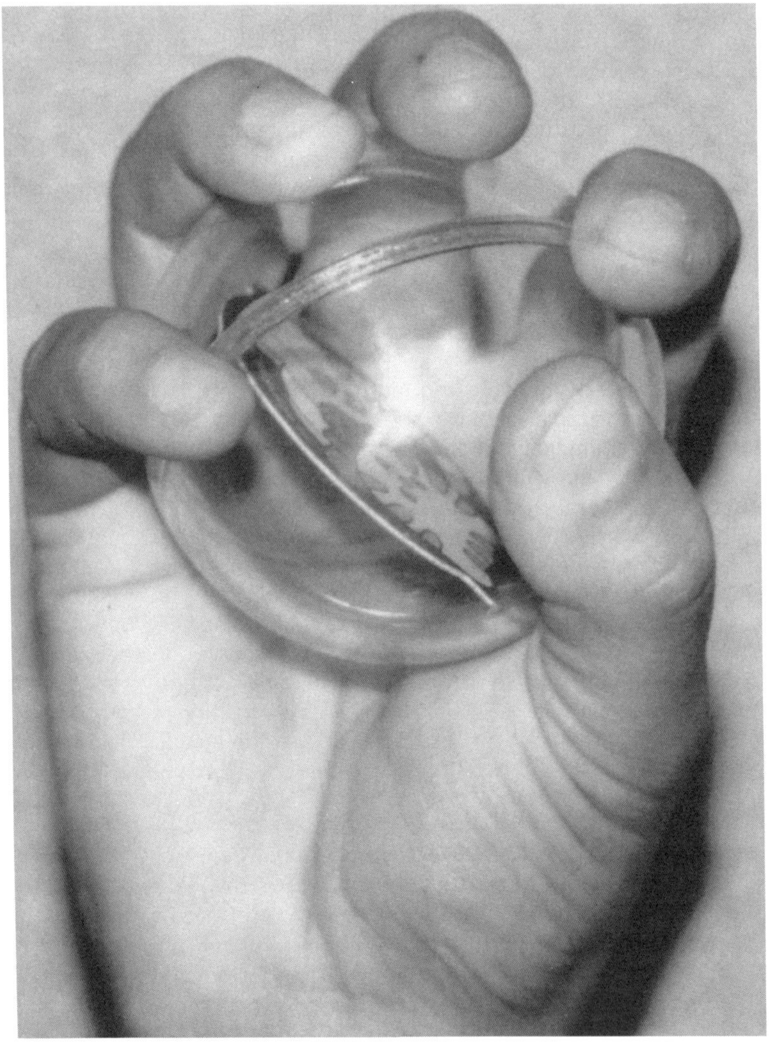

FIGURE 2.—Supination evident at the ring and small metacarpophalangeal joints while a spherical object is being held. (Courtesy of Krishnan J, Chipchase L: Passive axial rotation of the metacarpophalangeal joint. *J Hand Surgery [Br]* 22B:270–273, 1997.)

Results.—Analysis of variance demonstrated no effects of age or hand dominance. There was an effect of gender, as women had significantly greater ranges of lateral rotation in the middle, ring, and small finger MCP joints. Supination was significantly larger than pronation at each MCP joint. Supination was significantly different for each joint. The average range of supination was largest for the small finger MCP joint, followed by the ring finger, followed by the index finger, with the smallest range of supination in the middle finger MCP joint.

Conclusion.—The axial rotation of MCP joints allows adaptation of the hand when grasping an object. This report describes the range of passive rotation available for each MCP joint. This information will increase understanding of MCP joint function and contribute to the successful development of prosthetic devices.

► This study emphasizes the adaptive passive ability of MCP joints to conform to external forces placed on the fingers. This "essential" motion should be separated from the smaller conjunct rotation that occurs at the joint in flexion/extension and, more particularly, in radioulnar deviation. The greater passive supination, obviously, is an advantage in adjusting the fingers to grasp an object that is ovoid or cylindrical. This trait is consistent with the response of a 4-bar linkage to applied force. This would appear to be, in large part, a result of the greater obliquity of the ulnar collateral ligament as compared with the radial collateral ligament, as noted by Landsmeer.[1] It may also have some implications, in an evolutionary sense, for the physical anthropologists.

R.L. Linscheid, M.D.

Reference

1. Landsmeer JMF: *Atlas of Anatomy of the Hand.* Edinburgh, Scotland, Churchill Livingstone, 1976.

Ligamentomuscular Protective Reflex in the Elbow

Phillips D, Petrie S, Solomonow M, et al (Louisiana State Univ, New Orleans)
J Hand Surg (Am) 22A:473–478, 1997 1–17

Introduction.—The ligamentomuscular protective reflex has been demonstrated in the knee, shoulder, and ankle. It is uncertain, however, whether this reflex exists in all other major joints and which specific nerves, muscles, and ligaments are associated with the reflex in a given joint. Using a feline model, investigators sought to determine whether a ligamentomuscular protective reflex arc exists from the elbow ligaments to the associated muscles.

Methods.—Six anesthetized adult cats underwent dissection of each hindlimb. A bipolar stimulating stainless-steel electrode probe applied 100 μsec supramaximal pulses at a rate of 10 pulses/sec to the animals' articular nerve branches. Fine-wire electrodes were inserted into the muscle bellies to assess reflex activation of any muscles around the elbow joint. The M-wave discharge of each muscle was recorded, and the conduction time from application of the stimulus to the nerve to the appearance of the reflexive M-wave was calculated. The M-wave, or electromyographic response to each pulse, is the synchronous discharge of all active motor units in the muscle.

Results.—The feline model confirmed the existence of a reflex arc from the medial elbow ligaments to the forearm pronator muscles. Stimulation of the articular nerve elicited myoelectric activity in a number of monitored muscles: the flexor digitorum superficialis, flexor digitorum profundus, flexor carpi radialis, flexor carpi ulnaris, and pronator teres. The afferent nature of the articular nerve was confirmed by the disappearance of myoelectric activity in the muscles when this nerve was severed between the electrodes and the median nerve.

Discussion.—Findings in this feline model document the existence of a fast-acting reflex arc from sensory elements in the medial ligaments of the elbow to the flexor-pronator muscles of the forearm. This reflex is mediated by the median nerve and its articular branch. Elbow repair procedures should preserve the neural supply of the ligaments and elbow capsule.

► The authors demonstrate, in a feline model, that the medial collateral ligament of the elbow has afferent nerve fibers and a reflex arc involving protective muscle contraction. This confirms the existence of a physiologic basis for the close relationship between the medial collateral ligament and the muscles of the common flexor-pronator group. Implications for surgeons and sports medicine specialists include the fact that rehabilitation of the common flexor-pronator muscle group is important in the prevention and treatment of medial collateral ligament injuries as well as the postoperative rehabilitation after surgical reconstruction or repair. Additionally, surgery on the medial side of the elbow should attempt to preserve this intercapsular and ligamentous innervation. Afferent nerve fibers and protective reflex arcs have been demonstrated in the other major joints and, obviously, play a role in the normal function of the joint.

S.W. O'Driscoll, M.D.

Venous Pumps of the Hand

Simons P, Smith PC, Lees WR, et al (Rayne Inst, London; Univ College Med School, London)

J Hand Surg (Br) 21B:595–599, 1996 1–18

Introduction.—The mechanism of venous pumping of the lower limbs has been well investigated. However, few attempts have been made to describe this mechanism in the upper limbs. The venous pumping mechanism of the hand was quantitatively and objectively measured.

Methods.—Doppler ultrasound studies were performed; each vein in the hand was imaged at rest and at activation. The deep veins of the palm and the superficial dorsal and palmar venous systems were all activated by compression or isometric muscle contraction. Blood velocity was measured in the cephalic vein and the veins of the ulnar artery, and the mean increase during activation was determined. Venography was also performed using radiocontrast media. Four cadaver hands were dissected, and the diameter, number, and branching of the veins were examined.

Results.—Blood velocity was found to increase during activation in both the cephalic and ulnar collateral veins. The greatest increase in blood velocity was found when the hand was clenched and all 3 venous pumps were activated. At the ulnar vein, the mean increase in blood velocity was greater (7.46) than increases found for each activation separately. Palmar compression and adduction action produced similar increases in the ulnar veins (2.36 and 2.60, respectively). The smallest increase in blood velocity was observed with dorsum compression (1.90). Similarly, for cephalic vein measurements, mean increases were greatest when the hand was clenched and all 3 venous pump systems were activated (3.08). Adduction action and palm compression produced mean increases of 2.76 and 2.74, respectively. The lowest mean increase in blood velocity was found with dorsum compression (2.36). Dissection of the hand revealed a mean of 12.7 branches per hand and 17.8 branches in the hand and wrist. In venography, contrast media was found to flow from the superficial dorsal veins into the deep veins of the radial artery. In addition, contrast was observed to flow through the cephalic vein.

Conclusion.—Three independent venous systems were found: superficial palmar, deep palmar, and dorsal veins. When activated by fist clenching, these systems were found to act synergistically, producing a greater increase in blood velocity compared with each system independently.

▶ The authors have demonstrated that the venous systems of the hand are particularly well designed to work with the muscle systems to move blood out of the hand against a relatively high proximal venous pressure, itself a response to arm dependency. Various devices are now being marketed as assisting in the reduction of venous pooling in the hand after injury or surgery when the patient is unable or unwilling to produce the necessary intrinsic muscle contractions and cannot make a fist. Most devices are designed to compress either the palmar or the dorsal side. This study indicates the usefulness of compression on both sides.

V.R. Hentz, M.D.

Suggested Reading

Hurwitz PJ: Variations in the course of the thenar branch of the median nerve. *J Hand Surg (Br)* 21B:344–346, 1996.

▶ Knowledgable hand surgeons know they must heed not only median motor branches which penetrate the flexor retinaculum, but also those that may be multiple, or which course anterior to the retinaculum. An open approach to carpal tunnel release is no guarantee of a safe exposure. Anatomic variations always stand ready to trap the unwary.

P.C. Amadio, M.D.

Voche P, Merle M: Vascular supply of the palmar subcutaneous tissue of fingers. *Br J Plast Surg* 49:315–318, 1996.

▶ The authors demonstrate the anastomotic network in the palmar subcutaneous tissues in order to confirm the vascular reliability of a flap of subcutaneous tissue based on one or another of the digital arteries.

V.R. Hentz, M.D.

2 Diagnosis and Evaluation

The Hand Injury Severity Scoring System

Campbell DA, Kay SPJ (St James's Univ, Leeds, England)

J Hand Surg (Br) 21B:295–298, 1996 2–1

Background.—Scoring systems have proved useful in trauma management, both for prognostication and auditing purposes. Hand injuries constitute a major component of the trauma workload. A scoring system for the classification of hand injuries was used.

Development and Validation.—The system divides the hand, distal to the carpus, into the categories of integument, skeletal, motor, and neural, or ISMN. Each ray is examined for injury in each category. The total score is then multiplied by a weighting factor for each particular ray: 6 for the thumb, 3 for the long and ring fingers, and 2 for the index and little fingers. The scores are totaled to obtain a final Hand Injury Severity Score (HISS). The system can be modified to score for contaminated wounds.

The system was validated in 2 ways: by comparison with the severity ratings of experienced hand surgeons and by a retrospective study of actual hand injuries.

Results.—The original version of the HISS was modified to provide values comparable to the experienced hand surgeons' rankings. On review of the actual hand injuries, the HISS was significantly related to the time off work. Eighty-four percent of patients with a HISS of less than 20 points went back to work after 8 weeks, compared with just 38% of those with a HISS of greater than 20 points. The results suggested 4 grades of increasing severity: minor injury, HISS less than 20 points; moderate injury, 21 to 50 points; severe injury, 51 to 100 points; and major injury, 101 points or higher.

Conclusions.—The HISS is described as a system to grade the severity of hand injuries. It will permit comparison of injuries of similar severity. Although developed for research purposes, the HISS may serve as a useful immediate indicator of severity as well as a predictor of outcome.

▶ I like the tissue-oriented rationale behind this system because it parallels the method of analyzing a complex hand injury that I have tried to teach to the residents on my hand service during the past 20 years. The methodology does leave out an important element, circulation, and one assumes that the scoring system proposed is applied after exploration to assess structures and revascularization if necessary. Nonetheless, a scoring system that fails to take into account loss of 1 or both digital arteries despite a viable digit remains incomplete.

V.R. Hentz, M.D.

Ultrasound Characteristics of Five Common Soft-Tissue Tumours in the Hand and Forearm

Höglund M, Muren C, Engkvist O (Södersjukhuset [Hosp], Stockholm)
Acta Radiol 38:348–354, 1997 2–2

Background.—Benign soft-tissue tumors are common in the hand and forearm, although deep-seated lesions may be difficult to diagnose. There are few reports of soft-tissue tumors of the hand and forearm only and no comprehensive reports characterizing ultrasound findings of common soft-tissue tumors of the hand. The frequency of separate traits of 5 common soft-tissue tumors of the hand and forearm was identified to learn whether the individual tumors have specific ultrasound patterns.

Methods.—Ninety-six tumors of the hand and forearm in 33 males and 63 females aged 1–81 years were examined by ultrasound. There were 18 localized villonodular synovites, 26 hemangiomas, 14 lipomas, 27 peripheral nerve tumors, and 11 glomus tumors. Ganglions were not examined.

Results.—Vessels were observed in 7 circumscribed hemangiomas (Fig 3), and a capsule was found in 9 tumors. Findings were divided into 5 groups of characteristics important for differentiating tumors. These groups were then divided into subgroups. The 5 main groups were (1) growth pattern, with subgroups of pattern of growth and location; (2) echo pattern, with subgroups of echogenicity, echo enhancement, and echo structure; (3) capsule; (4) consistency, with subgroups of compressibility and characteristics of compression; and (5) vessels, with subgroups of presence or absence of vessels, and location. Up to 7 alternatives could describe each subgroup.

Discussion.—These findings verify prior intuitive knowledge of specific ultrasound characteristics of these 5 common lesions of the hand and forearm. Ultrasound provides specific information about the nature, localization, and extent of these tumors. These findings may help diagnosis and management.

► The authors describe a series of 96 benign soft-tissue tumors with histologic confirmation evaluated by ultrasound. Ultrasound features were able to differentiate among 5 common lesions with significant accuracy.

Ultrasound and MRI have long been used for evaluation of complex problems in the hand and wrist. Ultrasound, because of its lower cost, is an effective technique for evaluation of superficial tendon as well as other

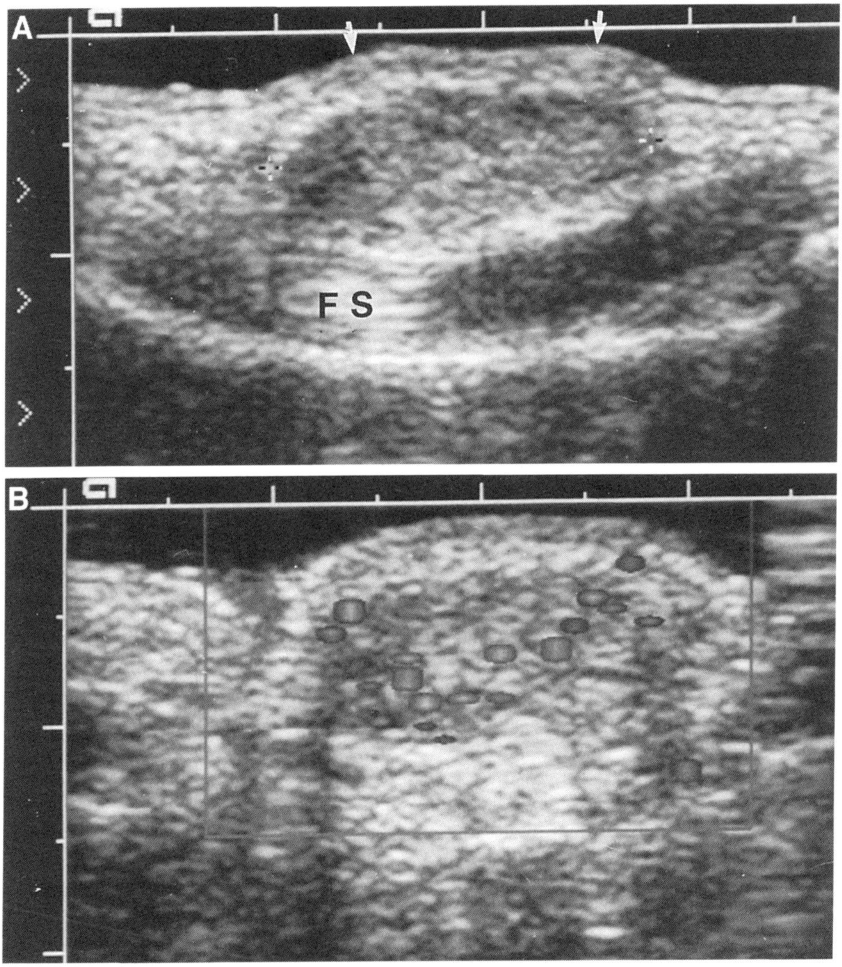

FIGURE 3.—A, volar longitudinal view of a proximal phalanx. Between the cutis (*arrow*) and the flexor tendon (*FS*), there is a high-echogenic, homogeneous, well-circumscribed mass. B, with color Doppler, vessels are seen in the tumor. This was a circumscribed hemangioma. (Courtesy of Höglund M, Muren C, Engkvist O: Ultrasound characteristics of five common soft-tissue tumours in the hand and forearm. *Acta Radiol* 38:348–354, 1997.)

disorders. This paper adds more credibility to the use of ultrasound for diagnosis of masses in the hand and wrist beyond the typical solid-cystic differentiation which is well-known in the literature. Therefore, ultrasound should be considered in patients with suspected benign neoplasms of the hand and wrist. It offers a less expensive alternative to MRI.

T.H. Berquist, M.D.

The Use of Routine Wrist Radiography in the Evaluation of Patients With Carpal Tunnel Syndrome

Bindra RR, Evanoff BA, Chough LY, et al (Washington Univ, St Louis; Mount Vernon Orthopaedic Clinic, Ill)

J Hand Surg (Am) 22A:115–119, 1997 2–3

Background.—Carpal tunnel syndrome (CTS) is the most common entrapment neuropathy. Wrist radiographs are routinely used as part of patient examination. The routine use of radiography is being reassessed in an effort to reduce health care costs. The importance of routine wrist radiography was evaluated in patients with CTS referred to a community-based hand surgery practice.

Study Design.—A retrospective review of charts and radiographs was performed for 300 consecutive CTS patients seen at a singe practice between 1993 and 1995. All patients completed a medical history questionnaire and underwent physical examination, electrophysiologic testing, and wrist radiography.

Study Group.—The study group consisted of 99 men and 201 women with 447 affected wrists. The average age at presentation was 59 years. Among the 153 patients with unilateral disease, the dominant hand was affected in 124 cases. The average symptom duration was 38 months.

Findings.—Abnormalities were detected in 33% of wrist radiographs in this patient group. Of these, 18.6% were abnormalities that might have contributed to the development of CTS but would not affect treatment. In only 2 of the 447 wrists were the radiographic findings of therapeutic significance. The radiography charges were calculated to be between $5,869 and $20,115 for each significant finding.

Conclusion.—The very low prevalence of therapeutically significant findings (0.4%) after routine wrist radiography in patients with carpal tunnel syndrome suggests that routine wrist radiography is not a cost-effective management strategy for these patients.

▶ The authors have used statistical analysis to recommend that radiographic examination of the hand not be used in the treatment of CTS. There is no question that this is a cheaper way to manage the patient, but the final question of quality of patient care is one with which we should be most concerned. In this article, the authors have proposed that a number of useless radiographs did not indicate the need for radiographic evaluation in patients with carpal tunnel syndrome.

In my own practice, I have identified a giant cell tumor (1 patient), Kienbock's disease (2 patients), and significant wrist arthrosis (a number of patients) as contributing to the presence of CTS. As the authors imply, these conditions may not affect the management of the actual CTS. However, I believe that radiographic evaluation produces an overall higher quality of medical care of the hand and wrist in patients presenting to the surgeon with CTS, and I cannot agree with the concept that the cheaper patient evaluation is associated with an equal quality of care.

R.D. Beckenbaugh, M.D.

Sensory Function Assessment: A Pilot Comparison Study of Touch Pressure Threshold With Texture and Tactile Discrimination

King PM (Univ of Wisconsin, Milwaukee)

J Hand Ther 10:24–28, 1997 2–4

Background.—Determining cutaneous sensibility involves determining sensory acuity and determining the function of a specific level of acuity. Threshold tests include those for the 4 classic cutaneous distinctions—pain, heat, cold, and touch-pressure—as well as for vibration. Whether there is a correlation between touch-pressure threshold testing and sensory discrimination function—specifically, tactile gnosis for texture and object recognition—was determined.

Methods.—Twenty-nine patients with carpal tunnel syndrome (CTS), as confirmed by electromyography or nerve conduction velocity tests, underwent the Semmes-Weinstein monofilament test, a texture discrimination test, and an object identification test. Texture and object recognition tests were normed in a group of 100 subjects with normal touch-pressure thresholds. The patients with CTS were grouped as normal, diminished light touch, or diminished protective sensation on the basis of their performance on the Semmes-Weinstein monofilament test. Each group's mean response times for identifying textures and objects were compared with normed response times.

Findings.—The patients identified all textures and objects accurately. There was a significant difference in response times between patients with CTS and diminished light touch in the identification of 4 of the 6 objects. Patients with diminished protective sensation had significantly longer response times in identifying the textures of cork, coarse and fine sandpaper, and rubber. These subjects also had significantly longer response times when identifying objects such as a screw and a button and the shapes of a square, a triangle, and an oval.

Conclusion.—Although the number of subjects in each impairment group was small, these findings reveal the significance of response time in the performance of sensory discrimination tasks by patients with diminished touch-pressure thresholds. These data are important for determining the true value of cutaneous sensibility and its associated implications for performance.

► King's Sensory Function Assessment Test is a springboard for dialogue and future studies that may correlate the results of Semmes-Weinstein monofilament testing to function and, for this reason, is an important contribution. Time identification is an important concept introduced by the author and one which has not yet been addressed in the literature in relation to filament/function correlation. The Limitations section is honest and points out problems with test instrumentation.

The functional tests used in the study are not reliable or valid. It would seem that age and intelligence would be factors with timed response testing, and these variables are not controlled in the study. Only 3 of 29 subjects given a diagnosis of CTS were in the *diminished protective sensation* range, so the author's finding that these 3 subjects who demonstrated significantly longer response times for identification of all textures and objects (with the exception of 2 textures and 1 object) is of limited value.

R.B. Evans, O.T.R./L., C.H.T.

Validation of Cutaneous Pressure Threshold Measurements for the Evaluation of Hand Function

Dellon ES, Keller KM, Moratz V, et al (Johns Hopkins Univ, Baltimore, Md; Children's Hosp for Reconstructive Surgery, Baltimore, Md)
Ann Plast Surg 38:485–492, 1997 2–5

Background.—Measuring hand function continues to be problematic. The validity of the pressure threshold measurements obtained with the Pressure-Specifying Sensory Device, using the Mayo Dexterity Test and the object recognition test, was investigated.

Methods and Findings.—The results of the Mayo Dexterity Test, which permits the use of vision, and a timed object recognition test, which does not, were correlated with the 1- and 2-point static and moving touch thresholds for the index finger pulp of 44 hands. The Pressure-Specifying Sensory Device was used for quantitative sensory testing. Cutaneous pressure threshold measurements with this device were significantly associated with the small-object subset of the Mayo Dexterity Test and with the object recognition test. Thus, the Pressure-Specifying Sensory Device proved to be a valid tool for assessing the sensory aspect of hand function.

Conclusion.—The cutaneous pressure threshold measurements made with the Pressure-Specifying Sensory Device are valid in the assessment of hand function. The relative merits of cutaneous pressure threshold testing in diagnosis or prognosis have yet to be established.

▶ Oftentimes we order hand function tests without thinking through what it is we want to measure—sensation, coordination, strength, activities of daily living function, or job abilities? Dellon et al. discuss the rationales for the various hand function tests quite cogently, particularly in relation to tests of sensation. The introduction section is worth reading if only to review these concepts of hand function measuring devices. The various office measurements of hand sensation are also put through intense scrutiny to determine what is actually being measured.

Two-point discrimination will still be the easiest and cheapest way of measuring gross sensation in the office setting. However, the pressure threshold device may eventually supersede the Semmes-Weinstein monofilament test as the test of choice for sensation threshold. Moreover, there are situations in which a simpler test of sensation alone (such as this cutaneous pressure threshold device) may be substituted accurately for a more lengthy hand function test.

K.A. Bengtson, M.D.

Suggested Reading

Drapé J-L, Idy-Peretti I, Goettmann S, et al: MR imaging of digital mucoid cysts. *Radiology* 200:531–536, 1996.

► This article demonstrates the capability of MRI technology in providing really exquisite detailed assessment of this common lesion. The methodology has little practical value except in unusual cases or perhaps for subungual lesions. However, the images are very good.

V.R. Hentz, M.D.

Jónsson Á, Laurin S, Karner G, et al: Spatial resolution requirements in digital radiography of scaphoid fractures: An ROC analysis. *Acta Radiol* 37:555–560, 1996.

► As picture archiving and communication systems become more common, familiarity with the potential as well as the limitations of use of digital radiography will also be useful to the hand surgeon. This article shows that for detection of subtle scaphoid fractures on digital images a pixel size of 0.17 mm was the best compromise between detection rate and scanning/transmission time/archive memory requirements.

Pixel size is calculated as the field-of-view (length and width of the radiographed area) divided by the matrix used on the display monitor. It therefore depends both on the size of the radiographic (for example a hand radiograph of 10 × 12 inches [25 × 30 cm]) and on the monitors used for viewing in the clinic, which usually have a resolution of "1 k" (1024 × 1024 pixels) or "high-resolution 2k" (2048 × 2048 pixels). A 10 × 12 inch hand radiograph displayed on a 1 k monitor will give a 0.25 × 0.30 mm pixel size, which is not sufficient for detection of subtle scaphoid fractures according to this paper; a better choice is a 2 k display monitor giving 0.13 × 0.15 mm pixel size.

Another important concept discussed in this article is "compression" of digital data. Several compression techniques are available, the purpose of which is to find the best compromise between providing economical storage of digital images with efficient transmission of data to users' monitors and maintaining a diagnostic quality image. Compression is usually performed after the initial interpretation of the digital image because an irreversible compression technique by definition introduces some loss of resolution when the images are viewed on a monitor. In this article, a compression rate of 10:1 using wavelet compression was found to not decrease detection of subtle scaphoid fractures significantly when a pixel size of 0.17 mm was used.

G. Bergman, M.D.

Josty IC, Tyler MPH, Shewell PC, et al: Grip and pinch strength variations in different types of workers. *J. Hand Surg (Br)* 22B:266–269, 1997.

► Those with more strenuous jobs have slightly more strength (12 vs. 10 kg pinch; 54 vs. 46 kg grip) and less dominant/nondominant strength difference. Little surprise here.

P.C. Amadio, M.D.

Sørenson J, Bengtsson M, Malmqvist EL-Å, et al: Laser Doppler perfusion imager (LPDI)—for the assessment of skin blood flow changes following sympathetic blocks. *Acta Anesthesiol Scand* 40:1145–1148, 1996.

▶ The laser Doppler perfusion imager is a new noninvasive modality which provides a spatial representation of laser Doppler fluxometry over a 12 × 12 cm area by a maximum of 4,096 laser Doppler measurements. In contradistinction to other laser Doppler fluxometry systems, this machine works without skin contact. This device allows the reproducible assessment of spatiotemporal microvascular events which heretofore have been unavailable. The documentation of the heterogeneity of microvascular perfusion throughout the upper extremity demonstrates the clinical difficulty in extrapolating single laser Doppler flux measurements and highlights problems in interpreting isolated temperature measurements in non-acral areas of skin.

L.A. Koman, M.D.

Strauch B, Lang A, Ferder M, et al: The ten test. *Plast Reconstr Surg* 99:1074–1078, 1997.

3 Skeletal Trauma and Reconstruction

Splinting in the Management of Proximal Interphalangeal Joint Flexion Contracture

Prosser R (St Luke's Hosp, Sydney, Australia)

J Hand Ther 9:378–386, 1996 3–1

Background.—Injury to the proximal interphalangeal (PIP) joint often involves rupture of the stabilizing structure, usually the volar plate and collateral ligaments. There have been no published descriptions of the quality of joint stiffness, objective measurements of passive extension in PIP flexion contracture caused by trauma, or how this is changed by treatment with a splinting program in a clinical setting.

Methods.—Twenty patients with PIP flexion contracture were included in a dynamic splinting program using either a Capener or low-profile outrigger splint. A 250-g force was applied to the distal end of the middle phalanx. The patients wore the splint 8–12 hours per 24 hours for 8 weeks, followed by a 2- to 3-week weaning period. Torque range-of-motion measures were used to objectively assess passive extension.

Findings.—The mean flexion contracture was 39 degrees before treatment; the final extension deficit improved by an average of 18 degrees. Total end-range time averaged 10 hours in a 24-hour period for a mean of 4.3 months. Splinting time was the only statistically significant variable affecting outcome.

Conclusion.—This small clinical study suggests that dynamic splinting is an effective treatment for PIP flexion contracture. Splinting duration was the most significant factor in flexion contracture resolution. Joints that were stiffer before splinting were still the stiffer joints after splinting. However, some improvement in passive extension was achieved in the stiffer joints.

► This study investigates the treatment outcomes and variables in a small sample of 20 subjects with PIP flexion contracture treated with dynamic splinting with either a finger-based Capener splint or a low-profile outrigger splint. The author concludes the following: greater PIP extension deficits and greater joint stiffness initially yield poorer final results; greater initial stiffness is predictive of continuing problems of joint stiffness at the end of treatment; the greater the flexion contracture, the stiffer the joint; the longer the contracture time, the stiffer the joint; and greater stiffness requires long-term splinting, often in excess of 4 months.

This study will be helpful to those in clinical practice because it supports the use of long-term splinting and formal supervision for this difficult problem, giving us some leverage as we deal with managed care organizations. The study also lends statistical support to the work of Flowers and LaStayo on the effect of *total end range time* on improving passive range of motion, in which they concluded that the increase in passive range of motion of a stiff PIP joint is directly proportional to the length of time the joint is held at its end range.[1] It is important to note that the forces applied with dynamic splinting were light and designed to allow for tissue reorganization without increasing inflammation. Torque on the PIP joint was controlled at between 100 and 250 g with dynamic splinting allowing extended wearing time.

I found it interesting that no flexion contracture completely resolved. Earlier therapuetic intervention (average intervention in this study was 12.8 weeks post injury) and serial finger casting,[2] in my clinical experience, yield better, faster results in terms of decreasing edema, decreasing inflammation, and the remodeling of tight connective tissues of the PIP joint compared with dynamic splinting. Interested readers may want to review the technique for objective measurement of passive range of motion, *torque range of motion,*[3] and the concept of *total end range time.*[1]

R.B. Evans, O.T.R./L., C.H.T.

References

1. Flowers KR, LaStayo P: Effect of total end range time on improving passive range of motion. *J Hand Ther* 7:150–157, 1994.
2. Bell-Krotoski JA: Plaster cylinder casting for contractures of the interphalangeal joints, in Hunter JM, Mackin EJ, Callahan AD (eds): *Rehabilitation of the Hand: Surgery and Therapy*, ed 4. St Louis, Mosby, 1995, pp 1609–1616.
3. Breger-Lee D, Bell-Krotoski J, Brandsma JW: Torque range of motion in the hand clinic. *J Hand Ther* 3:7–13, 1990.

A Comparative Mechanical Analysis of Plate Fixation in a Proximal Phalangeal Fracture Model

Lins RE, Myers BS, Spinner RJ, et al (Duke Univ, Durham, NC)
J Hand Surg (Am) 21A:1059–1064, 1996 3–2

Background.—Fractures of the proximal phalanx of the hand are common injuries that can result in functional impairment. A variety of implantable devices for open reduction and internal fixation of such fractures are currently available. The mechanical properties of hand and craniofacial plating systems commonly used in the treatment of proximal phalangeal fractures were compared.

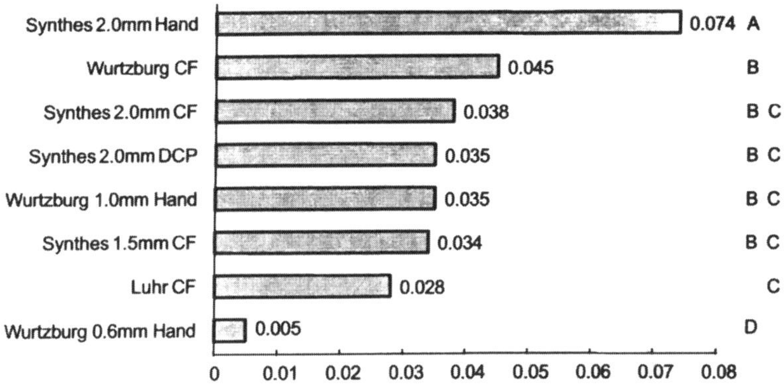

FIGURE 3.—Results of apex palmar bending stiffness testing. *Abbreviations: CF*, craniofacial; *DCP*, dynamic compression plate. (Courtesy of Lins RE, Myers BS, Spinner RJ, et al: A comparative mechanical analysis of plate fixation in a proximal phalangeal fracture model. *J Hand Surg [Am]* 21A:1059–1064, 1996.)

Methods.—A yellow-birch-dowel model of a proximal phalanx was used. A transverse cut was made in the middle of the dowel section to model a midshaft transverse osteotomy or fracture. Two plates of each of several systems were then mounted dorsally on the model. Torsional rigidity was achieved, and failure testing in apex palmar 4-point bending was assessed.

Findings.—Torsion varied by 1,600% among plating systems. The results of apex palmar testing varied by 1,500%. Apex palmar moment-to-failure testing varied by 1,000%, respresenting a 3.5% to 38% range of intact proximal phalangeal strength. In addition, this represented 12% to 128% of the maximum calculated in vivo bending moments of the proximal phalanx (Fig 3).

Conclusions.—The great variation in plate strengths and stiffness raises questions about the suitability of certain plating systems for early mobilization. Also, some systems were found to be mechanically weaker than the reported strengths of certain Kirschner wire fixation methods.

► Closed treatment of unstable phalangeal fractures frequently leads to unsatisfactory results. Rigid fixation is necessary to anatomically reduce the fracture and permit early mobilization, decreasing tendinous adhesions. The selection of a proper plate system is essential for a successful outcome. Four 0.028 in diameter K-wires were more rigid in apex palmar testing than was any plate configuration; however, all plating systems were stiffer in apex palmar testing than were 2 cross wires.

P. Dell, M.D.

A Comparative Biomechanical Analysis of Resorbable Rigid Fixation Versus Titanium Rigid Fixation of Metacarpal Fractures

Prevel CD, Eppley BL, Ge J, et al (Univ of Kentucky, Lexington; Indiana Univ, Indianapolis; PolyMedics Inc, Warsaw, Ind)

Ann Plast Surg 37:377–385, 1996 3–3

Background.—The clinical use of resorbable pins, screws, tacks, and rods has been reported in the treatment of hand fractures, ligament reinsertion, and joint arthrodesis. However, there has been no study of a resorbable plating system for the hand. The biomechanical stability of a new, resorbable, miniplate fixation system for the hand was described.

Methods.—The plates and screws studied were made of Lactosorb, a copolymer of polyglycolic (PGA) and poly-l-lactic (PLLA) acid. The plates were used in osteotomized fresh frozen human cadaveric metacarpal bones, which were then subjected to apex bending and torsional load testing. Data from this in vitro experiment were compared with data from an earlier study of low-profile titanium mini- and microplates and screws.

Findings.—In an analysis of variance, the linear-flat Lactosorb plate and screws were found to have apex dorsal rigidity and force-to-displacement measures equal to all but 2 of the titanium plates. The 3-dimensional-flat Lactosorb plate had the greatest torsional rigidity of the resorbable system. However, it was only moderately rigid, in both bending and torsion, compared with the titanium systems.

Conclusions.—These data suggest that the copolymer PGA–PLLA plating system may be better suited for metacarpal fractures than for proximal phalangeal fractures, since the demands of torsional loading are lower, compared to those of apex bending, in metacarpal fractures as compared to phalangeal fractures.

► Modern low-profile metal mini- and microplates are less likely than their predecessors to cause prominence and irritation under the skin, which would require their removal. Bone atrophy and osteoporosis as a result of plate stiffness are seldom, if ever, seen in metacarpal or phalangeal fractures treated with these plates. Problems with metal sensitization and carcinogenesis are indeed remote. Resorbable plates do not obviate the biggest problem of plate application, which is the dissection necessary for their application. A distinct disadvantage of resorbable plates is that they can not be contoured intraoperatively. Nevertheless, resorbable plates, screws, or combinations that adequately stabilize reduced fractures until they heal, support functional recovery, and then disappear without a trace or problem have distinct appeal. Resorbable implants seem especially suited to simple fractures. They have passed biomechanical testing. Clinical results are pending.

A.A. Freeland, M.D.

Fixation for Comminuted Phalangeal Fractures: A Biomechanical Study of Five Methods

Lu WW, Furumachi K, Ip WY, et al (Univ of Hong Kong)

J Hand Surg (Br) 21B:765–767, 1996 3–4

Introduction.—Not enough is known about comminuted fractures of the hand to recommend the best fixation method(s). The mechanical rigidities of 5 different methods of fixation for comminuted fractures of the proximal phalanx were compared to determine the best fixation method for early mobilization.

Methods.—A comminuted fracture model was used on 12 proximal phalangeal bones of index and middle fingers with similar width and length from embalmed cadaver hands to simulate comminuted fracture. The 5 fixation methods used were as follows: 4 Kirschner (4K) wires, lateral plating with 6 screws (LP6), lateral plating for the triangular butterfly fragment defect model (LPD), fixation with 2 screws (2S), and fixation with 2 crossed intramedullary K-wires (2CK) (Fig 1). Mechanical testing of compression, bending, and torsion was used to test each fixation method for intrinsic stability under varying loads.

Results.—The most rigid fixation technique for resisting torsion loads was LP6, (mean 3.5 N/mm) and the least rigid method was 2CK (mean 2.21 N/mm). A significant difference in resisting torsion loads was observed between LP6 and all other fixation methods. Compared with other methods, the LP6 (mean 3.5 N/mm) and 4K (mean 57.8 N/mm) were

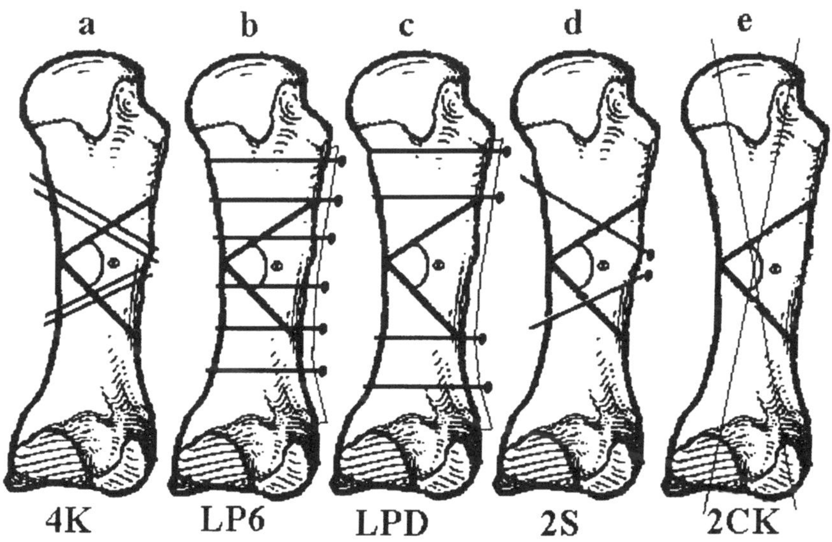

FIGURE 1.—Five fixation models used in the study. **A**, 4 Kirschner (K) wires; **B**, lateral plating with 6 screws; **C**, lateral plating for the triangular butterfly fragment defect model; **D**, fixation with 2 screws; and **E**, fixation with 2 crossed intramedullary K-wires. (Courtesy of Lu WW, Furumachi K, Ip WY, et al: Fixation for comminuted phalangeal fractures: A biomechanical study of five methods. *J Hand Surg [Br]* 21B:765–767, 1996.)

more rigid during bending tests. The 2S (31.5 N/mm) was the least rigid method during bending tests. For axial compression testing, most fixation methods were rigid enough to resist axial loads, but the LP6 (mean 82 N/mm) was significantly stiffer than the 2S (mean 76.3 N/mm).

Conclusion.—Overall, the LP6 was mechanically superior in resisting torsion, bending, and axial compression loads for fixation of comminuted fractures of the phalanges. The 4K was comparable to the LP6. The 2S had the least rigidity. As soft tissue damage must be considered when choosing a fixation method, the 4K method may be the best choice, as it requires less soft tissue dissection and periosteal stripping than the LP6.

► The authors have designed a model for a comminuted fracture by placing a uniform triangular osteotomy in the mid-diaphysis of the proximal phalanx (Fig 1). The triangle can be removed to create a bone defect.

Whereas biomechanical stability is only 1 parameter in the decision-making process, comminuted fractures usually require more stability than simple fractures. Because final functional outcome correlates highly with the severity of soft-tissue damage, both from injury and surgical exposure, the surgeon must weigh biomechanical stability against biological integrity. The intangibles of judgment and the individual surgeon's comfort, familiarity, experience, and skills with particular approaches, methodologies, and implants are equally important and are sometimes paramount.

The data provided in this study assist the surgeon in selecting the most secure fixation for either percutaneous or direct application. One must remember that in vivo results with an intact or restored periosteal and soft-tissue sleeve might produce different values.

A.A. Freeland, M.D.

External Fixation for Comminuted Phalangeal Fractures: A Biomechanical Cadaver Study

Fitoussi F, Ip WY, Chow SP (Univ of Hong Kong)

J Hand Surg (Br) 21B:760–764, 1996 3–5

Introduction.—Comminuted proximal digital fractures of the hand are frequently accompanied by significant soft tissue injuries, and the outcome is often unsatisfactory. A comminuted fracture model was used to compare 3 methods of internal and external fixation for proximal phalanges.

Methods.—Twenty-four proximal phalangeal bones from index, middle, and ring fingers from embalmed cadaver hands were used to test bending, compression, and torsion resistance of 3 different fixation techniques: 2 crossed Kirschner (K) wires, lateral plate with 7 holes, and external fixation using the Pennig Minifixator. Using varying loads, fixation techniques were evaluated in apex palmar bending, compression, and torsion.

Results.—When undergoing apex palmar bending testing and compression testing, the lateral plates were significantly more rigid, by a factor of roughly 1.5, compared with K-wires and external fixation. The K-wire was not significantly more rigid than external fixation in either bending testing or compression testing. In torsion testing, external fixation was significantly more rigid (3.7 N/mm) than the lateral plate (1.6 N/mm) or K-wire (1.4 N/mm) configuration.

Conclusion.—External fixation provided an acceptable rigidity. Future clinical testing is needed, as the effects of applied forces from muscles and ligaments during finger movement need to be understood before external fixation can be recommended for comminuted phalangeal fractures.

▶ This article is a companion to Abstract 3–4. The same fracture model is used. External fixation in an in vitro mid-diaphyseal fracture model achieves initial stability comparable to, or better than, plate fixation or crossed K-wires. This is attractive if the fixator can be applied without crossing a joint—especially the proximal interphalangeal joint—because soft tissue trauma would be less than with plate application. The clinical efficacy of the premise remains to be seen in terms of fracture healing, pin loosening, pin track problems, and functional recovery.

A.A. Freeland, M.D.

Effectiveness of the Chevron Arthrodesis in Small Joints of the Hand

Pribyl CR, Omer GE Jr, McGinty L (Univ of New Mexico, Albuquerque)

J Hand Surg (Am) 21A:1052–1058, 1996 3–6

Background.—Small-joint arthrodeses are generally performed in hands with a partially recoverable functional loss. The usual indications are pain and instability; function may be improved in hands with neurologic impairments. Various techniques of small-joint arthrodesis have been reported, with bone-cutting techniques including the flat cut and the chevron cut. The flat cut is the most commonly used—only 1 clinical series using the chevron technique has been reported. An experience with chevron arthrodesis for the small joints of the hand was reviewed.

Methods.—The review included 98 chevron arthrodeses performed distal to the wrist joint in 53 patients. The metacarpophalangeal joint was operated on in 53 cases and the proximal interphalangeal joint in 39. The patients underwent a total of 71 operations. They had a wide range of clinical indications, most frequently rheumatoid arthritis and trauma. The technique was fairly simple, with chevron cuts angled to the desired degree of flexion. The apex of the chevron pointed in a proximal direction, and the apex of the distal bone was angled perpendicular to the axis of the bone. Fixation was achieved using 2 or 3 crossed Kirschner wires. The patients were studied for an average of 33 months.

Results.—Successful fusion was achieved in all cases. In a radiographic review of 11 patients, the average time to union was 8 weeks. The average difference in flexion angle between the first and final postarthrodesis radiographs was 2 degrees. Pin removal was required in 34 patients, usually in the outpatient clinic. Aside from 2 infections, the only significant complication was malunion in a proximal interphalangeal joint that fused at 90 degrees. This patient and 1 other were unsatisfied with their results. There were no problems with pain at the arthrodesis site.

Conclusions.—The chevron cut technique provides good results in small-joint arthrodesis of the hands. As an alternative to the flat cut technique, the chevron cut provides a greater bone surface area for healing. However, the authors no longer use the chevron technique for arthrodesis of the distal interphalangeal joint because of concern regarding possible damage to the nail bed and resultant deformity.

► The recent literature concerning small-joint fusion in the hand has consistently demonstrated a high rate of success regardless of the type of bone cut or fixation technique. To ensure a solid fusion, surgeons have emphasized the importance of careful preparation of the surfaces to expose cancellous bone and to secure bony coaptation and fixation. The chevron arthrodesis follows these principles and, like other techniques, was found to be quite reliable. The authors advocate this technique because rotational alignment is controlled by the bone cuts and a larger area of cancellous bone is exposed than with flat or cup/cone bone preparations (theoretically leading to a higher union rate). However, one must keep in mind that this technique is unforgiving. If the bony cuts are not made precisely, it may be difficult to correct for malrotation or size discrepancies. Furthermore, as the authors point out, chevron arthrodesis requires bone shortening, which may be undesirable, particularly in situations such as arthritis mutilans where there is significant pre-existing loss of digital length.

P.J. Stern, M.D.

Traumatic Dislocation of the Thumb Carpometacarpal Joint: Early Ligamentous Reconstruction Versus Closed Reduction and Pinning

Simonian PT, Trumble TE (Univ of Washington, Seattle)

J Hand Surg (Am) 21A:802–806, 1996 3–7

Purpose.—Traumatic dislocation of the carpometacarpal (CMC) joint of the thumb is a rare injury. When instability is present, early reconstruction is recommended to prevent recurrent instability and long-term joint degeneration. Two approaches were used in the management of traumatic thumb CMC dislocations: closed reduction and percutaneous pinning vs. early ligamentous reconstruction.

Patients.—All patients had dorsal dislocations with substantial instability; passive adduction and flexion caused recurrent dislocation. The first 8 patients (group A) underwent closed reduction and percutaneous pinning with Kirschner wires. Four of these patients had recurrent subluxation an average of 6 weeks postoperatively. Repeated surgery was required for recurrent instability in 3 patients and for joint degeneration in 1.

Subsequently, 9 patients (group B) underwent early ligamentous reconstruction. The operation was done an average of 7 days after the injury. The reconstruction used the flexor carpi radialis according to the technique of Eaton et al. The average follow-up in this group was 42 months.

Outcomes.—Eight of the 9 group B patients were pain free at work, and the other had only occasional discomfort. Early ligamentous reconstruction preserved near-normal range of motion and grip strength. Thumb abduction was decreased by 20% in group A vs. 10% in group B. Pinch strength was decreased by 19% in group A and 13% in group B. One third of patients in group B had slight, asymptomatic narrowing of the joint space. In contrast, 5 of 8 patients in group A had degeneration of the CMC joint, and 3 had posttreatment symptoms.

Conclusions.—Early ligamentous reconstruction may help to prevent recurrent instability and posttraumatic joint degeneration in patients with traumatic dislocation of the thumb CMC joint. At follow-up, the patients are pain free with essentially normal strength and range of motion. It is uncertain what the primary stabilizing structure damaged after CMC dislocation is.

► The authors show that reconstructing the prime stabilizing ligament of the thumb CMC joint is effective in preventing instability of this joint after traumatic dislocation. The group treated with reconstruction (9 patients) had fewer problems than the 8 patients treated by closed reduction and pinning.

Why does closed reduction fail? Is there an analogy here to failure of closed reduction and immobilization of the dislocated thumb metacarpophalangeal joint, a "Stenner" lesion of the thumb CMC joint? This is not an easy joint in which to assess reduction, either by clinical or radiographic examination. Does inadequate closed reduction lead to recurrent instability? In what position should the thumb CMC joint be pinned? Moreover, ligament reconstruction is not a technically easy operation, as opposed to exposure of the flexor carpi radialis tendon in the context of the excised trapezium, for example, in CMC arthroplasty procedures. I have favored closed pinning with the metacarpal fully flexed and somewhat adducted and early secondary reconstruction when recurrent instability is recognized.

V.R. Hentz, M.D.

Lengthening of the Forearm by Callus Distraction

Abe M, Shirai H, Okamoto M, et al (Osaka Med College, Japan)

J Hand Surg (Br) 21B:151–163, 1996 3–8

Background.—The Wagner technique for ulnar lengthening yields satisfactory results but involves bone grafting, subsequent hardware removal, and prolonged hospitalization. The use of the callotasis method for forearm lengthening, which avoids such disadvantages, was described.

Patients and Outcomes.—Included were 5 girls and 5 boys aged 3 to 13 years. Indications for forearm lengthening included shortening or deformity from exostosis of the distal ulna, enchondroma of the distal ulna, growth disturbance after fracture of the distal radius, radial club hand, congenital amputation, and congenital dislocation of the radial head. Lengthening of the ulna was performed in 4 children, the radius in 1, and the radius and ulna in 5. Forearms were lengthened by a mean of 30 mm. Complications included pin track discharge in 3 patients, callus fracture in 5, delayed consolidation of the callus in 1, and no callus formation in 1. After 1–7 years of follow-up, improvement in appearance and function was satisfactory. Patients who had had tumorous conditions or traumatic epiphyseal arrest especially benefited from the procedure (Fig 4).

Conclusion.—Callotasis is a useful, reliable method for forearm lengthening, especially in children with epiphyseal injury or tumors. This procedure avoids the disadvantages associated with the Wagner technique.

▶ Forearm lengthening by callus distraction is a very useful technique for selected deformities. The authors have concentrated their effort on using a unilateral frame and correcting any angular deformity acutely. An alternative method which allows one more latitude in the correction of angular defor-

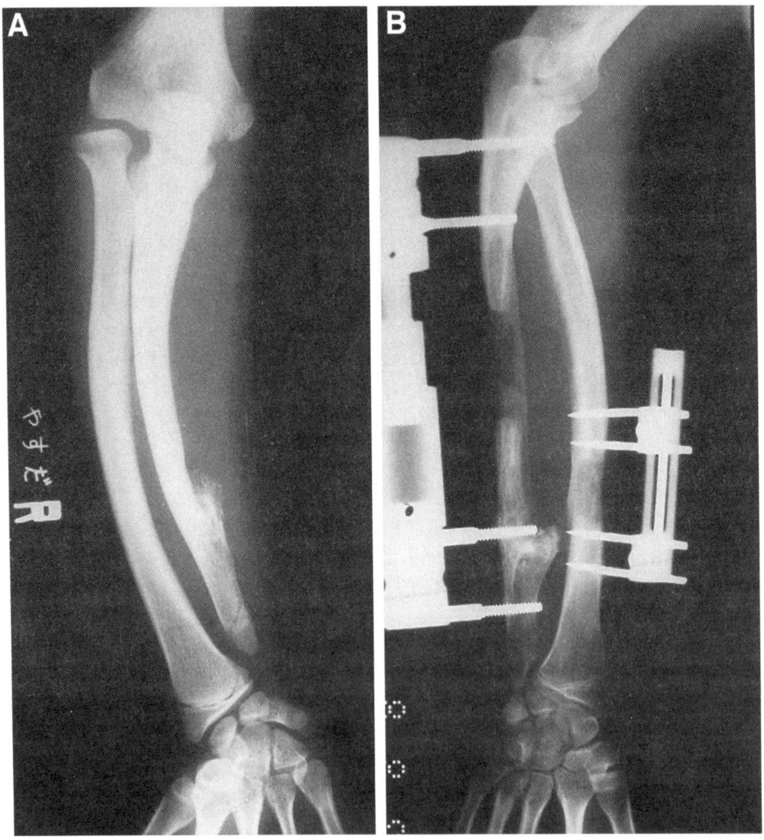

(Continued)

FIGURE 4 (cont.)

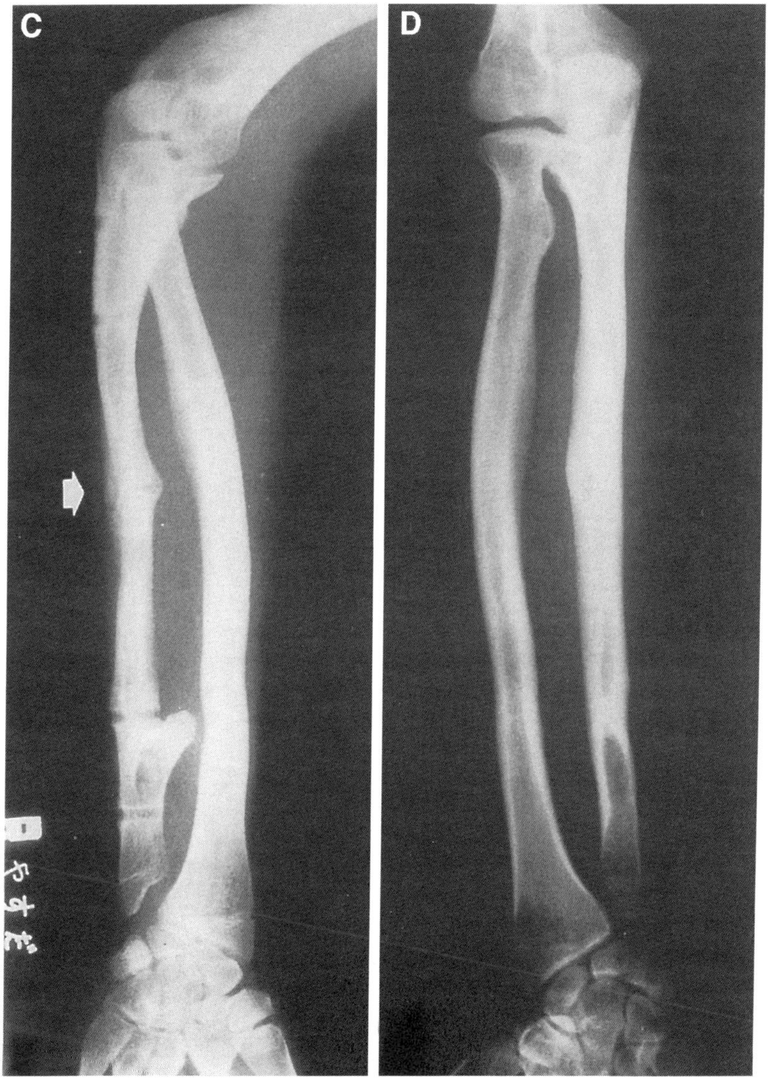

FIGURE 4.—Images of the forearm of a 12-year-old girl with shortening and bowing of the forearm caused by exostosis of the ulna. **A,** radiograph before lengthening. **B,** radiograph at 5 months after surgery. **C,** radiograph at 1 month after pin removal from the ulna (10 months after surgery). Note callus fracture in the regenerated callus without angular deformity. **D,** radiograph at follow-up (6 years 6 months after surgery). Note restored normal articulation of the humeroradial joint and no recurrence of the ulnar shortening. (Courtesy of Abe M, Shirai H, Okamoto M, et al: Lengthening of the forearm by callus distraction. *J Hand Surg [Br]* 21B:151–163, 1996.)

mities is to use a circular frame and the principles using hinges purported by Ilizarov. The authors are critical of circular frames, claiming a higher incidence of injury to nerves and more bulkiness. However, I have been very pleased using the pediatric circular frame fixation set, which is very lightweight and less bulky, and I have used the newer principle of a hybrid frame, that is, a circular wire with half pins. I recommend making an incision for insertion of these pins and, therefore, avoiding neurovascular compromise by visualizing these structures.

The authors have shown that one can predictably increase function in posttraumatic deformities such as epiphyseal arrests when the remaining soft tissues are normal, such as when an abnormally long ulna blocks rotation. On the other hand, correction of congenital deformities with length discrepancies, in which soft tissues have been contracted for a long time, may not result in increased function. This concept should be shared with patients carefully when selecting goals for lengthening, as lengthening procedures are long, tedious, and plagued by problems and complications. Nevertheless, lengthening does have its place and should be part of a hand surgeon's armamentarium for treating posttraumatic and congenital skeletal deformities.

R.M. Szabo, M.D., M.P.H.

Orthopaedic Management of Distal Forearm Fractures in Children: A 152 Cases Report [French]

Prévot N, Salanne P, Longis B, et al (CHU Dupuytren, Limoges, France)

Rev Chir Orthop 83:251–258, 1997 3–9

Introduction.—Distal forearm fractures in children are frequent. Management is conservative except in rare cases.

Materials and Methods.—A retrospective study was conducted of 152 distal forearm fractures in children aged 2 to 16 years (average age, 10 years). The average follow-up was 10.5 months (range, 6 to 48 months). Conservative treatment was undertaken in all cases but 5 in which surgical treatment was required at once. A clinical and radiologic assessment of fracture reduction was conducted immediately postoperatively and during follow-up. Initial angulation of the fracture was posterior or posterolateral in 92% of cases (average angulation, 28.5 degrees), 64% of which had instability criteria. Translation was present in 79 cases (52%) and rated 100% in 55 cases, between 50% and 100% in 11 cases, and less than 50% in 13 cases. In 8% (12 cases), initial angulation was anterior, with a translation greater than 50% in 6 cases and an angulation greater than 30 degrees in the remaining 6 cases.

Results.—Surgical treatment was necessary in 5 cases because of initial instability and/or irreducibility. In the remaining 147 cases, secondary displacement occurred in 43. Analysis of the potential causes of displacement—based on instability criteria, quality of reduction, quality of cast immobilization, and fracture location—showed that it occurred in 18 of 24 cases when reduction was incomplete, in 5 of 10 when cast immobilization was incorrect (and in 6 of 6 when both reduction and cast were incorrect), in 3 of 7 when the fractures was proximal, and in 6 of 6 when the cast was prematurely opened. Secondary reduction was judged necessary when the lateral angulation was greater than 10 degrees with associated distal radioulnar joint incongruity and when the dorsal angulation was greater than 20 degrees. A closed reduction was performed in 6 cases, an open reduction with wire pinning in 1, and secondary osteotomies in 2 cases after 2 and 5 months.

Discussion.—Closed reduction of distal forearm fractures is possible even when the initial displacement is significant. Secondary displacement is unlikely to occur if the initial reduction is perfect and cast immobilization is correct (i.e., a triple layer of stockinette, hyperflexion of the radiocarpal joint, and a closely molded cast with oval cross-section). When the fracture is irreducible (entrapment of pronator quadratus) or unstable (peroperative redisplacement with wrist flexion-extension maneuvres) or when reduction is not correct, surgery should be performed. The authors recommend a posterolateral intrafocal pinning.

► From the literature, criteria of instability of distal forearm fractures in children include the following:

1. major displacement (posterior or posterolateral translation greater than 50%),[1]
2. dorsal comminution,[2]
3. isolated fracture of the radius,[3]
4. perfect reduction of the ulna and imperfect reduction of the radius ("too good-looking" ulna),[2]
5. proximal fractures: between distal third and distal fourth.

In this series, it was found that secondary displacement occurred as follows: every time reduction and cast immobilization were imperfect, in 75% of cases in which reduction was not perfect but the cast was, in 50% of cases in which reduction was perfect but the cast was not, every time the cast was prematurely opened (either longitudinally split or changed), and in 43% of proximal fractures. The other clinical criteria did not influence secondary displacement in this series.

In other words, according to the authors, the best predictor of outcome of these fractures is the quality of reduction and of cast immobilization, regardless of the type of fracture or displacement.

C. LeClercq, M.D.

References

1. Mani GU, Hui PW, Cheng JCY: Translation of the radius as a predictor of outcome in distal radial fractures of children. *J Bone Joint Surg Br* 75:808–811, 1993.
2. Collet LM: Fractures of the distal 1/4 of the both bones of the forearm: Extremity fractures in children [French]. Montpellier, France, Sauramps Médical, 1990, pp 263–278.
3. Gibbons H, Woods DA, Pailthorpe C, et al: The management of isolated distal radius fractures in children. *J Pediatr Orthop* 14:207–210, 1994.

Open Reduction and Internal Fixation of Pediatric Forearm Fractures
Wyrsch B, Mencio GA, Green NE (Vanderbilt Univ, Nashville, Tenn)
J Pediatr Orthop 16:644–650, 1996 3–10

Background.—Closed reduction is the standard of care for fractures of the forearm bones in children. However, residual deformity from malunion in children may result in loss of motion and dysfunction. Open reduction and internal fixation (ORIF) is controversial in children because of fears of potential complications. The results of ORIF of unstable forearm fractures in skeletally immature patients were studied retrospectively.

Methods.—The medical records and radiographs of 26 skeletally immature patients who underwent ORIF of forearm fractures between 1986 and 1993 were reviewed. The patients had a mean age of 11.5 years. Their status was followed for an average period of 39 months. Subjective evaluations of pain and function and objective measures of function were reviewed.

Results.—The 26 patients had 17 closed fractures and 10 open fractures. All patients with closed fractures initially underwent closed reduction with unacceptable results. The 10 patients with open fractures underwent primary treatment with ORIF. Stabilization was provided with plate fixation in 22 patients and with intramedullary fixation in 4 patients. All fractures healed, with an average time to union of 3.5 months. All but 3 patients had full range of motion. Six patients had preoperative nerve deficits; these were completely resolved within 4 months in 5 patients. There were 3 complications: deep infection in 1 patient, initial nonunion in 1, and cross-union in 1.

Conclusion.—Although closed treatment is still the treatment of choice for pediatric forearm fractures, ORIF can be safe and effective treatment for unstable forearm fractures in children and may facilitate soft-tissue management in children with open fractures. Either compression plating or intramedullary techniques provide reliable fixation in children. Open reduction and internal fixation is most likely to be needed for fractures of the proximal third of the radius and ulna and high-energy displaced or comminuted fractures.

► The authors provide indications for and results of ORIF of forearm fractures in children. Their results are very good, with restoration of normal forearm rotation in 89% of cases. Their complication rate of 11% (3/27) is higher than the adult complication rates cited in their article, but it is acceptable considering that they used ORIF only for open fractures or those that failed closed reduction.

Because of thick periosteum, children's forearm fractures are usually closed, and closed reduction does not often fail (the series presented in this article represented less than 2% of pediatric forearm fractures seen by the authors). Because of their remodeling abilities, closed reduction in children under the age of 8 years does not have to be perfect. But, when an acceptable closed reduction cannot be maintained or when the fracture is open and, therefore, inherently unstable, this well-written article provides needed support to the surgeon planning ORIF.

M.A. James, M.D.

Single-bone Fixation of Both-bone Forearm Fractures
Flynn JM, Waters PM (Children's Hosp, Boston)
J Pediatr Orthop 16:655–659, 1996 3–11

Background.—Recent studies have reported that internal fixation can be succcessful after failed closed reduction of forearm fractures in children. Another approach, involving the internal fixation of either the radius or ulna, was developed to treat pediatric diaphyseal both-bone forearm fractures. The outcome of children treated with this approach was studied retrospectively.

Methods.—Seventeen children aged 5–14 years underwent single-bone fixation of a both-bone forearm fracture since 1989 at 1 institution. There were complete fractures of both bones in 13 patients and a complete fracture of 1 bone with a greenstick fracture of the other bone in 4 patients. Whenever possible, the ulna was fixed with an intramedullary pin; then the forearm was manipulated to reduce and stabilize the radius, and the arm was placed in a long-arm cast. When closed reduction of the radius was not possible, it was fixed with a tubular plate or intramedullary fixation; then the forearm was manipulated to reduce and stabilize the ulna. The status of the patients was followed until the fracture was healed and function was either normalized or stable.

Results.—Complete follow-up results were available for 16 of the 17 children. Healing was completed by 8 weeks for all fractures. Two children had a loss of 5 degrees of pronation; full motion of the elbow, wrist, and forearm was regained otherwise. No patients had infections, nonunions, malunions, synostoses, or refractures. Two patients had complications: 1 keloid and 1 transient superficial radial nerve neurapraxia.

Conclusion.—In children with failed closed treatment of both-bone diaphyseal forearm fractures, single-bone fixation is a safe and effective treatment involving the stabilization of 1 bone and the rotation and reduction of the other bone. This approach avoids the need for repeated anesthetics and prevents malreduction without the need for plating of both bones. Intramedullary fixation is preferred because it is easier and safer to place and remove.

▶ The authors provide a succinct but thorough literature review supporting their premise: unstable or open both-bone forearm fractures in children should be treated with an effective, minimally invasive method of internal fixation. Their surgical protocol makes sense and their results are excellent. Their only complications were from hardware removal in 2 cases in which plating of the radius was the single-bone fixation used. From this they conclude that intramedullary nailing is preferred, when possible, instead of considering the possibility that hardware removal may be unnecessary.

M.A. James, M.D.

Reconstruction of Forearm Bone Loss by Cubitalization of the Radius (One Bone Forearm): Comments on Six Clinical Cases [French]

Bessy H, Leemrijse Th, Cadot B, et al (Hôpital Bichat, Paris)

Ann Chir Main 15:199–211, 1996 3–12

Background.—Bone loss of the forearm is difficult to treat. When lesions of the interosseous membrane at radioulnar articulations are present, these authors have had success with cubitalization of the radius to form a 1-bone forearm. The functional and aesthetic results with the 1-bone forearm formation in 6 patients were reported.

Methods.—In 4 of the 6 patients, cubitalization of the radius was performed because of severe trauma; Volkmann's syndrome and bone loss resulting from tumor were the causes in the other 2 patients. Patient ages ranged from 32 to 78 years, and bone loss ranged from 6 to 15 cm. In all 6 patients, the proximal ulna was fixed to the distal radius via a vascular or cutaneo-osseus transfer.

Findings.—Pronation of the forearm after surgery ranged from 10 degrees to 20 degrees. Use of the hand was maintained in all cases. Bone consolidation was evident at follow-up (range, 5–12 months).

Conclusion.—When forearm rotation cannot be restored in cases of severe bone loss, cubitalization of the radius will salvage function. Bone consolidation occurs in a matter of months, resulting in a stable restoration. Fixation of the forearm in a slightly pronated position provides an aesthetic restoration as well as a functional one.

► Transfer of the distal radius to the proximal ulna is a reasonable option when there is significant forearm bone loss, particularly when the complexity of the injury is such that a significant functional deficit in the hand and forearm will remain. In such cases, it seems much more reasonable to construct a single-bone forearm than to attempt to reconstruct, by microsurgical or other means, a 2-bone forearm that will have limited function, even if the bony surgery is successful.

P.C. Amadio, M.D.

Early Excision of Heterotopic Ossification About the Elbow Followed by Radiation Therapy

McAuliffe JA, Wolfson AH (Cleveland Clinic Florida, Fort Lauderdale; Univ of Miami, Fla)

J Bone Joint Surg (Am) 79-A:749–755, 1997 3–13

Introduction.—Heterotopic ossification, characterized by the formation of bone in periarticular regions, can lead to severely limited motion in the affected joint. Excision of heterotopic bone about the elbow is reported to be a successful treatment, but recurrence is common. This review of 8 patients with heterotopic ossification about the elbow demonstrated the benefits of early excision followed by radiation therapy.

Methods.—Heterotopic bone was excised in these patients at an average of 7 months after the initial injury. Five patients had a neurologic injury (the spinal cord in 3 cases and the head in 2), and 3 had a local injury of the elbow. Heterotopic bone was predominantly posteromedial in all patients. Excision was performed under tourniquet control, and the ulnar nerve was transposed anteriorly at the end of the procedure. The nerve must be identified for it to be protected as deeper bone is excised. Radiation therapy consisted of 5 fractions, started on the first postoperative day and administered over a 7-day period. The total dose was 1,000 cGy. Therapist-supervised active and assisted range-of-motion exercises were begun on the first postoperative day.

Results.—The average arc of motion was 103 degrees at latest follow-up (average, 46 months), which compared favorably with that attained intraoperatively (average, 121 degrees). Two patients had residual motor deficits; their arcs of motion were 50 degrees and 70 degrees. When these 2 cases were excluded from analysis, the average arc of motion was 118 degrees in those with normal motor function. No patient had substantial recurrence of ossification, and no complications resulted from radiation therapy.

Discussion.—Heterotopic ossification occurs in approximately 1% of patients with burn injury, 3% with local injury of the elbow, and 11% with head injury. Prophylaxis using pharmacologic agents or radiation therapy has disadvantages, and it is difficult to identify patients in whom heterotopic ossification will develop. Early excision followed by radiation therapy was successful in restoring elbow function in this small series of patients. There appears to be no advantage in delaying treatment for 2–18 months after the injury to allow for maturation of heterotopic bone.

▶ This paper carries several important messages. First, patients who have lost motion as the result of formation of heterotopic bone should have the bone excised, as there is a high probability of functional return in the elbow. Second, the results in patients with head injury who have persistent neuromuscular deficit are inferior to those in patients with no residual neurologic or muscular dysfunction. Third, and very importantly, early excision is possible and information is accumulating to suggest that it may be preferred.

Many experienced elbow surgeons are currently recommending early excision at 3–6 months and rarely waiting 9 months or longer, as used to be recommended.

Although radiation in 5 divided doses was used postoperatively, the majority of such operations are now performed by most surgeons without the use of using postoperative radiation, and recurrence of the heterotopic bone is rare. Furthermore, the radiation can be given in a single dose without an apparent increase in complications. This certainly facilitates postoperative management. The indication for radiation usually involves a patient who is considered to be at high risk of reocurrence, rather than every patient who has heterotopic bone. Meticulous attention to surgical detail—such as draping out the surgical field when bone dust may be dispersed, profuse irrigation to eliminate bone dust, and the use of hand instruments rather than powered instruments to minimize bone dust—is recommended.

S.W. O'Driscoll, M.D.

Suggested Reading

Morgan R, Molnar J, Prevel CD, et al: Biomechanical testing of titanium self-tapping versus pretapped lag screw fixation of spiral metacarpal fractures. *Ann Plast Surg* 37:34–40, 1996.

▶ Screws ranging from 1.5 to 2.3 mm in outside diameter and 0.8 to 1.6 mm in core diameter were tested in adult human cadaver metacarpals. Failure torque and bending loads were similar regardless of screw size, suggesting that there is little difference in stress riser effect between any of these size screws.

P.C. Amadio, M.D.

4 Soft-Tissue Trauma and Reconstruction

Closure of Wounds in the Upper Extremity Using a Skin Stretching Device
Stahl S, Har-Shai Y, Hirshowitz B (Rambam Med Ctr, Haifa, Israel)
J Hand Surg (Br) 21B:534–537, 1996 4–1

Introduction.—In the presence of a skin deficit, such as after open fasciotomy, a gunshot wound, or removal of a skin tumor, closing the wound may be problematic. Some techniques to close such a wound are split-thickness skin grafting, wide undermining, and distant or free flaps. A skin-stretching device exploits the viscoelastic properties of the skin, allowing it to stretch rapidly with little recoil. Healthy skin can stretch from 20 to 40 minutes, whereas skin affected by edema and fibrosis can take 2–3 days. In 20 patients, a skin-stretching device was used in the upper extremity.

Methods.—Twenty patients with skin deficits in the upper extremity were treated with a skin-stretching device. The 2 women and 18 men had wounds from gunshot and shrapnel; wounds with exposed bone, joints, or tendons; open fasciotomy; scar revisions; and tumor excision. The device has 2 straight intradermal needles and a tension-regulating system composed of 2 U-shaped arms, which have hooks and a central screw bar. After the device is positioned, stretching occurs in increments, with a stretching force of up to 3 kg on the skin margins. When the wound margins are closed, the wound is sutured.

Results.—Complications included necrosis of skin edges, local infection, hypertrophic scars, and slight partial dehiscence, but overall complications were few. There was no need for further surgery. Average healing time was 2.5–4 weeks. One 20-year-old patient had a gunshot wound in the left arm. After initial excision and débridement, the stretching device was used 4 days later on the defect measuring 6 × 10 cm. Closure, using local anesthesia, occurred in 40 minutes, and complete healing was achieved (Fig 1).

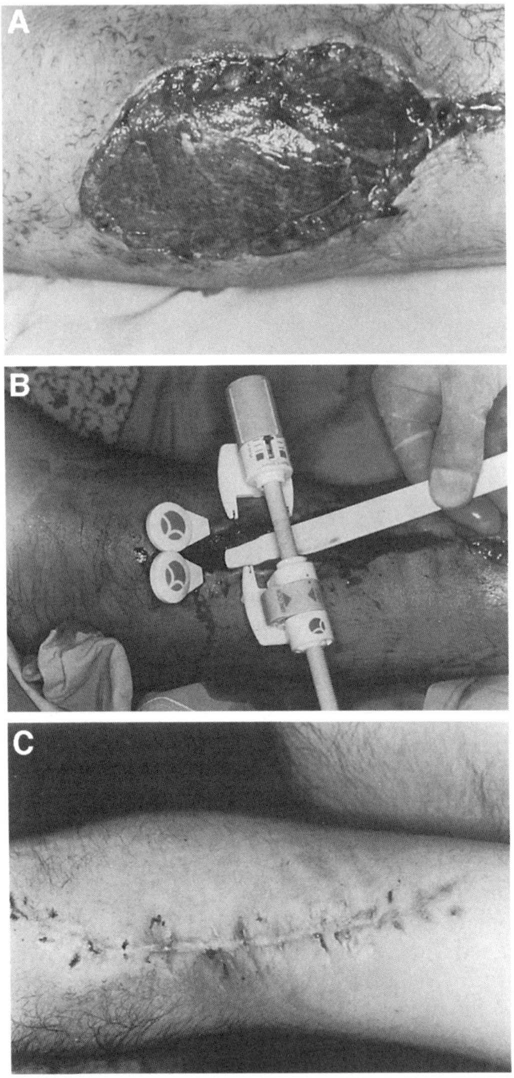

FIGURE 1.—Gunshot wound in arm and forearm. **A**, 6 × 10-cm skin deficit. **B**, skin-stretching device was applied; a plastic ruler prevented the deep soft tissue from bulging outward. C, 3 weeks after operation. (Courtesy of Stahl S, Har-Shai Y, Hirshowitz B: Closure of wounds in the upper extremity using a skin stretching device. *J Hand Surg [Br]* 21B:534–537, 1996.)

Conclusion.—The skin-stretching device reduces the need for more complicated surgical procedures like grafts or flaps, is simple to use, and can be used at the bedside with local anesthesia.

▶ There are currently 4 techniques available to increase the amount of local skin that can be used to close a wound: use of an implanted tissue expander, presuturing, load cycling, and continuous skin stretching. There are different though sometimes overlapping indications for each. This paper presents the authors' experience with the use of a commercially available skin-stretching device for closure of upper extremity wounds, most resulting from trauma, in a series of 20 patients.

The reader should keep in mind 2 separate aspects of this presentation: the biological process, and the device used to attain it. The process relies on realignment of dermal collagen fibers and redistribution of ground substance resulting in mechanical creep and stress relaxation of the skin in response to continuously applied tension. This may occur within minutes or may require hours or days depending on the freshness or chronicity of the wound, and is limited by the state at which dermal collagen fibers have become parallel, and by skin viability. The skin is not undermined. Presuturing relies on this same process. The device, in which at least 1 of the authors has a financial interest, has been refined to include a 3-kg tension gauge and safety clutch, and has been produced commercially since the earlier report of its use by Hirshowitz et al.[1] in 1993.

This technique is a useful addition to the armamentarium for wound repair, and the device is a convenient tool to apply the technique. Some cautions are in order. This is a utilitarian approach to wound closure, which may in some cases avoid the need for more extensive surgical undertakings. The visible scar with this type of repair often spreads or hypertrophies; it is not a procedure that produces a fine-line minimal scar. Also, in some cases this procedure, although able to close the wound successfully, will result in a scar that is in an unfavorable position or orientation for recovery of function, or for later reconstructive procedures. In such cases other methods of repair should be used.

J.M. Markley, Jr., M.D.

Reference

1. Hirshowitz B, Lindenbaum E, Har-Shai Y: A skin-stretching device for harnessing of the viscoelastic properties of skin. *Plast Reconstr Surg* 92:260–270, 1993.

Reconstructive Surgery After Traumatic Amputation of the Thumb [French]

Foucher G (Clinique du Parc, Strasbourg, France)
Ann Chir Plast Esthét 41:197–207, 1996 4–2

Review.—Replantation or reconstruction of a thumb after traumatic amputation requires careful consideration of the patient's functional needs and aesthetic sensitivities. This paper is an extensive review of the literature on the many available surgical thumb repairs, including the classic procedures that have been and still are popular, those that are no longer performed, and those currently favored. The author used a 200-point rating scale, which was applied to each reviewed study to standardize evaluation of the results and compare outcomes.

► This review of the art of thumb reconstruction after amputation is the standard for clarity and completeness. Guy Foucher humbly begins with a tribute to the original masters in the field and includes a valuable list of their references. He makes the following points:

1. The patient's functional and aesthetic goals must be established.
2. In the acute situation, a sensible attempt at replantation given proper indications will, if successful, give excellent results, with 92% of patients resuming their previous jobs. However, multiple attempts to save a hopelessly crushed thumb—with arterial rerouting, skin grafts, and vein grafts, which ultimately prove to be in vain—are not to be recommended; they lead to difficult donor site scars, which make secondary reconstruction more difficult.
3. The qualities that define a "good thumb" are painlessness, sensation, mobility, stability of bone and soft tissue in areas of friction, length poroportional to the opposable fingers, and, finally, good cosmetic appearance.
4. Certain techniques have lost favor, e.g., the "cocked hat" because of distal bone resorption and phalangization, although web deepening is still helpful in distal thumb loss.
5. Osteoplastic reconstruction—when modified by island finger flap for sensation and to prevent bone resorption, or by the various composite pedicle or free osteocutaneous flaps—is still useful, but the many shortcomings include multiple operations that lead to local and donor scars, lack of the nail, thumb stiffness, and poor appearance.
6. Lengthening techniques include the single-episode type with a bone graft placed in a metacarpal osteotomy, with length limited to 25 mm maximum, or progressive lengthening of the metacarpal osteotomy by external fixator, with an axial pin to prevent angulation; possible limiting complications are loss of distal sensation or circulation or intolerable pain. After several weeks of distraction, an iliac bone graft or a second metacarpal-interosseous muscle pedicle graft is used to fill in the distraction site. Problems to be prevented are distal web creep and angulation of the distal fragment toward the first web via muscle forces. The author is not very happy with these methods and believes that their 1 advantage is in thumb sensation.
7. Pollicization is the 1 classic method still often indicated. In pollicizing a healthy index, middle, or ring finger, the ring finger is to be preferred, supplemented by added venous return by a single-donor dorsal vein microsurgical anastomosis to the recipient site. Island transfer of a damaged finger is to be preferred, with at least 1 digital artery intact and good ulnar sensation, with free pollicization or neurotization possible.
8. In toe transfers, the great toe should no longer be used; despite good strength and motion, the donor problems of force transfer to the second toe—even with preservation of the metatarsal head and sesamoids—and poor cosmetic look outweighs the benefits. The second toe is to be pre-

ferred because the metatarsophalangeal joint can be transferred. Problems are persistent interphalangeal joint flexion and, thus, limited extension and a poor cosmetic match because of narrowness. There is the possibility of doing a proximal transfer to the anterior aspect of the distal radius to take advantage of radiocarpal motion, supplementing the toe with tendon transfers.

The author points out that, for amputation near the metacarpophalangeal joint, use of a great-toe free neurovascular wrap-around flap over a free iliac bone graft is helpful cosmetically, but there is some resorption of bone. A modified wrap-around flap that includes a portion of distal phalanx and, thus, better nail function is to be preferred. The "twisted 2 toes" method includes simultaneous free transfer of the interphalangeal joint and tendons of the second toe and a wrap-around flap, including distal phalanx and nail from the great toe. The "tailored" great-toe transfer—which includes half the width of distal phalanx and excision of fat and skin, with or without web deepening—is preferred for distal amputations, but distal reconstruction is only necessary in patients, such as musicians, needing nail function.

He ends by cautioning about patient selection. Age older than 40 years leads to poor nerve reconstitution. Diabetes, tobacco use, and Raynaud's disease are contraindications. Patients with unrealistic cosmetic expectations will be disappointed even if function is good. Having explained the microsurgical procedures available, he stresses that classic techniques still have a place, and that microsurgery poorly carried out and with improper indications represents the worst situation.

J.M. Failla, M.D.

Dorso-Ulnar Thumb Flap: Anatomical Study and Clinical Application. Report of Twenty-Two Cases [French]

Brunelli F, Brunelli G, Vigasio A (Université René Descartes, Paris; Università di Brescia, Italy)

Ann Chir Plast Esthét 41:259–268, 1996 4–3

Purpose.—The arterial vascularization of the thumb differs from that of the other fingers. The princeps pollicis artery, derived from the first intermetacarpal web, surfaces at the volar side of the thumb at the level of the metacarpophalangeal flexion crease. This relatively distal point of emergence limits the availability of pedicled flaps. Based on the findings of an anatomical study, a pedicled dorso-ulnar flap was designed to treat traumatic thumb injuries involving distal skin loss or distal pulp loss.

Methods.—For the anatomical study, the dorsal vascular supply of 25 fresh cadaver thumbs was dissected after arterial injection of colored latex. All dissections showed that there is an artery on the dorso-ulnar side of the thumb that connects the head of the first metacarpal bone with the dorsal arcade of the nail matrix. Two flaps were designed: a dorso-ulnar flap distally based on the matrix arcade and intended for coverage of tissue defects at the more distal part of the thumb, and a dorso-ulnar flap pedicled at the anastomosis between the palmar and dorso-ulnar arteries for coverage of a more proximal tissue defect.

Patients.—Between 1990 and 1995, a dorso-ulnar pedicled flap was used in 22 patients with hand injuries, 18 of whom had thumb injuries. Of the 18 thumb reconstructions, 4 were for coverage of a defect on an amputation stump at the interphalangeal level (Fig 9), 11 were for pulp reconstructions, and 3 were for covering a dorsal skin defect. In the other 4 patients, a dorso-ulnar flap was used on an injured index finger as a cross-finger flap. There were no major complications, and all flaps survived.

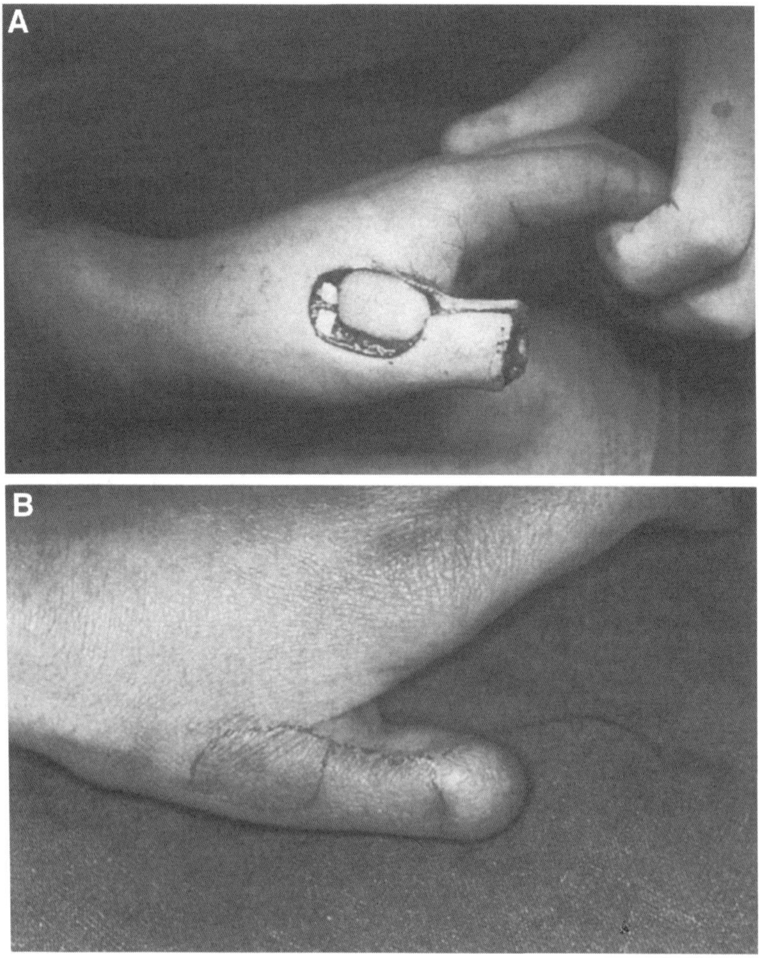

FIGURE 9.—**A**, failure of a thumb replantation at the interphalangeal level. Harvesting of the flap and proximal identification of the nerve of the flap (terminal branch of the radial nerve). **B**, final result. (Courtesy of Brunelli F, Brunelli G, Vigasio A: Dorso-ulnar thumb flap: Anatomical study and clinical application. Report of twenty-two cases [French]. *Ann Chir Plast Esthét* 41:259–268, 1996.)

Conclusion.—The dorso-ulnar thumb flap is extremely useful for the repair of important distal skin defects or pulp losses of the thumb. The technique can also be used to create a cross-finger flap for the repair of distal skin loss of the index finger.

► The authors describe a useful small flap from the dorso-ulnar aspect of the metacarpophalangeal joint area. Their study of the various vascular anastomoses about the thumb has identified a constant dorsal vascular arcade at the level of the nail matrix, which allows retrograde rotation of the flap on its subcutaneous pedicle. The flap can be used to cover defects of the distal thumb and also as a cross-fingerflap.

V.R. Hentz, M.D.

Boomerang Flap: A Real One-stage Cross-finger Pedicle Flap [French]

Legaillard P, Grangier Y, Casoli V, et al (Hôpital du Tondu, Bordeaux, France)

Ann Chir Plast Esthét 41:251–258, 1996 4–4

Background.—The availability of reverse flow island flaps to cover dorsal finger defects has greatly improved the outcome of such hand injuries. However, cross-finger flaps are still indicated for the repair of dorsal defects that are distal to the proximal interphalangeal (PIP) joint because an adequate blood supply is not available. A new 1-stage cross-finger flap, called a boomerang flap, for the repair of dorsal digital injuries distal to the PIP joint was described.

> *Surgical Technique.*—The boomerang flap is made possible in part because of interdigital bifurcations that are always present between dorsal collateral arterial networks and in part because of the anastomoses between dorsal and palmar collateral networks that are staggered along the fingers all the way up to the PIP joint. The flap is raised on the dorsolateral aspect of the first phalanx of the second, third, or fourth normal finger adjacent to the injured finger. A 5-mm band of fatty connective tissue in the shape of a boomerang is raised on the underlying dorsal collateral pedicle and rotated to cover any dorsal defect on the adjacent finger located between the PIP joint and the fingertip.

Patients.—Six men (mean age, 35.6 years) who had sustained traumatic finger injuries were treated with the boomerang flap. Three flaps were raised on the middle finger, 2 on the index finger, and 1 on the ring finger. After an average follow-up of 11 months, there had been no flap failures.

Conclusion.—The single-stage pedicled boomerang flap is raised on the healthy finger adjacent to the injured finger from where it can be rotated for the repair of digital defects all the way up to the fingertip. Although this procedure is a true cross-finger flap, it avoids all of the drawbacks of the classic cross-finger flap technique.

▶ The authors expand on previous descriptions of retrograde dorsal intermetacarpal flaps by describing how the surgeon can take advantage of the rich vascularity of the dorsal tissues overlying the proximal phalanx to create a dorsal flap from an adjacent uninjured digit to cover a defect too distal to be covered by the standard intermetacarpal flap. This flap is analogous to the volvar retrograde flap described by Elliot Rose[1] in which a lateral or volar skin flap based on a proper volar digital artery is transferred to an adjacent digit by dissecting the adjacent proper digital arteries and dividing their common digital vessel.

V.R. Hentz, M.D.

Reference

1. Rose EH: Local arterialized island flap coverage of difficult hand defects preserving donorsite and digit sensibility. *Plast Reconstr Surg* 72:848–853, 1983.

Pulp Neurovascular Island Flap for Finger Amputation

Lanzetta M, St-Laurent J-Y (Université de Montreal)

J Hand Surg (Am) 21A:918–921, 1996 4–5

Background.—In 1980, Srivastava and Kahl described a technique for covering the stump remaining after elective amputation at the proximal interphalangeal joint with an island neurovascular flap from the fingertip. Until the present report of eight case studies, this technique had not been further reported.

Technique.—The pulp flap is marked, the pneumatic tourniquet is inflated, and the digital neurovascular bundles are dissected bilaterally (unilaterally if 1 is injured) from proximal to distal. The perineurovascular fat tissue is conserved to preserve venous drainage through the venae comitantes. The flap is lifted, and the finger is amputated (Fig 1, C). The flap is positioned (without twisting) to lie mostly on the volar surface of the stump, with care taken not to apply compression to the redundant neurovascular bundles (see Fig 1, D). A loose dressing is applied, the tourniquet is relaxed, and hand elevation is maintained for 48 hours. Hand and finger mobilization begins immediately after surgery; follow-up includes a sensory reeducation program.

Patients and Results.—The flap procedure was performed for 8 men (mean age, 33 years), 7 of whom underwent elective amputation of a stiff, painful finger and 1 of whom had extreme, fixed-flexion Dupuytren's

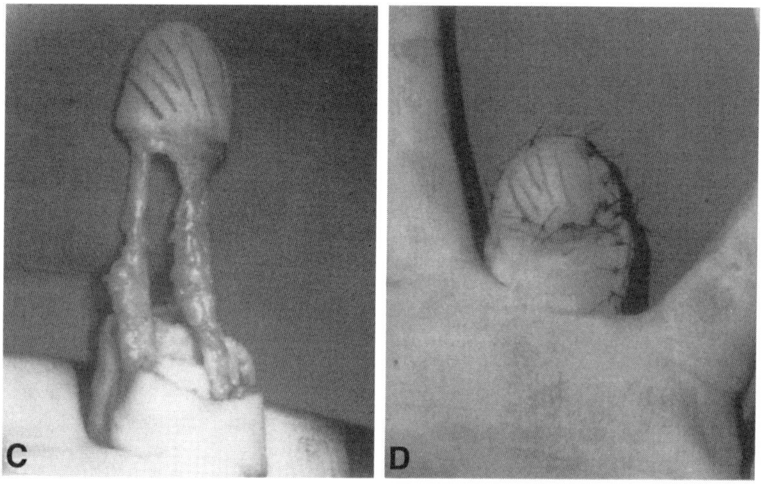

FIGURE 1.—Pulp neurovascular island flap for severe proximal interphalangeal joint flexion contracture of the ring finger. C, amputation has been carried out at the joint level. The flap is ready to be inserted. D, the stump is covered by the flap. Two short lateral incisions are used to accommodate the redundant neurovascular bundles in the subcutaneous tissue. (Courtesy of Lanzetta M, St-Laurent JY: Pulp neurovascular island flap for finger amputation. *J Hand Surg [Am]* 21A:918–921, 1996.)

deformity. After surgery, normal fingertip sensibility was retained at the stump for all 8 patients; no neuromas occurred.

Conclusions.—Pulp neurovascular island flap surgery is an alternative to conventional finger amputation. Sensation in these patients at first involved misinterpretation of the real length of the finger, but with an organized program of sensory education, this interpretation was eventually fully overcome. The best indication for this surgery is amputation through the middle phalanx distal to the flexor superficialis tendon insertion.

▶ The authors present their experience with a series of 8 neurovascular island transfers of the distal digital palmar skin and soft tissue for resurfacing of amputations of the same digit at the middle or proximal phalangeal levels, following up on a single case report of this specific use of the digital neurovascular island technique by Srivastava and Kahl in 1980.[1] The indication for amputation in 7 of these cases was severe posttraumatic functional impairment of the digit, and severe Dupuytren's contracture with proximal interphalangeal joint osteoarthritis in the eighth.

The authors correctly note that the indications for the use of this technique are to provide improved sensibility for the digital amputation stump and to avoid painful neuromas. I have used this maneuver with satisfying results and believe that the avoidance of painful neuroma is by far the more important feature and that it alone justifies the additional time and surgical expertise and effort necessary to do the island transfer. Indeed, I think the technique deserves more frequent application than it probably currently has.

Two technical features of the procedure that are critical to its success deal with the management of the neurovascular bundles. As with all digital neurovascular island flap transfers, whether homo- or hetero-digital, great care must be taken to maintain a circumferential layer of soft tissue around each digital artery and nerve to preserve the fine network of tiny veins adjacent to them. Second, the bundles must be carefully positioned without kinking or torsion in the soft tissue proximal to the flap.

In this series, all patients underwent postoperative sensory re-education for the flaps and all are reported to have gained spatial relocalization to the more proximal location within 8 weeks. I suspect that relocalization perception would occur in time with use alone as the flap remains with its original digital ray but would likely require more time than when assisted by formal sensory re-education.

In discussing the use of this flap relative to various levels of amputation, the authors suggest that with a ray amputation, the flap could be de-epithelialized and buried in the palm to avoid painful neuromas, although none of their cases involved amputation at this level. This remains speculative but is, I think, a good suggestion, as neuroma pain and dysesthesia are the most common problems resulting in poor functional results of ray amputations. However, it is of great importance whatever the level of amputation to be certain that the flap skin to be transferred has normal or near-normal sensibility and is not painful, dysesthetic, nor allodynic.

J.M. Markley, Jr., M.D.

Reference

1. Srivastava RK, Kahl JB: Shifting neurovascular island flap for the reconstruction of amputated digital stump. *Plast Reconstr Surg* 66:301–302, 1980.

Arterialized Venous Flaps From the Thenar and Hypothenar Regions for Repairing Finger Pulp Tissue Losses

Iwasawa M, Ohtsuka Y, Kushima H, et al (Nagano Red Cross Hosp, Japan)

Plast Reconstr Surg 99:1765–1770, 1997 4–6

Introduction.—For repair of digital pulp defects, various skin flaps have been used. The use of distal-based arterial island flaps has increased, but they require extensive vascular dissection and skin grafts to the donor site. A previous report showed that an arterialized venous flap from the volar forearm was helpful in the repair of finger tissue loss; however, the skin quality was not sufficient. A new arterialized venous flap with durable skin of appropriate texture was used for finger pulp reconstruction.

Methods.—The surgical technique involved the lateral side of the metacarpophalangeal joint for the thenar venous flap and the lateral side of the hypothenar region for the hypothenar flap. A dorsal cutaneous vein located close to the volar surface of the hand was where the flaps were based (Fig 1). Microvascular anastomoses were performed between a digital artery and dorsal vein. There were 3 flaps of the A-A type where the

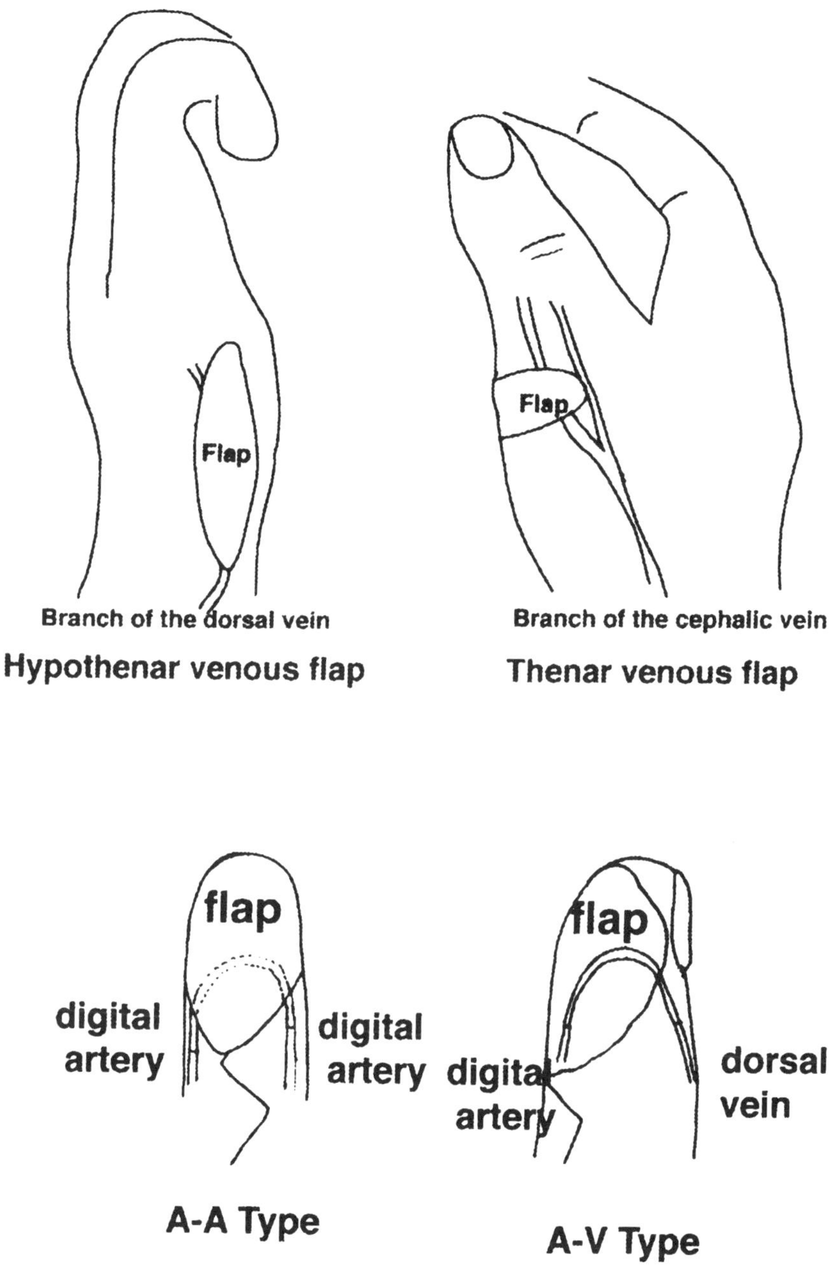

FIGURE 1.—*Top*, schematic diagram showing the design of the thenar and hypothenar venous flaps based on the dorsal cutaneous vein, which is located close to the volar surface of the hand. *Bottom*, drawing of inset technique regarding anastomoses. (Courtesy of Iwasawa M, Ohtsuka Y, Kushima H, et al: Arterialized venous flaps from the thenar and hypothenar regions for repairing finger pulp tissue losses. *Plast Reconstr Surg* 99:1765–1770, 1997.)

vascular inflow derived from the digital artery with outflow to a digital artery, and there were 12 flaps of the A-V type with vascular inflow derived from the digital artery with outflow to a dorsal vein. The average operating time was 90 minutes. To maintain patency of the vascular anastomoses, prostaglandin E_1 solution of 60 µg/day was injected intravenously.

Results.—In the treatment of 13 patients, 15 flaps were transferred, with 11 thenar venous flaps and 4 hypothenar venous flaps. There was complete survival of 13 flaps. One flap was completely necrotic and 1 flap had partial necrosis at the periphery with reinnervation apparent 3 months after the operation. At follow-up, all the flaps that survived exhibited stable coverage and good texture. Because the mini-Brunner skin incision was used and because the amount of vascular dissection was small, there was no loss in range of motion related to vascular dissection.

Conclusion.—For replacement of finger pulp defects, the thenar and hypothenar skin is durable and of appropriate texture. For repairing the tissue loss of the fingers, an average flap size of 2 × 3 cm was adequate. Although these were not sensory flaps, they exhibited useful sensory recovery within 6 months of the operation. For the repair of finger pulp tissue losses, the arterialized venous flap is a useful alternative.

▶ The authors have presented a pretty nice series of fingertip reconstructions using flow-through venous flaps, either arterial or arteriovenous, for pulp loss with the donor site on the thenar or hypothenar eminence. They have done 15 cases, all with local anesthesia with an average operating time of 1½ hours. Although I have very limited experience with venous flow-through flaps, and no one has been able to explain the physiology of their survival to me appropriately, the authors' results are very nice, including reasonable return of 2-point discrimination postoperatively, which also is surprising in a noninnervated flap. The results are excellent with 1 partial loss that healed and 1 full loss out of 15 cases. I think that it is an interesting article and should be included and, perhaps, the technique would prove useful in chronic or acute fingertip wounds. The downside is that it requires a fairly sophisticated microsurgical team.

N.B. Meland, M.D.

Salvage of Fingertip Amputated at Nail Level: New Surgical Principles and Treatments

Hirase Y (Jikei Univ, Tokyo)

Ann Plast Surg 38:151–157, 1997 4–7

Background.—Recent reports suggest that replantation surgery should be done in all patients needing it, if possible, especially if the patient wishes it. Surgical principles for the treatment of fingertip amputation at the nail level, according to the anatomical level of amputation, have been developed.

TABLE 1.—Surgical Procedures for Zone DP-I, IIA, IIB, and III Amputations

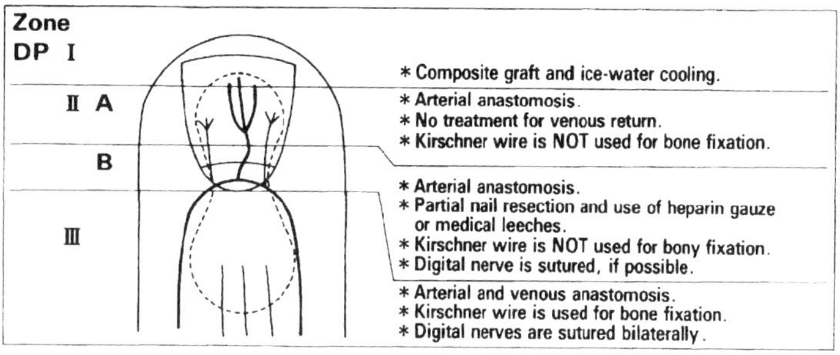

(Reprinted from *Annals of Plastic Surgery*, courtesy of Hirase Y: Salvage of fingertip amputated at nail level: New surgical principles and treatments. *Ann Plast Surg* 38:151–157, 1997, by permission of Little, Brown and Company, Inc.)

Methods and Findings.—One hundred fifty replantations in 137 patients performed between 1987 and 1992 were reviewed; 49 fingertip replantations in 45 patients operated on consecutively by 1 surgeon were included in the analysis. The distal phalanx (DP) of the finger was categorized as zone DP-I, IIA, IIB, or III, from distal to proximal. The classification system was based on the difference in surgical treatment as well as amputation level. For zone DP-I amputations, extending from the fingertip to the most distal dividing point of the digital artery, the amputated part is attached without vascular anastomosis. The whole finger is then wrapped in aluminum foil and cooled in ice water for 3 days. For zone DP-IIA and IIB amputations, anastomosis of the digital artery is done in the central part of the palmar region of the finger. However, Kirschner wire fixation is not done, to avoid disturbing the venous drainage through the medullary cavity. For DP-IIA amputations, no special treatment is needed for venous congestion. For zone DP-IIB amputations, partial resection of the nail is performed if necessary. Venous anastomosis is needed to salvage zone DP-II amputations. Using this classification system, the overall final survival rate was 91.5% (Table 1).

Conclusion.—Unlike previously published classification systems, the system described here is based on both the anastomotic level of the digital artery and the surgical treatment for reattachment. This system has been found to be very useful.

► This article provides a new and descriptive classification system for distal fingertip amputations. More importantly, associated with each division in the classification system there are prescribed treatment modalities and an algorithm of management that relates to each specific level. Although at times this appears to be a triumph of technology over reason, especially in the Western world, there may be times when distal fingertip amputation is indicated; this article provides useful organization concepts.

C.H. Johnson, M.D.

The Lateral Forearm Flap: An Anatomic Study

Lanzetta M, Bernier M, Chollet A, et al (Univ of Milan, Italy; Univ of Montreal)

Plast Reconst Surg 99:460–464, 1997 4–8

Background.—The lateral arm flap appears to be reliable in the coverage of small and medium-sized defects in the extremities and head and neck region. The distal limit of the posterior radial collateral artery in the forearm was studied, together with possible anastomoses of the posterior radial collateral artery with other arteries of the forearm. Also studied was whether a true forearm flap can be raised safely and successfully based on this pedicle.

Methods and Findings.—Twelve fresh cadaver arms were studied with methylene blue and latex injections and arteriography. The posterior radial collateral artery divided constantly into 2 terminal branches—an anterior and a posterior division. The anterior division serves as the nutrient vessel for the flap, the artery extending significantly beyond the lateral epicondyle of the elbow into the lateral aspect of the forearm. The mean length is 15 cm, with a range of 13–18 cm. Thus, the fasciocutaneous flap in the proximal forearm can be raised with a much longer vascular pedicle than the classic lateral arm flap.

Conclusion.—The lateral forearm flap has several advantages over the classic lateral arm flap, including very thin skin and subcutaneous tissue and less sensory deficit at the donor site. The primary indication for this flap is the need for soft, thin, pliable skin to cover small-to-medium–sized defects.

▶ The anatomical basis upon which the extended lateral arm flap exists is clearly described in this exquisite anatomical injection and dissection study. It is recommended reading for the hand and upper extremity surgeon, as the lateral arm flap is a useful workhorse in reconstructive efforts.

C.H. Johnson, M.D.

Neurocutaneous Island Flaps in Upper Limb Coverage: Experience With 44 Clinical Cases

Bertelli JA (Joana de Gusmão Children's Hosp, Santa Catarina, Brazil; Université René Descartes, Paris)

J Hand Surg (Am) 22A:515–526, 1997 4–9

Background.—The vascularity of the cutaneous nerve of the upper limb and that of the skin are closely connected. Perforators of the main arteries vascularize both skin and nerves. Small longitudinal paraneural vessels in close contact with the cutaneous nerves connect these perforating arteries. A clinical experience with 44 neurocutaneous island flaps for upper-limb coverage was evaluated.

Methods and Findings.—The flaps were supplied by the vessels around and inside cutaneous nerves. These flaps, which were as large as 4 × 10 cm, provided reliable coverage of skin defects in the upper limb. The proximally based flaps, free flaps, and flaps based distally on the dorsal side of the hand were extremely safe. Necrosis developed in 1 flap based distally on the medial antebrachial cutaneous nerve of the forearm and in 3 flaps used to reconstruct the thumb.

Conclusions.—Neurocutaneous island flaps are reliable, versatile, and easy to dissect. Major vessels, such as the radial, ulnar, and posterior interosseous arteries, are preserved. The donor site may be closed primarily in most patients, with minimal donor site morbidity.

► This study contains an excellent discussion of the cutaneous blood supply to the skin of the upper extremity with particular reference to the use of neurocutaneous island flaps. The rationale for the reliability and clinical use of these flaps is clearly delineated. Additionally, surgical technique as it pertains to raising a neurocutaneous flap is well discussed. The surgical results after 34 neurocutaneous island flaps raised from the upper limbs of 33 children as well as 11 neurocutaneous flaps raised from the upper limbs of 11 adults are then reported. The flaps were raised as proximally based flaps, distally based flaps, and as free flaps. Flap survival was excellent with only 1 incident of marginal necrosis occurring in the group of proximally based flaps and free flaps. Distally based flaps did nearly as well, with only 1 partial flap loss. The clinical cases, which are well documented, demonstrate use of the neurocutaneous flaps in difficult coverage problems. Although use of these flaps has not undergone the "test of time," their reliability, in this series, predicts their widespread use in the not so distant future.

A.A. Smith, M.D.

Comparison of Free and Reversed Pedicled Posterior Interosseous Cutaneous Flaps

Shibata M, Iwabuchi Y, Kubota S, et al (Niigata Univ, Niigata-shi, Japan)
Plast Reconstr Surg 99:791–802, 1997 4–10

Introduction.—The posterior interosseous cutaneous flap (or reversed pedicled flap) is versatile and can be used to cover small and medium hand and distal arm defects. Flap survival was compared in patients in whom the posterior interosseous flap was used as a free flap vs. a reversed vascular pedicled flap.

Methods.—Of 28 patients with soft-tissue defects in the hand and forearm, 17 received free flaps and 11 received reversed vascular pedicled flaps. Free flaps were used primarily in reconstruction of the digits, and reversed vascular pedicled flaps to repair soft-tissue defects of the proximal hand.

Results.—Sixteen of 17 free flaps survived completely, and in the remaining 1, partial necrosis caused by late thrombosis developed. In 2 reversed vascular pedicled flaps, partial necrosis developed, and a second

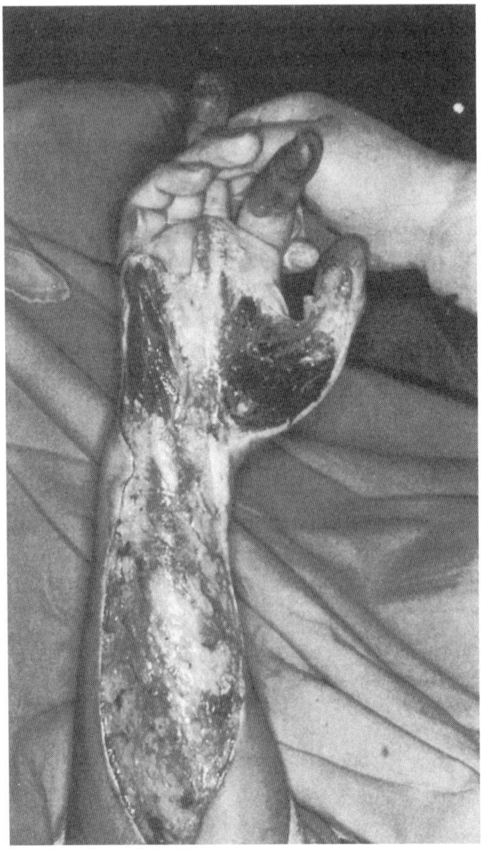

FIGURE 13.—After débridement. (Courtesy of Shibata M, Iwabuchi Y, Kubota S, et al: Comparison of free and reversed pedicled posterior interosseous cutaneous flaps. *Plast Reconstr Surg* 99:791–802, 1997.)

surgical procedure was performed for coverage of the defect. In another 2 reversed vascular pedicled flaps, epidermal necrosis developed. Three flaps that were combined with the lateral arm flap survived completely, as did another flap in which the proximal posterior interosseous artery was anastomosed to another artery. The operative times for simple coverage averaged 3 hours 41 minutes and 3 hours 5 minutes, respectively, for free and pedicled flaps. All patients had return of protective sensation, without parathesias.

Case Report.—Man, 39, had a heat press machine injury to his right hand and forearm. After débridement, he had a wide defect (Fig 13). He received a reversed vascular pedicled flap combined with a lateral arm flap (13 × 29 cm) that was elevated (Fig 14). The posterior radial collateral artery was anastomosed to the fourth common digital artery (Fig 15). The flap survived completely.

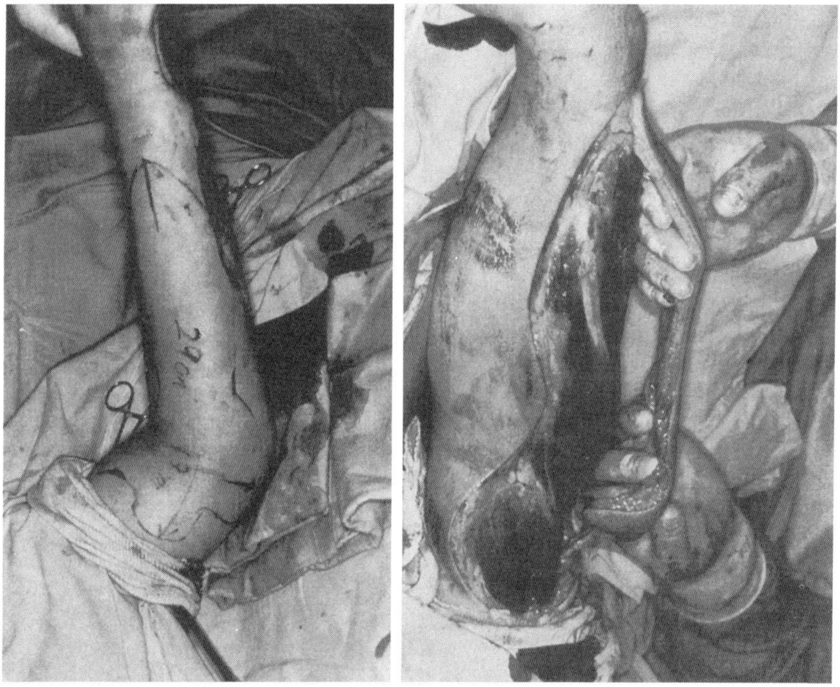

FIGURE 14.—*Left*, design of posterior interosseous and lateral arm flaps. *Right*, elevation of combined flap with reversed posterior interosseous vessels and posterior radial collateral vessel (29 × 13 cm). Later, posterior radial collateral vessels were severed. (Courtesy of Shibata M, Iwabuchi Y, Kubota S, et al: Comparison of free and reversed pedicled posterior interosseous cutaneous flaps. *Plast Reconstr Surg* 99:791–802, 1997.)

Conclusion.—The posterior interosseous flap is useful for reconstruction of defects of the forearm, hand, and digits. Findings suggest that free flaps may be more reliable than reversed vascular pedicled flaps.

► I feel the significant contribution here is the recognition that the posterior interosseous flap can be combined with the lateral arm flap, and this combined reverse flap can be used to cover extensive defects of the upper extremity. This was used in 3 of the 11 pedicled reverse flaps with posterior radial collateral artery (the inflow vessel to the lateral arm flap) anastomosed in the hand to "supercharge" this reverse flap.

A.A. Smith, M.D.

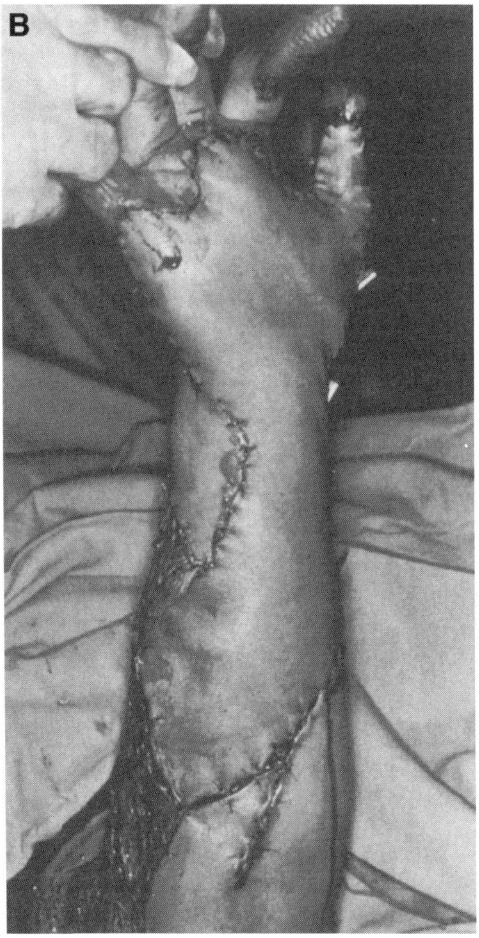

FIGURE 15.—After coverage with combined flap. The flap was turned around based on the reversed posterior interosseous vessels. The posterior branch of the radial collateral artery was connected to the radial artery in the snuff box for "supercharging" the large flap. (Courtesy of Shibata M, Iwabuchi Y, Kubota S, et al: Comparison of free and reversed pedicled posterior interosseous cutaneous flaps. *Plast Reconstr Surg* 99:791–802, 1997.)

The Arterialized Antebrachial Skin Flap for Hand Reconstruction

Reynoso R, Espinosa A, Mendoza M, et al (Instituto Nacional de Ortopedia, Mexico City)

J Reconstr Microsurg 13:267–275, 1997 4–11

Background.—Studies of experimental and clinical flaps, replants, and revascularizations based on arterioarterial, venovenous, and arteriovenous perfusion have appeared in the literature often in the last few years. Both conflicting survival rates and highly successful outcomes have been reported. The arterialized antebrachial skin flap for hand reconstruction was described.

Methods.—Twenty microvascular flaps based on arteriovenous perfusion were done. The flaps were harvested from the distal anterior forearm and configured in 3 different ways. The flap was used for small palmar, dorsal, and commisural defects; when other, conventional procedures could not be done; for problematic cases of open reduction internal fixation with skin defect; and when aggressive rehabilitation was necessary. Follow-up ranged from 6 to 28 months.

Findings.—All flaps showed some degree of vascular congestion. Those changes were classified in a progressive form. For 75% of the flaps, coverage was judged to be stable, thin, and pliable. Aggressive rehabilitation was begun promptly when possible. On average, an additional 2.4 hours were needed to perform the original procedure.

Conclusion.—The arterialized antebrachial skin flap for hand reconstruction requires little technical expertise when used by a microsurgery surgeon. No important donor vessels are sacrificed. Follow-up of this flap should consist of simple palpation of the pulse, Doppler auscultation, or plethysmography.

► Venous flap reconstruction, no matter where the donor site originates, continues to be a method that, I believe, is searching for a use. In this study, the defects shown and subsequently treated with venous flaps all had other viable local or regional flaps available, which, in my mind, would supercede venous flaps as a method of reconstruction.

The physiology of flap survival continues to be puzzling. The need for neovascularization and inosculatory ingrowth cannot be disputed, and beds that appear to be favorable with respect to this need generally produce better survival data when venous flaps are placed in this setting. Not coincidentally, these same types of beds with good healthy, well-vascularized underlying tissue, or a healthy, robust granulation bed, are also those that promote the receipt and subsequent take of a composite or full-thickness skin graft. Interestingly, as venous flaps begin to adhere and "heal," they show remarkable similarity to composite and full-thickness skin grafts in the sense that they often show marked congestion, edema, and epidermolysis before proceding to full consolidation and "healing."

There is no doubt about the role of the adequate bed. As evidence of this fact, I have yet to see the clinical circumstance or a clinical report of a flap placed across multiple digits which shows the intervening segment of the flap not in contact with an underlying bed (i.e., "free floating") and with subsequent survival of this intervening portion of the flap. I believe it is important to have the venous flap—especially with adequate multiple venous outflow sites—as a part of the overall microsurgical armamentarian, but, in my mind, its use continues to be relegated to second-line defense.

C.H. Johnson, M.D.

The Distally Based Ulnar Artery Island Flap in Hand Reconstruction

Grobbelaar AO, Harrison DH (Mount Vernon Hosp, London)

J Hand Surg (Br) 22B:204–211, 1997 4–12

Background.—The distally based ulnar artery island flap can be very useful in reconstructing the hand. This technique and its outcomes in 6 patients were described.

The Distally Based Ulnar Artery Island Flap.—The flap, based on the ulnar artery distal to the common interosseous branch, provides thin, pliable, hairless skin. It may be used as a composite flap, including tendon and bone. It also provides an ideal tunnel for tendons to glide in. As a fasciocutaneous or fascial flap, it can be rotated easily to the dorsum of the hand by opening Guyon's canal. The palm, dorsum of the hand, and fingers are easily reached. The flap was used successfully in 5 women, aged 26–45 years, and in a 15-year-old boy, with some patients achieving full range of motion postoperatively. If marked venous congestion occurs intraoperatively, a superficial venous anastomosis should be made.

Conclusion.—The distally based ulnar artery flap is the authors' first choice for reconstructing large soft-tissue defects of the hand. This flap can be raised in about 45 minutes. It is versatile, and the 360-degree rotation permits adequate coverage of all zones of the hand. To minimize morbidity at the donor site, a fascial flap can be used to provide a large flap, maintaining the possibility of primary wound closure at the same time.

▶ This article provides one of the more clear, concise discussions of the ulnar artery forearm flap, including its uses, specifically the advantages it has with respect to design in a distally based fashion. I, personally, believe, however, that the discussion of which vessel is "dominant" in the hand is sometimes irrelevant. In the vast majority of patients, all 5 digits can be supported on the perfusion of a single major vessel of the hand, be it the radial or the ulnar artery.

In this group of patients, my own preference, when considering forearm flaps, involves the determination of where the pivot point would be best placed with respect to the necessary coverage. In this case, the ulnar artery does have distinct advantages because it can be placed at a more distal location on the extremity, with the resultant larger—and, therefore, more useful—arc of rotation. The non–hair-bearing skin is certainly an advantage as well. I find the fact that the ulnar nerve must be dissected free from the flap during harvest to be an insignificant problem and not adding a great deal of time to the dissection.

All things being equal, and the circulation to the distal fingertips being able to draw support from either the radial or the ulnar artery, my choice of which forearm flap to base the flap on, with respect to radial or ulnar circulation, is dependent on the following: the geometry and location of the defect, the placement of the pivot point needed, the issue of hair-bearing or non–hair-bearing skin, and the location of the osseous portion of the flap to be transferred (should bone need to be carried with the flap). I do not have a first choice regarding a radial- or ulnar-perfused, distally based flap in hand reconstruction, but rather let the individual circumstances and geometry of the problem—as well as perfusion of the hand—dictate the choice of donor site.

I also believe that, in certain circumstances, consideration should be given to placing a vein graft for reconstruction of the hand. Although we do this rarely, I have been impressed by the number of people who live in extremes of climate who have experienced cold intolerance after harvesting of the radial or ulnar artery. Because most perfusion to the hand is thermoregulatory in nature, this intuitively makes sense. Recently, I have given stronger consideration to this issue. It is probably only pertinent, however, when one's hand is exposed to the extremes of winter weather.

C.H. Johnson, M.D.

The Lateral Arm Fascial Free Flap for Resurfacing of the Hand and Fingers

Chen H, El-Gammal TA (Chang Gung Mem Hosp, Taipei, Taiwan)

Plast Reconstr Surg 99:454–459, 1997 4–13

Purpose.—The lateral arm flap is widely used for reconstruction of the head and extremities. Its use as a fascial or fasciocutaneous flap has been described as well. Results with the lateral arm fascial free flap for resurfacing of the hand and fingers are reported.

Methods.—The experience included 12 patients with either degloving injuries of the fingers or skin loss of the dorsum of the hand with tendon and bone exposure. The flap was harvested using a curvilinear excision or an H-shaped incision if a fascial flap wider than 6 cm was needed. The scar on the lateral arm was easily covered by clothing. The osteofascial flap included a 1- × 5-cm segment of distal humerus above the lateral epicondyle. The periosteum was supplied by septal perforators from the posterior radial collateral artery, which were protected by leaving behind a muscular cuff of the triceps and brachioradialis.

In the first stage of the operation, the patients underwent débridement and coverage with the lateral arm free fascial flap. The wound was covered with porcine skin. Reconstruction of a missing phalanx, using part of the distal humerus, was also performed at this time if needed. Once the flap was stable, redundant tissue was removed and a split-thickness graft was placed.

Results.—The flap survival rate was 100%, and there were no cases of partial flap loss. Complications consisted of 2 cases of arm numbness and 1 case of complete and 1 of partial loss of the split-thickness skin graft.

Conclusions.—The lateral arm fascial skin flap is useful for resurfacing of the hand and fingers. This flap permits harvesting of a large area of tissue while allowing the donor site to be closed primarily. The thin, pliable fascia conforms to the shape of the fingers. It is not so bulky that it gets in the way of finger motion, and its undersurface provides a gliding surface for the tendons. In the authors' experience with this flap, the success rate is high and complications are few.

▶ The authors present 12 cases of digital reconstruction using the lateral arm free fascia flap with skin grafts. One included the lateral portion of the humerus for a vascularized bone graft. The article discusses anatomy, blood supply, harvesting, and then the case reports of patients undergoing lateral arm fascia free flap resurfacing. The bibliography contains only 6 references.

I agree with the authors' conclusions that free fascia flaps with skin grafts are an excellent way to reconstruct digital defects with bone or tendon exposure. Six of the 12 patients in this series had circumferential degloving injuries to a digit, and these patients ended up with no motion in the proximal interphalangeal joints and basically a covered, nonfunctional digit. I am not convinced that I agree with the authors' patient selection regarding this. Nevertheless, I agree with the authors' conclusions that free fascia flaps should be skin grafted in a delayed fashion as they, because of prolonged bleeding and venous hypertension, show very poor initial skin graft take when done immediately. Waiting a few days to maintain motion in the digit to allow granulation tissue to form for skin grafting is a good suggestion and one that we follow in our practice. I do believe that the lateral arm free fascia flap certainly is a high priority flap for fascial tissue in comparison with other donor sites as mentioned by the authors, but I disagree with its use in some of the specific patient selections, primarily its use in a degloving injury of a digit.

N.B. Meland, M.D.

Limiting Donor Site Morbidity by Suprafascial Dissection of the Radial Forearm Flap

Chang SC-N, Miller G, Halbert CF, et al (Chang Gung Med College, Taipei, Taiwan; Northern Gen Hosp, Sheffield, England; Univ Hosps of Cleveland, Ohio)

Microsurgery 17:136–140, 1996 4–14

Introduction.—Complications of the radial forearm donor site are primarily related to a lack of understanding of the anatomical relation between the superficial and the deep fascia. A technique of suprafascial flap elevation to prevent donor site problems was described.

Technique.—The blood supply for the type C fasciocutaneous radial forearm flap is provided by the radial artery. The dissection proceeds toward the radial vessels in a suprafascial plane, preserving the superficial radial nerve and the lateral antecubital nerve and allowing the 2 layers of deep fascia to remain conjoined. Radial artery, venae comitantes, overlying intermuscular septum with septocutaneous vessels, and the radially located lateral antecubital nerve are elevated together; vascular structures are dissected; the pedicle is cut to length; and the donor site is closed, usually with a thick split-thickness skin graft.

Results.—More than 400 forearm flaps had been prepared when donor site problems required a revision of the dissection protocol. A prospective review of 49 patients receiving flaps by the new protocol revealed 100% skin "take" and normal tendon excursion in all of them with little or no numbness.

Conclusion.—A thorough knowledge of anatomy eliminates many intraoperative problems that have plagued the donor site of radial forearm flaps.

▶ This well-illustrated article describes a technique of radial forearm flap harvest that limits deep dissection to the radial vessels while preserving fascial cover over adjoining muscle compartments and sparing significant cutaneous nerves. A limited prospective study of this technique showed no skin graft loss, no tendon adhesions, and minimal sensory disturbances. The anatomical issues raised in this article deserve consideration by any surgeon using this flap.

W.L. Lineaweaver, M.D.

Free and Island Flap Transfer for Soft Tissue Defects in the Hand and Forearm

Yajima H, Tamai S, Fukui A, et al (Nara Med Univ, Kashihara, Japan)

Microsurgery 17:150–154, 1996 4–15

Background.—Soft-tissue injuries of the hand are common. Repair of large skin defects with distant flaps is complicated by prolonged fixation and the need for a 2-stage operation. A review of patients receiving free- and island-flap transfers and indications for flap transfers in the hand and forearm were presented.

Methods.—Between 1973 and 1994, 220 patients (45 women), aged 6–86, received 82 free (79 patients) and 144 (141 patients) island-flap transfers to the thumb (74), fingers (117), hand (30), and forearm (5) (Table 7). Thumb reconstruction required sensory flaps in 73 of 74 transfers.

Results.—Five free flaps (3 dorsalis pedis) failed and 77 (93.9%) survived. Failures involved arteriovenous fistula in 2 patients, a degloving injury, and a thumb amputation. Four island flaps, all reverse-flow, failed, and 140 (97. 2%) survived. Four of 5 radial forearm reconstructions using tendocutaneous flaps were satisfactory.

Conclusion.—Island-flap transfers are favored more than free-flap transfers when time and success rate are considered. Radial forearm and dorsal metacarpal flaps are reliable and can be used to cover composite tissue defects. Free-flap transfers are superior for thumb and finger defects

TABLE 7.—Indications for Island- and Free-Flap Transfers

Location	Defect	Flap
Thumb	Total	Wraparound, radial forearm (OC)
	Distal	Voral advancement, NVIF
	Volar	NVIF, hemipulp
	Dorsal	Digital island, FDMA
Fingers	Total	Dorsalis pedis, radial forearm (S)
	Distal	Volar advancement, oblique triangle
		Reverse digital island
	Other	Reverse dorsal metacarpal, Rose, DMF
Hand	Volar	Dorsalis pedis, radial forearm
	+ Nerve	Peroneal (+ sural nerve)
	Dorsal	Posterior interosseous, radial forearm
	+ Tendon	Radial forearm (TC), dorsalis pedis (TC)
	First web	Posterior interosseous
Forearm		Latissimus dorsi, peroneal, scapular

Abbreviations: OC, osteocutaneous; *S*, sensory; *TC*, tendocutaneous; *NVIF*, neurovascular bundle island flap; *FDMA*, first dorsal metacarpal artery flap; *DMF*, dorsal middle phalangeal flap.

(Courtesy of Yajima H, Tamai S, Fukui A, et al: Free and island flap transfer for soft tissue defects in the hand and forearm. *Microsurgery* 17:150–154.

and for large defects. Radial forearm tendocutaneous flaps are preferred for tendon defects of the back of the hand.

▶ The authors present a large series of hand and forearm reconstructions after trauma. Microsurgical flaps (82) and island flaps (144) were used with similar success rates (93.9% and 97.2%, respectively). Sensory reconstruction was achieved in most cases. Microvascular flap failures consisted mainly of dorsalis pedis flaps, and island-flap failures occurred with dorsal reverse-flow flaps (2 posterior interosseous flaps and 2 digital island flaps).

The authors present a scheme for choosing between microsurgical flaps and island flaps. Although arguable in details, their scheme demonstrates how many surgeons may organize their flap strategies for specific problems, thereby coherently integrating their reconstructive repertoires.

W.L. Lineaweaver, M.D.

Revascularization of Degloving Injuries of the Limbs

Waikakul S (Mahidol Univ, Bangkok, Thailand)

Injury 28:271–274, 1997 4–16

Introduction.—Degloving injuries involve severe damage to skin and subcutaneous tissue and may also affect bones, joints, fascia, muscles, and other soft tissues. Management of these injuries is based upon debridement and covering of the defects with split-thickness or full-thickness skin grafts. Treatment approaches for 3 types of degloving injuries were illustrated in a study of 32 patients.

Methods.—All patients had degloving injuries of the limbs: 14 in the forearm, 10 in the leg and foot, and 8 in the hand. Twelve patients had industrial injuries and 20 were involved in motorcycle accidents. Six patients required immediate treatment for associated fractures and joint injuries, 5 had muscle and tendon repair, and 10 underwent decompression of the compartment. The degloving or avulsed flaps were then examined under the operating microscope and categorized according to type.

In type I injuries (9 patients), most flaps were severely damaged, with some area of laceration, abrasion, and burn. Most of the flap was moderately damaged in type II injuries (13 patients); subcutaneous veins were still identifiable and there was no venous backflow. The flaps in type III injuries (10 patients) were moderately damaged, with only small areas of burn; skin was not severely crushed and subcutaneous veins were still intact. Management was based upon the type of degloving injury. In type I, patients were treated by extensive debridement and the flaps were used for free full- and split-thickness skin grafting. Arterialization of the venous system of the flaps was performed in type II and venous anastomoses in type III.

Results.—Patients with type I injuries needed further debridement and had split-thickness skin regrafting. Those with injuries of the leg and foot had good function of the knee and ankle. Four patients with hand and forearm injuries needed further reconstructive surgery because of limited movement of nearby joints. The average hospital stay in type I injuries was 28.2 days. Arterialization of the venous system of the flaps was performed in type 2 injuries, and 9 of 13 patients had successful reperfusion. The 4 patients with partial reperfusion underwent further debridement and split-thickness skin grafting. The average hospital stay was 10.6 days for those with complete reperfusion and 43.1 days for those with partial reperfusion. Venous anastomoses yielded good results in all patients with type III injuries; their average hospital stay was 4.2 days.

Conclusion.—Revascularization of flaps in types II and III degloving injuries yielded good results, minimizing the raw surface in need of skin grafting and decreasing morbidity and length of hospitalization. Venous anastomoses should be performed in type III injuries to prevent venous congestion.

► The author offers a classification scheme based upon the injury to the skin, subcutaneous tissue, and subcutaneous veins of the degloved skin envelope in extremity degloving injuries. Operative treatment of the degloved skin envelope is then stratified, based upon the classification scheme. Predictably, results were least predictable when the degloved skin envelope was ischemic and required microsurgical arterial revascularization as well as venous reconstruction. Results were excellent when the degloved skin envelope lacked only venous outflow. The author's recommendations for handling the degloved skin envelope which has arterial inflow but no venous outflow merit review.

A.A. Smith, M.D.

Suggested Reading

Bakhach J, Martin D, Baudet J: The ulnar parametacarpal flap: Experience with ten clinical cases. *Ann Chir Plast Esthet* 41:269–276, 1996.

▶ The authors describe the utility of a skin and subcutaneous tissue flap raised from the dorsoulnar aspect of the hand and vascularized by the artery that accompanies the dorsal ulnar sensory branch. This flap can be rotated on either a proximal or a distal vascular pedicle, with a large axis of rotation. Distally based, it can provide cover for the tip of the little finger. Proximally based, it can cover the palm and distal forearm.

V.R. Hentz, M.D.

Emerson ET, Krizek TJ, Greenwald DP: Anatomy, physiology, and functional restoration of the thumb. *Ann Plast Surg* 36:180–191, 1996.

▶ I recommend to you this review paper which includes a good recounting of anatomy and function of the thumb as well as the options for thumb reconstruction after amputation.

R.A. Chase, M.D.

Foucher G, Rostane S, Chammas M, et al: Transfer of a severely damaged digit to reconstruct an amputated thumb. *J Bone Joint Surg (Am)* 78-A:1889–1896, 1996.

▶ This is a timely article not because the ideas presented are novel, but because it is a necessary reminder that not everything injured needs reconstruction. The concept of the salvage of amputated or badly damaged parts as a resource for the reconstruction of a missing part or function cannot be overemphasized.

V.R. Hentz, M.D.

Kumar VP, Satku K, Liu J: The Brunelli reversed flow pedicle flap from the thumb. *Plast Reconstr Surg* 98:1298–1301, 1996.

▶ This case report demonstrates another of the very versatile reversed flow flaps that can be utilized in the reconstruction of distal digital injuries. This flap, based on the dorsoulnar collateral vascular supply to the thumb, can be rotated at its pivot point near the thumb's metacarpophalangeal joint to reach almost any area of the hand. It may be possible to elicit some sensation if a small branch of the dorsal sensory radial nerve is included and this branch then connected to a recipient nerve near the zone of injury. Today, the need to bury an injured digit into a chest or groin pedicle flap donor site is rare indeed.

V.R. Hentz, M.D.

Lyall H, Elliot D: Total middle ray amputation. *J Hand Surg (Br)* 21B:675–680, 1996.

▶ This paper presents results of 8 cases—2 for malignancy and 6 for trauma—of middle finger ray amputation by removal of the entire third metacarpal (including the base) and soft tissue repair. The authors believe this technique allows improved narrowing of the second-to-fourth metacarpal gap with less resultant digital scissoring than when the third metacarpal base is preserved. They contend that this method is technically easier, with no risk of non- or malunion, than index to middle transposition. It is a small series, and no comparative data with the other techniques are presented. The results presented appear satisfactory. The authors indicate that ECRB function is maintained by preservation of the third metacarpal base periosteum plus some existing ECRB insertion into the second metacarpal, but no measurements or functional data are presented to confirm this.

J.M. Markley, Jr., M.D.

Wolff K-D, Ervens J, Hoffmeister B: Improvement of the radial forearm donor site by prefabrication of fascial–split-thickness skin grafts. *Plast Reconstr Surg* 98:358–362, 1996.

► The authors build upon the work of others in attempting to minimize the cosmetic deformity associated with harvesting a radial forearm flap. In an initial procedure, through a relaively small incision, the fascia is covered with a skin graft. The incision is closed leaving the skin graft on the fascia and under the skin flaps. Two weeks later, after revascularization of the graft, the incisions are reopened, extended if necessary for appropriate pedicle length, the fascia and radial artery are mobilized in a conventional manner, and the flap is transferred. This technique yields a thin flap perhaps more applicable for intraoral reconstruction; it also has a place in upper extremity reconstruction.

V.R. Hentz, M.D.

5 Tendon Trauma and Reconstruction

Sagittal Band Reconstruction

Watson HK, Weinzweig J, Guidera PM (Connecticut Combined Hand Service, Hartford; Yale Univ, New Haven, Conn; Univ of Massachusetts, Worcester; et al)

J Hand Surg (Am) 22A:452–456, 1997 5–1

Background.—The occurrence of extensor tendon subluxation at the metacarpophalangeal joint in patients without rheumatoid arthritis is rare. In almost all such patients reported, disruption of the radial sagittal band with ulnar subluxation of the extensor tendon was noted. A technique for sagittal band reconstruction was described that effectively recentralizes and stabilizes the extensor tendon by using the deep transverse metacarpal ligament, the normal volar attachment of the sagittal band, thus avoiding the need to distort normal collateral ligament or lumbrical anatomy.

Methods and Outcomes.—Twenty-one sagittal band reconstructions were done in 16 patients. There were 18 cases of ulnar subluxation caused by radial sagittal band disruption and 3 of radial subluxation caused by ulnar sagittal band disruption. The technique involved weaving a retrograde segment of extensor tendon on itself after passing it through the deep transverse metacarpal ligament. The procedure eliminated pain in all patients. No recurrences of extensor tendon subluxation were documented.

Conclusion.—The technique described effectively produces a stable mechanism for maintaining the centralized position of the extensor tendon without disrupting normal anatomy or limiting the range of motion of the metacarpophalangeal joint. It involves weaving a retrograde segment of extensor tendon on itself after passing it through the deep transverse metacarpal ligament, which serves as a pulley.

► In nonacute cases of sagittal band rupture in which direct repair is not feasible or is ill advised because of the condition of the tissues, this technique represents an anatomical and stable reconstruction that satisfies the criteria of recentralization, sufficient strength, and anatomical rebalancing. I have used this technique with similar success.

C.H. Johnson, M.D.

Optimization of the MGH Repair Using an Algorithm for Tenorrhaphy Evaluation

Wasserman RJ, Howard R, Markee B, et al (Univ of South Florida, Tampa)
Plast Reconstr Surg 99:1688–1694, 1997 5–2

Objective.—The benefits of early mobilization after tenorrhaphy are controversial. Early mobilization can enhance healing and increase strength, or it can result in gap formation or rupture. Optimum results should be surgeon independent. An algorithm was developed to assess the biomechanical performance of the modified Becker (MGH) and the modified Kessler repairs using a dynamic human cadaveric model for evaluating strength, toughness, and glide after zone II flexor digitorum profundis repairs.

Methods.—Three surgeons performed 7 repairs each in 14 fresh frozen human cadaver hands using the 2 techniques. Pull to rupture measurements were made in the dynamic hand model, and results of the 2 techniques were compared statistically.

Results.—Compared with the modified Kessler technique, the MGH technique was significantly stronger (79 vs. 64 newtons) and significantly tougher (92 vs. 78 newtons). The glide efficiency of the MGH technique was 32%, similar to that of the Kessler technique (33%). Whereas strength was operator independent for the MGH technique, strength of the modified Kessler repair depended significantly on the individual surgeon. The MGH 2-cross configuration was significantly more gap resistant than the 0-, 1-, 3-, or 4-cross configurations.

Conclusion.—The algorithm demonstrates that the MGH technique for zone II tenorrhaphy results in a significantly stronger and tougher repair that is significantly more gap resistant than other configurations and is operator independent.

▶ There is increasing evidence that the lateral trap suture (MGH) is an improvement over the benchmark Kessler repair. What is needed now is a prospective, comparative, clinical study of the 2 repairs in humans.

P.C. Amadio, M.D.

Tensile Strength of Flexor Tendon Repairs in a Dynamic Cadaver Model

Komanduri M, Phillips CS, Mass DP (Univ of Chicago)
J Hand Surg (Am) 21A:605–611, 1996 5–3

Introduction.—As a method of assessing wound strength and healing, measurement of tensile strength has been used since 1928. The first week after repair is considered the most crucial period in tendon healing. Traditionally, the recommendation was to place sutures at the palmar aspect at the repair site because this avoids strangling the primarily dorsal blood supply in the human profundus tendon. The validity of the hypothesis that dorsal placement of classic suture repairs will enhance tensile strength was studied.

Methods.—The study included 26 fresh-frozen cadaver hands with 78 tendons that had sharp zone II profundus tendon transection and repair with Bunnell, Kessler, Kessler with circumferential epitenon, or epitenon-alone sutures. Sutures were randomly placed either at the dorsal or palmar aspect within the flexor tendon. There were 10 trials of each placement and suture type. To test the strength, flexion of the repair digit was performed at a constant excursion rate until the tendon ruptured.

Results.—Significantly more tensile strength was provided by the sutures placed at the dorsal aspect than at the palmar aspect in all cases. Over a prolonged time, epitenon curves had a stepwise failure. Maximum tensile strengths generated by Kessler core sutures with epitenon repairs were significantly stronger than the other repairs to dorsal without an epitenon repair. When compared to equivalent linear pulls, the use of a dorsal Kessler core suture with or without an epitenon suture in the curvilinear model demonstrated significant increase in strength.

Conclusion.—Because of their increased strength, a dorsally placed core suture and circumferential epitenon repair should be considered for zone II profundus repairs. An anatomical curvilinear model should be used to test future tendon repairs because it simulates the specific biomechanical conditions unique to the flexing digit.

► The authors have studied sharp zone II profundus tendon transection and repair in a cadaveric model with Bunnell, Kessler, Kessler with circumferential epitenon, or epitenon-alone sutures to test whether dorsal placement enhances tensile strength. They conclude that dorsal placement of core suture (Kessler with circumferential epitenon repair) had significantly increased repair strength compared to palmar core sutures.

The authors correctly state that further testing of these results in an in vivo animal model is necessary before recommendations can be made. I totally agree. The milieu of the healing tendon is complex. In this study, the dorsal placement of sutures potentially places at risk the tendon blood supply, a fact which the authors acknowledge. Although tendon viability is not totally dependent on vascular supply, however, it does play a role, as evidenced by studies that indicate that when vincula remain intact after injury, recovery is enhanced. The authors of this study have also not given any information on tendon excursion except to mention that their values were within physiologic ranges. If there were any significant differences among the various repairs with both palmar and dorsal placement, we are not aware of this. Further, any significant restrictions of tendon excursion may suggest the potential formation of adhesions. For example, Noguchi et al.[1] have shown that the Savage repair has a greater tensile strength than that reported by the present authors with superior excursion.

In general, the authors have presented a carefully done study, but, as they point out themselves, the final word on dorsal placement of zone II tendon sutures must await future animal and clinical studies.

M.A. Badalamente, Ph.D.

Reference

1. Noguchi M, Seiler JG III, Gelberman RH, et al: In vitro biomechanical analysis of suture methods for flexor tendon repair. *J Ortho Res* 11:603–611, 1993.

Colour Doppler Ultrasound Examination of Hand Tendon Pathologies: A Preliminary Report

Buyruk HM, Stam HJ, Laméris JS, et al (Erasmus Univ Rotterdam, The Netherlands)

J Hand Surg (Br) 21B:469–473, 1996 5–4

Introduction.—All of the imaging modalities used to examine the musculoskeletal system provide only static images; they provide no direct information about the function of the musculoskeletal system. Color Doppler imaging (CDI) is used mainly for the study of blood flow. Its imaging characteristics suggest that it might be useful in studying the movement of the tendons and muscles of the wrist and hand. The CDI findings of the flexor and extensor tendons on injured and uninjured hands were assessed.

Methods.—Color Doppler imaging was done in 5 patients with various unilateral pathologic conditions of the hand. The function of the flexor and extensor tendons was evaluated as the patient continuously flexed and extended the fingers. Scanning was done at the level of the wrist, the metacarpus, and the proximal phalanx.

Findings.—All muscle and tendon displacements were recognized by CDI. The sliding tendon appeared blue during contraction and red during relaxation or contraction of the extensor. Nonmoving structures appeared gray. Transverse scans showed no apparent pathology. The CDI scans showed the absence of adhesions in a hand with restricted mobility, the recovery of muscle function after an injury, progressive adhesion of a forearm flap to the extensor tendons, connected displacement of 2 tendons after hand surgery, and tendon pathology responsible for trigger thumb.

Conclusions.—Color Doppler imaging is a promising technique for studying pathologic conditions of the flexor tendons of the hand. More research is needed to optimize the imaging and quantitative aspects of CDI examination of the locomotor system.

► Most of us are familiar with CDI of the blood vessels. Perhaps we ask our ultrasound experts to help assess a mass as solid or fluid-filled or to locate a foreign body. The current study, while limited to only certain areas of the limb because of technical constraints, invites additional research into the possibilities of using CDI to determine whether a contracted finger after tendon repair cannot be extended because of adhesions, too short a tendon, or stiffness of the joint. Is it the tendon or the joint that is snapping? This technology bears watching.

V.R. Hentz, M.D.

Corticosteroid Responsive Tenosynovitis Is a Common Pathway for Limited Joint Mobility in the Diabetic Hand

Sibbitt WL Jr, Eaton RP (Univ of New Mexico, Albuquerque)
J Rheumatol 24:931–936, 1997 5–5

Introduction.—Stiff hand syndrome, diabetic palmar flexor tenosynovitis, trigger finger, and syndrome of limited joint mobility are some typical diabetes-associated hand conditions. Digital flexion contractures and mechanical dysfunction of the hand occur in virtually all diabetic hand conditions, supporting the concept that diabetic hand conditions may represent different clinical manifestations of essentially one pathogenic disorder. With therapy specific for tenosynovitis, such as a corticosteroid injection of the palmar flexor tendon sheath, it was determined whether the syndrome of the limited joint mobility and diabetic trigger finger could be reversed.

Methods.—After Dupuytren's contracture, hand neuropathy, carpal tunnel syndrome, and arthritis were excluded, adult patients with diabetes mellitus and syndrome of limited joint mobility were evaluated. To obtain a baseline, patients were observed for 3 months. Ten mg of methylprednisolone acetate or 10 mg triamcinolone acetonide were injected into the palmar flexor tendon sheaths and the sheaths were reassessed at 1, 3, and 12 months.

Results.—There was a 94% response rate at 1 month, defined by complete resolution of digital contractures and trigger after corticosteroid injection. At 3 months, the response rate was 76%, and at 12 months, the response rate was 61%; all were significantly different from preinjection. Although there was a trend for earlier recurrence with methylprednisolone, no appreciable differences between methylprednisolone acetate and triamcinolone acetonide were observed.

Conclusion.—In patients with syndrome of limited joint mobility or diabetic trigger finger, corticosteroid injection is a safe and effective therapy that should be considered. Diabetic tenosynovits is a common pathway in diabetic hand conditions, as is evidenced by the excellent response to injection.

▶ It is often said that diabetic trigger fingers and diabetic finger flexion contractures do not respond to nonsurgical treatment. This article, which seems to be nicely done, suggests otherwise. I believe it is reasonable to treat such patients initially with steroid injection. If relief is not provided, then trigger finger release and local synovectomy may be indicated to address triggering and contracture, respectively.

P.C. Amadio, M.D.

Independent Index Extension After Indicis Proprius Transfer: Excision of Juncturae Tendinum

Kitano K, Tada K, Shibata T, et al (Osaka Univ, Japan; Kansai Rosai Hosp, Osaka, Japan)

J Hand Surg (Am) 21A:992–996, 1996 5–6

Introduction.—Patients who have undergone transfer of the extensor indicis proprius (EIP) tendon may experience a loss of independent extension of the index finger. To preserve the motion of independent index extension, the variations of the juncturae tendinum (JT) and extensor digitorum communis (EDC) muscle and its innervation were examined.

Methods.—Twenty-seven hands were dissected in a cadaveric study to determine the variations of the JT between the index and long fingers and EDC muscle. The JTs between the index finger and the long finger were classified into 2 groups (von Schroeder IA and IB) and the EDC muscle of the index finger was examined for innervation and independence from the other muscle. In a clinical study, 13 hands of 12 patients who had EIP transfer for a variety of reasons were inspected for the appearance of the JT. Classification of the JT was done as in the cadaveric study. Patients had the digit involved in the transfer immobilized for 3 weeks.

Results.—In the cadaveric study, 16 (59%) of 27 hands were von Schroeder type IA: the JT consisted of fascia that looked like membrane without bands (identical to von Schroeder's "absent" JT). Eleven hands (41%) had von Schroeder type IB: JT were much more substantial, with filamentous bands (identical to von Schroeder's type I JT). Ten of 13 hands in the clinical study were classified as type IB JT, and 3 were type IA JT. Independent index finger extension was retained at follow-up in all 13 hands.

Discussion.—Because of its ease of exposure, appropriate length and exposure, and retention of function, the EIP muscle is often transferred to restore mobility to a variety of hand movements. Some patients, however, may lose independent extension of the index finger. This problem may be prevented if the hood is preserved, or repaired if disrupted, and if the JT (whether type IA or IB) is excised.

▶ This article and its set of references, plus the article that immediately precedes it in the November 1996 *Journal of Hand Surgery,*[1] present the state of current information about the anatomy and physiology af the digital extensors over the dorsum of the hand and metacarpophalangeal joints as effecting and affecting independent extension of the index finger, particularly after transfer of the EIP. It is worthy of review by those engaging in tendon transfer surgery.

The authors have unfortunately complicated the nomenclature, however, by introducing an unnecessary modification of von Schroeder's classification of juncturae. The type IA of Kitano et al. is the same as von Schroeder's fascia-only, and Kitano type IIB is von Schroeder's type I. The important finding is the confirmation anatomically of evidence for neuromuscular independence of the EDC of the index finger from that of the middle, ring, and small fingers.

J.M. Markley, Jr., M.D.

Reference

1. Gonzalez MH, Weinzweig N, Kay T, et al: Anatomy of the extensor tendons to the index finger. *J Hand Surg (Am)* 21A:988–995, 1996.

Patterns of Cellular Activation After Tendon Injury

Khan U, Edwards JCW, McGrouther DA (Univ College, London)

J Hand Surg (Br) 21B:813–820, 1996 5–7

Background.—The adhesions and scar tissue that can form after flexor tendon surgery of the hand interfere with treatment success. The mechanisms that lead to these disabling lesions were investigated in a rabbit model.

Methods.—A transverse laceration was made through 50% of the tendon on the flexor aspect of the flexor digitorum profundus tendon of the rabbit. The synovial sheath was kept intact. Monoclonal antibodies to proliferating cell nuclear antigen, macrophages, the vascular cell adhesion molecule (VCAM-1), transforming growth factors-β (TGF-β), basic fibroblast growth factor, epidermal growth factor receptor, and uridine diphosphoglucose dehydrogenase (UDPGD) were used to follow the response of the synovial sheath, epitenon, and endotenon at various times after injury.

Results.—There was no staining for proliferating cell nuclear antigen in normal or sham-operated tissue. After injury, positive cells were detected in the synovial sheath and epitenon. Macrophages were present in normal synovial sheath and epitenon, but were rare in the endotenon. Within 3 days of injury, macrophages had increased in all 3 compartments. The VCAM-1 was present in normal synovial sheath and epitenon. Staining increased after injury, even in uninjured areas. The active form of TGF-β was present in normal epitenon. Three days after injury, positive staining occurred in the epitenon matrix and was not cellular. After 28 days, cells of the epitenon and endotenon were labeled. There was no significant change in labeling for UDPGD after injury.

Conclusions.—The normal epitenon and synovial sheath were shown to contain fibroblasts and macrophages, which can interact via VCAM-1. Cells in the uninjured synovial lining proliferated more rapidly and extensively than those of the injured endotenon. There was increased expression of TGF-β by synovial sheath and epitenon after injury. After tendon injury, the synovial lining, even if uninjured, appears to play a dominant role in the scarring response.

▶ The authors have performed a very good study based on the idea that 1 component of a tendon may be relatively more reactive than other components with respect to scar formation after injury. In a rabbit model, the flexor digitorum profundus tendon was lacerated through 50% of the tendon but the tendon sheath was not injured, such that the injured tendon was returned to glide below a normal sheath. The authors studied cell proliferation, macrophages, VCAM-1, and certain growth factors.

An important finding was that the synovial sheath, although uninjured, and the epitenon have fibroblasts and macrophages that interact with one another via VCAM-1. Tendon injury induces synovial fibroblasts to proliferate in preference to endotenon fibroblasts. Although the injury to the synovial sheath was minimal in this study, as it was exposed but not injured, this is an important concept consistent with the literature, which shows that injury to the sheath is critically important to the formation of adhesions. Similarly, increased TGF-β_1 expression has been shown in synovial sheath and epitenon fibroblasts, which is also important to cell proliferation and synthesis of extracellular matrix proteins.

It is becoming increasingly clear from the work of many authors that the "intrasynovial" and "extrasynovial" tendon environments may be different in their injury/repair responses. Studies such as this work by Drs. Khan, Edwards, and McGrouther add significantly to our knowledge of the cell biology of the injury/repair response in tendons, such that, in the future, potential therapies may be available to prevent scarring and adhesions.

M.A. Badalamente, Ph.D.

Cyclic Stress Testing After In Vivo Healing of Canine Flexor Tendon Lacerations

Pruitt DL, Tanaka H, Aoki M, et al (Washington Univ, St Louis)
J Hand Surg (Am) 21A:974–977, 1996 — 5–8

Introduction.—Healing after repair of lacerated flexor tendons is often complicated by the formation of restrictive adhesions. Early passive motion has been found to be the most effective means of preventing adhesion formation. However, passive motion may cause repetitive cyclic stress on the site of repair. This type of stress has been associated with gap formation in recently repaired cadaver tendons. The effects of cyclic stress testing on canine flexor tendon lacerations after repair and in vivo healing were evaluated.

Methods.—After anesthesia, forepaw tendons of adult mongrel dogs were surgically lacerated and then repaired. The animals were killed after 3, 7, 10, 21, and 30 days of healing, and the operated and contralateral unoperated tendons were removed for testing. The contralateral tendons were lacerated and repaired in the same manner as the test tendons and served as controls (0 days of healing). Tendons were repetitively stressed on a cyclic testing machine, and gap formation at the repair site was measured.

Results.—After 3 days of healing, the final gap formation was found to be 1.14 mm and was significantly greater than final gap formation observed at later healing times. At 7 days, the final gap value was 0.88 mm; at 10 days, 0.63 mm; at 21 days, 1.10 mm; and at 30 days, 0.65 mm. A final gap of 0.75 mm was found in control tendons tested immediately after repair.

Conclusion.—Gap formation in repaired tendon lacerations was found to occur for up to 30 days after repair following repetitive cyclic stressing. Gap formation was greatest on postoperative day 3.

▶ The authors investigated the effects of cyclic tensile force applied to completely lacerated and repaired canine flexor tendons. The study found that gap formation was observed after periods of healing of up to 30 days. The authors have stated that although the results of this study cannot be directly applied to humans, it would be reasonable to protect a flexor tendon repair site from *strong* repetitive tensile forces for at least 30 days to limit gap formation.

Most will certainly agree that protection from strong forces, repetitive or otherwise, is critical to the healing process of flexor tendons to prevent adhesions and improve gliding. This study used only 1 value (250 g) of applied tensile force although the rate of cyclic tension was high at every 1.5 seconds. We do not know the force in newtons that was actually applied, nor do we know the stress in megapascals applied; these values were not reported. As the authors themselves state, the clinical importance of gap formation is not entirely clear. Some reports suggest that gaps greater than 3 mm are associated with increased adhesion formation. Other reports disagree. Although it is not a direct analogy, a recent survey by McCarthy[1] of 591 American Society for Surgery of the Hand member respondents showed that protected mobilization of partially lacerated tendons begins very early, within the first 48 hours. If one considers a partially lacerated tendon as having a gap, then this would argue for early, gentle motion. Until a range of forces can be defined as inducing clinically significant gaps of known values after flexor tendon repair, recommendations on rehabilitation protocols should not be made.

M.A. Badalamente, Ph.D.

Reference

1. McCarthy CK: *ASSH Correspondence Newletter*. American Society for Surgery of the Hand, 1996.

Suggested Reading

Foucher G, Binhamer P, Cange S, et al: Long term results of splintage for mallet finger. *Int Orthop* 20:129–131, 1996.

▶ The authors reinforce the notion that prolonged and continuous splinting (8 weeks) of the distal interphalangeal joint in full extension is the preferred treatment for closed mallet finger injuries with or without bone avulsion involving less than 30% of the joint surface. A dorsal splint that reduces the likelihood of skin maceration (a perforated plastic splint) increases patient acceptance and compliance with splint use for the long duration. The result at 6 months will be maintained for the long term. My preference is closed splinting almost regardless of the size of the fracture fragment, provided that there is not palmar subluxation of the joint.

V.R. Hentz, M.D.

Gahankari D, Tambwekar S, Rana R: Flexor carpi radialis opponensplasty *Br J Plast Surg* 49:401–403, 1996.

▶ Surely every muscle tendon unit in the forearm and hand has been used at one time or another to substitute for the paralyzed median innervated thenar muscles, a testament to the inherent quality of the design of the carpometacarpal joint. Witness another choice.

V.R. Hentz, M.D.

Kubota H, Aoki M, Pruitt DL, et al: Mechanical properties of various circumferential tendon suture techniques. *J Hand Surg (Br)* 21B:474–480, 1996.

▶ This study was designed to evaluate mechanical properties of 6 different peripheral circumferential tendon suture techniques. Tensile strength, gap strength, and work of flexion (WoF) were measured as independent variables. Seventy-two human cadaver flexor profundus tendons were used and the 6 sutures were (1) simple, (2) simple locking, (3) Lembert mattress, (4) Halsted mattress, (5) cross-stitch, and (6) Lin-locking. In the study, 6/0 propylene monofilament suture material (Prolene; Ethicon, Somerville, NJ) was used for all techniques. Work of flexion was determined on the wooden frame, using a 25 g counterweight and a tensile testing machine. This work of flexion was calculated in Newton meters as the area under the force-excursion curve. Postoperative repair values were compared to control values to determine a delta WoF. Load-to-failure testing was performed cut across-head speed of 5 cm/min.

The authors found that in terms of tensile strength, the Lin-locking technique was stronger than the other techniques tested. The simple technique had the strongest gap strength. This study also looked at the effect of varying numbers of strands across the repair site. The increased number of strands produced increased tensile strength values. This was also true for gap strength. The work of flexion did not, however, seem to be influenced by the factor of suture strand numbers. The Lin-locking technique had the most increased work of flexion and also had the most exposed sutures outside of the tendon. These were increased 33% to 36% compared to the other techniques, which increased the work of flexion from 6% to 22%.

In conclusion, the strongest circumferential peripheral sutures also had the most deleterious effect in terms of increasing work of flexion. These sutures also have the most complex pattern in terms of surgical technique (Lin-locking). The cross-stitch, the Halsted, and the Lembert had reasonable tensile and gap strength values with reasonably modest increased work of flexion values as well. The authors recommended these techniques over the simple and the simple-locking method.

In my opinion, this is another in a series of excellent studies by established investigators looking at several of the conventional suture methods available for the peripheral circumferential suture. The methodology is sound and the conclusions that are drawn help answer the question of "what is the ideal suture?"

Although it does not fully answer this question, it points out mechanical advantages and disadvantages of each type.

E. Diao, M.D.

LeHuec JC, Moinard M, Liquois F, et al: Distal rupture of the biceps. *J Bone Joint Surg (Br)* 78-B:767–770, 1996.

► MRI is useful not only to assess the degree of retraction after complete rupture, as reported here, but also to investigate cases of partial rupture, for which surgery is also often indicated.

P.C. Amadio, M.D.

6 Nerve Trauma and Reconstruction

Tubular Versus Conventional Repair of Median and Ulnar Nerves in the Human Forearm: Early Results From a Prospective, Randomized, Clinical Study

Lundborg G, Rosén B, Dahlin L, et al (Univ of Lund, Malmö, Sweden)

J Hand Surg (Am) 22A:99–106, 1997 6–1

Introduction.—The regeneration of an injured peripheral nerve involves local synthesis and release of key neurotrophic factors. These include nerve growth factor, brain-derived neurotrophic growth factor, and ciliary neurotrophic factor. The authors have been using a principle of tubulization, that is, encasing the 2 cut ends of the nerve to allow neurotrophic factors to accumulate. Early results of a randomized trial of this approach for the repair of transected nerves in the human forearm are reported.

Methods.—Eighteen patients with transected median or ulnar nerves of the distal forearm were studied. All of the transections were located at the wrist or within 10 cm of the wrist. They were randomized to tubulization or conventional microsurgical repair. In the tubulization group, the 2 cut ends were attached to the inside wall of a silicone tube, with a 3–4-mm gap left between the ends. The patients were followed up closely for 1 year, and the follow-up included tests of motor and sensory function.

Results.—At follow-up, the 2 groups were similar in most measures of recovery, including the Tinel's sign, the results of tactilometry, and tactile gnosis. The exception was touch perception as measured with the Semmes–Weinstein monofilaments, which was better at 3 months in the tubulization group. One patient underwent surgical re-exploration to remove the tube at 11 months. In this case, the gap between the proximal and distal nerve ends had been replaced by regenerated nerve tissue. The replacement was so complete that it was impossible to pinpoint the location of the previous injury.

Conclusions.—Good early results are reported with a tubulization approach to the repair of transected peripheral nerves. This technique emphasizes the intrinsic healing capacity of the cut nerve and provides an optimal environment for nerve healing while minimizing surgical trauma. The results are comparable with those achieved with conventional microsurgical repair. The authors plan further studies to refine their approach, including the development of bioresorbable materials that will not interfere with the axonal regeneration process.

▶ Nerves will regenerate across short gaps and will make directional changes to find distal nerve tissue. However, as this study has demonstrated, nerve regeneration across a controlled nerve gap is not superior to an excellent microsurgical nerve repair. At a 1-year follow-up, there was no difference between these 2 techniques. Thus, the enthusiasm of the 1980s that suggested the possibility that a nerve gap could enhance the results of a standard nerve repair appears not to be warranted. However, reconstruction of a nerve injury using a tubulization technique can be considered as an alternative to a short nerve graft or a direct nerve repair if the topography of the proximal distal nerve is not known. The authors, recognizing that, in time, a circumferential silicone tube will likely result in compression neuropathy, emphasize the need for a bioabsorbable material. In time, nerve conduits will likely find a role in the clinical management of a short nerve injury.

S.E. Mackinnon, M.D.

Reference

1. Evans PJ, Bain JR, Mackinnon SE, et al: Selective reinnervation: A comparison of recovery following microsuture and conduit nerve repair. *Brain Res* 559:315–321, 1991.

Determining the Maximal Length of a Vein Conduit Used as an Interposition Graft for Nerve Regeneration

Strauch B, Ferder M, Lovelle-Allen S, et al (Albert Einstein College of Medicine, Bronx, NY)

J Reconstr Microsurg 12:521–527, 1996 6–2

Introduction.—Autogenous nerve grafting is currently used to repair severed peripheral nerves when other techniques cannot be used. However, nerve grafts result in donor sensory deficits, prompting investigators to search for alternative conduits. Recent studies have found some success with the use of autogenous venous nerve conduits (AVNC) for nerve regeneration for short gaps (3 cm or less) in sensory nerves. The use of AVNC in nerve gaps between 1 and 6 cm was studied.

Methods.—Sixty male PF New Zealand white rabbits were used in the experiment. After anesthesia, the common peroneal nerve was separated and an excision (less than or equal to 6 cm) of a mixed motorsensory nerve was made. In 3 groups of animals, the nerve defect was repaired with either a 1-cm, 3-cm, or 6-cm AVNC graft (groups 1, 2, and 5, respectively). In 2 groups of animals, a 1-cm or 3-cm proximal nerve or vein repair only was used (groups 3 and 4, respectively). In the remaining group (group 6), the 6-cm defect was repaired with a 6-cm nerve graft; this group also served as a control. Electromyography and motor nerve conduction tests were performed periodically for up to 12 months. Animals were then killed; neurol regeneration was quantified as full (100%) growth, moderate (50%), sparse (25%), rare (10%), or none (0%). In a second, similar investigation, 36 rabbits received either a 3.75-cm, 4.5-cm, or 5.25-cm autogenous vein graft to the left peroneal nerve. The animals were examined clinically and then killed after 12 months to assess neuronal regeneration.

Results.—Moderate to abundant nerve regeneration was observed at 6 months in animals in groups 1 and 2. Axonal regeneration, with distal nerve myelinization and organization, were found on neurohistologic examination. Denervation potential was found in the AVNC at 6 months, but not at 3 months. Rare axonal growth was found in animals in groups 3 and 4. Axonal regeneration was also rare at 12 months in animals in group 5. Excellent axonal regeneration was found in animals in group 6, with action potentials observed at 1 year. In the second investigation, histologic examination was performed on 26 nerve specimens. Midpoint axonal growth was sparse in animals who received 3.75-cm grafts, with rare distal propagation. In the 4.5-cm group, a 35% midpoint regeneration was found, with 8.3% distal growth. Sparse propagation was observed in the 5.25-cm group, whereas the distal growth was rare. No evidence of muscle reinnervation was shown by electromyograph.

Conclusion.—The use of AVNCs of up to 3 cm were associated with nerve growth that exceeded 50% of normal. Autogenous venous nerve conduits longer than 3 cm were found to have less capacity for nerve regeneration.

► In a rabbit model, the authors confirm the findings of others that approximately 3 cm is the maximum distance that axons, guided through an artificial membrane, will grow. To extend the distance and thus make the concept of an artificial nerve graft a reality, the guide must contain both neurotrophic and neurotropic substances or must contain substances that promote the production of the proper chemicals by the sprouting axons and accompanying Schwann cells.

V.R. Hentz, M.D.

Changes in the Structural Properties of Peripheral Nerves After Transection

Toby EB, Meyer BM, Schwappach J, et al (Univ of Kansas, Kansas City)

J Hand Surg (Am) 21A:1086–1090, 1996 6–3

Introduction.—Although many advances have been made in microsurgical techniques, the functional and sensory results after peripheral nerve repair remains poor. Timing of the repair of peripheral nerve injuries is controversial. Structural property changes in peripheral nerves over time after transection were assessed.

Methods.—After anesthesia, the sciatic nerves of Sprague-Dawley rats were surgically exposed and completely transected; the nerve on the contralateral side of each test animal was not transected and served as a control. Ten animals were killed every week for 5 weeks, and the distal stump on each side was resected. Each nerve was mechanically stretched until failure, and the force required was recorded. Stiffness and toughness of each nerve were then calculated and compared between transected and intact nerves.

Results.—At weeks 1 and 2, transected nerves had a 15% greater linear elastic stiffness than did intact nerves; this difference was statistically significant. At weeks 3, 4, and 5, transected nerves had 6.5%, 4.8%, and 3.9% greater stiffness than intact nerves, respectively. These differences, however, were not significant. At weeks 2–5, transected nerves also showed significantly greater failure elongation than did intact nerves. Toughness was significantly greater in the transected nerve; the maximum difference was 50% at week 4. At each week tested, the transected nerves had a 21% or greater increase in failure load than did the intact nerves.

Conclusion.—Elastic stiffness was found to be increased at 1–2 weeks after nerve transection when compared with intact nerves. This could result in increased tension at the suture line if repairs of transected nerves are delayed.

► This is an uncomplicated study of the alterations in several biomechanical properties of the peripheral nerve distal to the site of transection. The relative simplicity of the experimental design is not carried through in terms of interpreting the findings and in applying the data to the clinical situation. In the rat, stiffness of the distal nerve increases rapidly after transection, remains high during the first 2 weeks (increase of 15% over control), and then decreases, again rapidly, during the next 3 weeks (3.9% increase over control at 5 weeks.) The study examined nerves only up to 5 weeks after transection. Does stiffness continue to decrease during the next several weeks? Increased tension is required to re-elongate the nerve (i.e., to overcome increased stiffness) if an end-to-end repair is to be performed. Repair at 1–2 weeks after transection seems, in the rat, to be associated with overcoming great stiffness. From the data, one can conclude that waiting an additional few weeks reduces tension at the repair site. However, many questions remain. What is the effect on delay in repair on the proximal side of the injury? Are the same effects observed in primates, which have significantly more connective tissue composing the nerve? If you pull too hard on the distal stump and diminish its blood supply, does it become, in essence, a nerve graft? Signal the rats! They are still needed.

V.R. Hentz, M.D.

Injection Injury to the Median Nerve

Fremling MA, Mackinnon SE (Washington Univ, St Louis)

Ann Plast Surg 37:561–567, 1996 6–4

Purpose.—Injection injury of a peripheral nerve is an uncommon but potentially serious injury. It is especially likely to occur during administration of local and regional anesthetics. Prevention of these injuries relies on knowing the anatomy and instructing the patient to provide feedback during anesthetic injection. An illustrative case of injection injury to the median nerve was reviewed.

Case Report.—Woman, 68, was undergoing incision and drainage of an abscess on the medial aspect of her upper arm. Skin anesthesia was provided with 1% lidocaine, but a deeper infiltrate was given because of persistent pain. This injection resulted in persistent loss of sensation in the thumb, index finger, and long finger and loss of flexion in the thumb and index finger. Surgical inspection of the median nerve, done 2 days later, found no overt signs of injury. During the next 6 months, the patient had severe pain that persisted despite treatment with amitriptyline, clonidine, and desipramine. Results of nerve conduction studies suggested severe median nerve injury.

When seen at 7 months after the injury, the patient had severe hyperalgesia and no functional sensibility or appreciable motor function in the distribution of the median nerve. The tentative diagnosis of injection injury to the median nerve was made, and surgical exploration with nerve grafting was recommended. The nerve was thickened and firm for a distance of 5 cm, with a normal nerve action potential proximal to the injury but no electricity across or distal to the lesion. The damaged area was resected, leaving a 7-cm gap that was reconstructed with four 8-cm sural nerve grafts. The resected area was grossly damaged, which was confirmed on histologic examination. The patient's motor and sensory problems persisted after surgery. Eighteen-month follow-up showed partial relief of pain.

Discussion.—Injection injury to the peripheral nerves is a serious iatrogenic complication. Many different nerves are vulnerable to injection injury, usually during local anesthetic procedures. The damage produced depends on several factors, the most important of which is the injection site: intrafascicular injection with a toxic agent produces severe nerve injury. During local or regional anesthetic procedures, the patient should be told to alert the physician if there is any paresthesia. If so, the injection should be stopped and redirected. This measure of protection is lost if the patient is already anesthetized or sedated.

▶ The authors report on 1 case and review the literature as it relates to the pathologic effects of inadvertent intraneural injury. Almost any substance, injected intraneurally, carries the potential to damage the nerve. In the awake patient, we are able to recognize whether the needle has struck the nerve or whether the injection is being administered intraneurally because the patient will tell us. If we listen to the patient, we can redirect the needle and avoid a complication. However, our anesthesiology colleagues are routinely asking the surgeon to either infiltrate the operative site or perform a peripheral nerve block before commencing surgery but after the administration of general anesthesia, to decrease spinal cord bombardment and to reduce the amount of anesthetic agent that needs to be administered. Perhaps it is in our and our patients' best interests to consider performing a peripheral nerve block before the patient goes under general anesthesia.

V.R. Hentz, M.D.

Long-term Follow-up Evaluation of Cold Sensitivity Following Nerve Injury

Collins ED, Novak CB, Mackinnon SE, et al (Washington Univ, St Louis)
J Hand Surg (Am) 21A:1078–1085, 1996 6–5

Background.—Patients often report cold sensitivity after nerve injury. Although some authors have suggested that this sequela declines with time and with the return of sensibility, few have reported the long-term outcomes of patients with cold sensitivity associated with nerve injury. The long-term follow-up of 50 patients with upper-extremity peripheral nerve injuries was documented.

Patients and Findings.—The 36 men and 14 women, aged 24–82 years, were followed up for 5–42 years after injury (mean, 10 years). Cold sensitivity was the most common persistent symptom, reported by 38 patients. Thirty-three of these patients described moderate or severe symptom intensity. Typically, cold sensitivity developed within months of the initial injury. It resolved in only 2 patients. The incidence of this symptom did not differ significantly between patients with subjectively normal sensation and those with abnormal hand sensibility. Cold sensitivity severity scores were associated with patients' subjective ratings of cold sensitivity intensity and change in job status or occupation because of injury. The incidence of cold sensitivity was unrelated to age, mechanism of injury, smoking, and level of nerve injury. Cold sensitivity was significantly associated with digital amputation injuries (Fig 5).

Conclusions.—Cold sensitivity is a common sequela of nerve injury that usually does not diminish with time. Patients should be cautioned about this symptom and advised to reduce their exposure to cold temperatures.

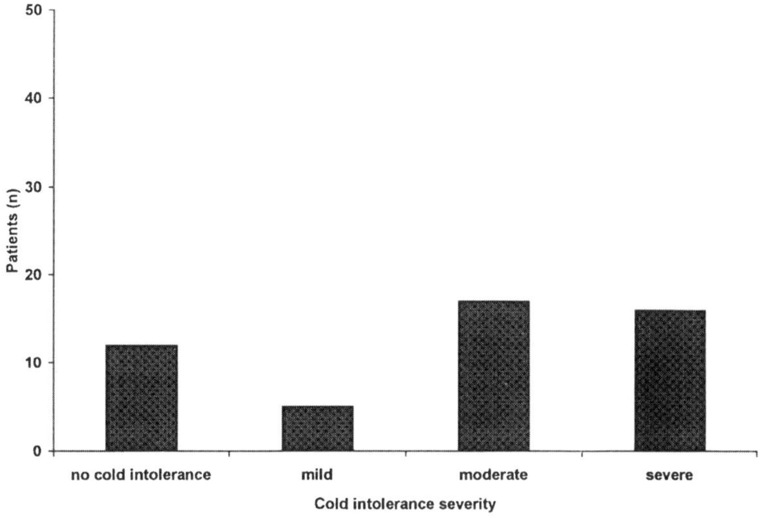

FIGURE 5.—Subjective rating of cold sensitivity severity. In the 50 study patients, 12 reported no cold sensitivity and 38 reported persistent cold sensitivity. In these 38 patients, 5 rated the cold sensitivity as mild, 17 rated it as moderate, and 16 rated it as severe. (Courtesy of Collins ED, Novak CB, Mackinnon SE, et al: Long-term follow-up evaluation of cold sensitivity following nerve injury. *J Hand Surg [Am]* 21A:1078–1085, 1996.)

► This manuscript highlights the magnitude of cold sensitivity after peripheral nerve injury in a select patient group that required multiple surgical procedures, including nerve grafting, proximal transposition of neuromas, digital amputations with proximal nerve transposition, digital amputations with nerve grafting, and nerve repair. These data provide important insights into the negative effects of painful neuromas or neuroma incontinuity or both on the health-related quality of life. This information cannot be extrapolated directly to end-to-end nerve repairs (n = 31) or nonpainful neuromas. However, painful neural injury and associated cold sensitivity or intolerance has a negative impact on the health-related quality of life.

L.A. Koman, M.D.

Non-traumatic Paralysis of the Posterior Interosseous Nerve
Hashizume H, Nishida K, Nanba Y, et al (Okayama Univ, Japan)
J Bone Joint Surg (Br) 78B:771–776, 1996 6–6

Background.—Nontraumatic paralysis of the posterior interosseous nerve is a rare condition associated with a variety of disorders, including entrapment by the edge of the supinator, a space-occupying lesion, inflammatory changes, and neuralgic amyotrophy. The best management for this condition is unclear. One experience with patients with moderate-to-severe symptoms was reviewed.

Patients and Findings.—Thirty-one patients with nontraumatic paralysis of the posterior interosseous nerve were treated during 15 years. They were 21 women and 10 men, aged 17–71 years. Surgery was performed in 25 patients. In the remaining 6 patients, treatment was conservative. Entrapment occurred at the supinator in 14 patients. Three of these patients had double compression at the entrance and exit from the muscle. Entrapment was caused by a ganglion in 4 patients, a lipoma in 1, a dislocated radial head in 1, and marked constriction in the nerve of unknown cause in 2. In the remaining 3 patients neuralgic amyotrophy was diagnosed retrospectively, the only observable change at surgery being slight nerve edema. The paralysis resolved 2–18 months postoperatively in 24 of the 25 patients. The last patient subsequently had a tendon transfer.

Conclusion.—Patients with entrapment neuropathy may recover spontaneously. However, if recovery has not occurred within 6 weeks, decompression should be performed. Surgery may be delayed for up to 6 months if neuralgic amyotrophy is suspected. Surgery may also be done early, as the risk to the patient is minimal, and release of the arcade of Frohse may provide improvement in some patients.

▶ This clinical article details the experience of 1 orthopedic surgery department with 31 patients with idiopathic or nontraumatic paralysis of the posterior interosseous nerve. Paralysis was complete in 21 of 31 patients and incomplete in 10. Twenty-five patients went on to operation, and 24 of 25 improved clinically. Six patients who did not undergo operation but had conservative management were used as the control group. All 6 of these patients went on to recovery with conservative therapy.

It is difficult to understand the significance of the posterior interosseous nerve relief given that conservative therapy also resulted in resolution of the paralysis. In fact, among patients treated operatively, some required 18 months for recovery. Several of the patients who underwent operations had space-occupying lesions such a a ganglion or a lipoma, and 2 had clear constriction of the nerve. The remaining patients had varying causes for their paralysis. Of interest is the discussion of patients having Parsonage-Turner syndrome, which is a very interesting problem seen in patients after minor infectious or traumatic preceding events. This is not an uncommon problem, and even outside the context of the posterior interosseous nerve, it can be found with isolated paralysis of a distal branch of the upper extremity or other limb, and can range from a single branch paralysis to total paralysis of the brachial plexus. Management of these problems is challenging but can be very rewarding as well.

S.M. Shenaq, M.D.

Intrinsic Muscle Flaps: The Treatment of Painful Neuromas in Continuity

Rose J, Belsky MR, Millender LH, et al (Eastern Virginia Med School, Norfolk; Tufts Univ, Boston)

J Hand Surg (Am) 21A:671–674, 1996 6–7

Background.—Neuroma in continuity in a digital nerve on the palmar surface of the hand is a difficult problem to treat; goals are relief of pain and preservation and improvement of sensory function, if possible. Eight patients were successfully treated with neurolysis and coverage with local rotation flaps of intrinsic muscles (abductor pollicis brevis, adductor pollicis, and lumbrical muscles).

> *Technique.*—Lumbrical muscle flap coverage is performed for the injured digital nerve at the base of the finger. The injured nerve is exposed through a zig-zag palmar incision. External (not internal) neurolysis is performed. The extent of the nerve damage and tender area are identified, then dissection proceeds proximally to the nearest lumbrical muscle (avoiding damage to the common digital nerve branches and arteries). The muscle is mobilized by 1 of 2 methods: separation from the profundus tendon in the palm or release of the lumbrical tendon at the level of the metacarpophalangeal joint. The lumbrical flap may then be either proximally or distally based. The adductor muscle is used for injured ulnar digital nerves; the abductor pollicis brevis muscle is used for injured radial digital nerves.

Patients.—Eight men (average age, 29 years) each with hypersensitivity at the site of a nerve injury resulting in significant disability were included. Four patients with damaged digital nerves in the thumb were treated with neurolysis and intrinsic muscle flap coverage. Lumbrical muscle flaps were used to cover digital nerves in the palms of 4 patients; 2 of the flaps were distally based. Tenderness was decreased or absent over the nerve, and pain was decreased for all 8 patients. All patients indicated that, subjectively, sensibility had improved or had not worsened. No deficits as a result of the surgery were identified.

Discussion.—Relief from pain and contact tenderness may have been caused by the muscle serving as a barrier to mechanical compression, or the muscle along with neurolysis may have somehow altered the pathophysiology of the neuroma in continuity. Intrinsic muscle flaps are recommended as an adjunct to neurolysis for the treatment of painful digital nerves in which preservation of intact nerve function is vital.

► This paper presents a technique intended to relieve contact pain resulting from a digital neuroma in continuity. The series is built on an idea of Dr. Millender's to treat a painful bowler's thumb over 16 years ago. The current paper describes 8 cases, 4 of which used lumbrical muscle rerouting after external neurolysis to cover painful digital neuromas in continuity of the index or middle fingers. The technique for the lumbrical flap is discussed in detail. The other 4 cases used either the abductor pollicis brevis or the adductor pollicis to cover neuromas in continuity of the radial or ulnar digital nerve of the thumb. Unfortunately, the thumb technique is not discussed. Dr. Belsky has told me that in these cases, the abductor pollis brevis or adductor pollicis was detached at its tendon of insertion, rerouted to cover the neuroma after neurolysis, and reinserted by repair of the tendon of insertion, with subsequent preservation of normal function of the transferred muscle. The interested reader should peruse Belsky and Millender's 1980 paper.[1]

Improvement of sensibility was a secondary goal in this study; indeed only 4 of the 8 patients had preoperative and postoperative quantitative sensory evaluation. All 4 of them had improved two-point sensibility postoperatively, better results than expected by external neurolysis alone.

This technique for relieving in-continuity neuroma pain is worthy of further use. It should be more critically evaluated with a uniform functional and sensory testing protocol.

Finally, this is among the last published works of Dr. Millender, a fine hand surgeon and teacher whom we shall miss because of his untimely recent death.

J.M. Markley Jr., M.D.

Reference

1. Belsky MR, Millender LH: Bowler's thumb in a baseball player. *Orthopedics* 3:122–123, 1980.

Suggested Reading

Carr MM, Boyd JB, Bowen CVA: Riche-Cannieu connection in median nerve injuries. *Can J Plast Surg* 4:117–120, 1996.

▶ This interesting paper highlights and explains a common clinical scenario following sharp injury to the distal forearm. Anesthesia in the median nerve distribution in combination with functioning thenar musculature is seen quite commonly in clinical practice, and knowledge of the frequent connection between the recurrent branch of the median nerve and the deep branch of the ulnar nerve is important both in diagnosis and treatment of these injuries. In addition to explaining the seemingly contradictory physical findings, knowledge of the Riche-Cannieu connection can also assist in decision-making at the time of surgery when a badly scarred median nerve without good fascicular separation is encountered. Isolation of a clear motor branch for preservation in the face of a functioning thenar eminence is difficult. This paper also gives a brief summary of the Martin-Gruber connection along with its similar clinical significance. It would have been of interest if the authors had included a summary of other frequent connections between digital nerve branches in the hand, which can often explain various unusual paresthesia findings in patients having undergone endoscopic or open carpal tunnel surgery.

S.M. Shenaq, M.D.

Gaur SC, Swarup A: Radial nerve palsy caused by injections. *J Hand Surg (Br)* 21B:338–340, 1996.

► This is a series of 56 cases of this iatrogenic injury collected over a period of 13 years. More than half the cases failed to recover, and ultimately required tendon transfers. Early exploration seemed helpful in cases of partial or progressive paralysis.

P.C. Amadio, M.D.

McAllister RMR, Gilbert SEA, Calder JS, et al: The epidemiology and management of upper limb peripheral nerve injuries in modern practice. *J Hand Surg (Br)* 21B:4–13, 1996.

► This study of 813 patients with 1,111 nerve injuries indicates that, in this area of the UK, the most common reason for nerve grafting was failure to recognize a nerve injury in the acute injury period and thus delay in recognizing the need for and referral for treatment.

V.R. Hentz, M.D.

Prochazka A, Gauthier M, Wieler M, et al: The Bionic Glove: An electrical stimulator garment that provides controlled grasp and hand opening in quadriplegia. *Arch Phys Med Rehabil* 78:608–614, 1997.

► The Bionic Glove is another step in the improvement of Functional Electrical Stimulation (FES). This device succeeds where other FES devices fail largely because the subjects have somewhat preserved tactile touch and proprioception in the involved body part. Many gait-aid FES devices have complications because they attempt to move an insensate limb.

However, the most pertinent question is how this device compares with the alternative functional solutions. For example, tendon transfer surgery is often quite effective in these same patients and has a reasonably low complication rate. Also, the hand/wrist tenodesis splint is an alternative prosthetic device that has been used for years. This is lightweight, simple to don and doff, relatively inexpensive, and has essentially no complications. At this time these two alternatives are still much more attractive than the newer myoelectric device for practical reasons. However, with further technological advances, the Bionic Glove or its successors may compete with tendon transfers and simpler splints.

K.A. Bengtson, M.D.

7 Compression Neuropathy

Carpal Tunnel Release With Short Incision
Serra JMR, Benito JR, Monner J (Hosp Clinic of Barcelona)
Plast Reconstr Surg 99:129–135, 1997 7–1

Background.—The long incision approach to carpal tunnel release leaves a painful or tender scar, loss of grip strength, scar hypertrophy, and "pillar" pain. Endoscopic procedures have improved this but require extensive training and cannot visualize the carpal tunnel and nerve. Results using a short incision and a new guide to protect the carpal contents combine the best parts of both the open and closed techniques.

Methods.—Dissection of 21 cadaver hands revealed where the incision should be made to avoid injuring the vascular arch and the median and ulnar nerves.

> *Technique.*—A 1.5- to 2-cm incision is made proximal to the transverse palmar line. Two Senn-Miller retractors are positioned, and the incision is deepened by a scalpel, guided by a blunt, rounded tipped instrument, to the carpal ligament. A third retractor positioned at the proximal edge of the incision helps visualization of the carpal ligament, which is then sectioned (Fig 4). The carpal tunnel is examined, and an epineurotomy can be performed, if required. The wound is sutured.

Results.—The technique was used on 153 hands in 112 patients (16 men aged 31–70 years). Results of electrophysiologic and grip strength testing were satisfactory at 3 and 12 months postoperatively. At 1 year, 107 patients had complete relief. There were no hypertrophic scars. Six patients still had pillar pain at 1 year. Only 8 patients were unable to return to work by 3 weeks postoperatively.

Conclusion.—The short-incision technique for carpal tunnel release eliminates many of the complications resulting from long incisions and gives results similar to those obtained from endoscopic release procedures.

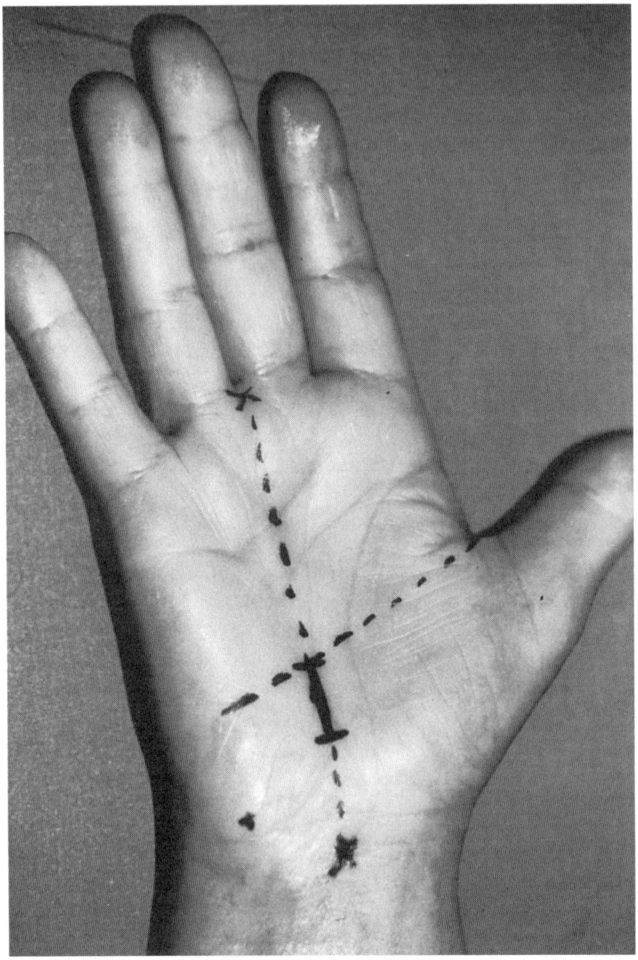

FIGURE 4.—Preoperative view with the incision design. (Courtesy of Serra JMR, Benito JR, Monner J: Carpal tunnel release with short incision. *Plast Reconstr Surg* 99:129–135, 1997).

► The authors, reporting from Barcelona, Spain, describe a technique for dividing the transverse carpal ligament using a short palmar incision. They report their experience in 112 patients so treated. Most returned to work by the third week. This is the latest article (as of this writing) to describe how to divide this structure with a minimal incision. The goal of surgery now seems less directed toward ensuring complete decompression of the nerve and more directed toward minimizing the sequellae of surgery, e.g., tender scars.

A recent analysis of the incidence of major complications associated with so-called "open" carpal tunnel release carried out by Andrew Palmar (unpublished as of this writing) suggests that the hand surgery literature significantly underreports complications and that the incidence of complications may be increasing. One might reasonably argue that this suspected increase is a consequence of the desire of today's surgeons to perform this task through as minimal an incision as possible in the pursuit of emulating the presumed benefits of endoscopic release, i.e., minimizing operative site sequellae. How ironic!

V.R. Hentz, M.D.

Flexor Carpi Radialis Approach for Carpal Tunnel Release
Weber RA, Sanders WE (The Hand Ctr, San Antonio, Tex; Texas A&M Univ, Temple)
J Hand Surg (Am) 22A:120–126, 1997 7–2

Introduction.—The endoscopic approach to repairing carpal tunnel syndrome is replete with complications. It is important to find a method for dividing the carpal ligament that minimizes palmar disruption and surgical complications. The flexor carpi radialis (FCR) approach to carpal tunnel repair (CTR) is described and results are reported in 87 hands (74 patients) operated on.

Surgical Technique.—A 3-cm incision is made over the distal FCR tendon, slightly toward the radial side of the tendon to avert medial nerve damage. The FCR tendon is exposed and dissected from its sheath. If the volar branch of the radial artery is small, it is divided; if it is large, it is mobilized and preserved. The thenar muscles are dissected off the transverse carpal ligament at its insertion, and the ligament is divided at its bony insertion. With the FCR tendon retracted radially, an incision is made in the floor of the FCR sheath that angles about 45 degrees toward the flexor pollicis longus (FPL) tendon. With the carpal tunnel now open, the PFL tendon is identified and retracted ulnarly. Under direct vision, the proximal half of the deep leaf of the TCL is divided as it passes between the FPL and FCR. Median nerve damage can be averted by sliding the back of the blade along the FPL tendon and aiming the belly of the blade 45 degrees toward the FCR tendon, away from the nerve. With the deep leaf partially divided, ulnar retraction of the FCR and volar retraction of the proximal portion of the superficial leaf allow direct viewing of the remaining leaf. This is transsected in its entirety so that the superficial leaf is completely separated. The remaining undivided deep leaf is then sectioned, releasing the TCL. Any remaining bands are divided. The median nerve is inspected, and epineurotomy and tenosynovectomy can be performed while visualized.

Results.—There was complete relief of preoperative signs and symptoms in 66 hands (76%), and incomplete but substantial relief in 13 hands

(15%). Eight patients (9%) did not experience relief or worsening of symptoms (all 8 patients were seeking compensation).

Conclusion.—The FCR approach to CTR provides direct visualization of carpal tunnel contents and reduces disruption of palmar skin and soft tissues while decreasing pillar pain.

▶ The authors provide an approach to arthroscopic repair of the triangular fibrocartilage complex (TFCC) and demonstrate a technique for repair of peripheral injuries to the TFCC that provides pain relief and improved work performance in a large percentage of patients. Mechanical and clinical evidence supports the beneficial effects of repair of TFCC injuries. The authors' approach appears appropriate; however, a larger series with more extensive follow-up is necessary to fully delineate the exact indications for TFCC repair. This manuscript demonstrates the advantages of arthroscopic repair and provides data that support reconstruction when possible.

L.A. Koman, M.D.

The Role of Epineurotomy in the Operative Treatment of Carpal Tunnel Syndrome

Leinberry CF, Hammond NL III, Siegfried JW (St Joseph Hosp, Reading, Pa; Lankenau Hosp, Wynnewood, Pa)

J Bone Joint Surg (Am) 79A:555–557, 1997 7–3

Introduction.—Reports vary regarding the benefit of epineurotomy in the surgical treatment of patients with carpal tunnel syndrome. The effect of epineurotomy of the median nerve on the outcome of operative treatment of chronic median nerve compression in the carpal canal was prospectively evaluated in 50 hands (44 patients).

Methods.—Patients were randomized to receive either operative decompression of the median nerve by longitudinal incision of the transverse carpal ligament alone (group 1) or release and adjuvant epineurotomy of the median nerve (group 2). An electrophysiologic evaluation and physical examination by a blinded physician were performed at 12 months postoperatively.

Results.—At 12-month follow-up, 15 and 14 group 1 and group 2 hands, respectively, were free of symptoms related to the median nerve. There were no significant between-group differences in measures of 2-point discrimination, strength of the abductor pollicis brevis muscle, or average sensory latency. Six hands in group 1 and eleven hands in group 2 had a positive Tinel's sign. Symptoms were elicited by the Phalen maneuver in 2 group 1 hands and 4 group 2 hands.

Conclusion.—There were no significant differences between outcomes of hands treated with division of the transverse carpal ligament alone and hands treated with release and adjuvant epineurotomy of the median nerve.

▶ This was a prospective, randomized study. That's good. Forty-four patients were randomized to have carpal tunnel release with or without epineurotomy. That's not so good. There are few who advocate indiscriminate epineurotomy; the real issue is whether epineurotomy might be indicated in cases of severe epineurial fibrosis. The selection criterion here—fibrillation potentials on electromyography—is certainly evidence of denervation but not necessarily of epineurial fibrosis. Outcomes measured were 2-point discrimination, Tinel's sign, Phalen's sign, and electrodiagnostic studies. That's also not so good. These measures are less sensitive than patient-completed functional status and symptom measurements like the Brigham carpal tunnel questionnaire.

So, what have we learned? Is epineurotomy indicated for routine use with carpal tunnel release? Clearly not. Is it indicated if the physical examination or electrodiagnostic studies are particularly severe? Probably not. Might epineurotomy be indicated in cases in which intraoperative findings include significant fibrosis? We still don't know. What is needed is a prospective study with intraoperative randomization to epineurotomy or not, based on a finding of epineurial thickening, and follow-up by more sensitive clinical measures such as the Brigham carpal tunnel questionnaire. Any takers?

P.C. Amadio, M.D.

The Hypothenar Fat Pad Flap for Management of Recalcitrant Carpal Tunnel Syndrome

Strickland JW, Idler RS, Lourie GM, et al (St Vincent Hosp, Indianapolis, Ind; Indiana Hand Ctr, Indianapolis; Hand Treatment Ctr, Atlanta, Ga; et al)

J Hand Surg (Am) 21A:840–848, 1996 7–4

Background.—Open carpal tunnel decompression is unsuccessful in 10% to 25% of patients. Recurrence often results from the tethering of a median nerve in the carpal canal. Soft-tissue flaps have been used to alleviate residual compression and adherence of the median nerve in the carpal canal. However, many of the procedures described are technically demanding and involve the use of tissue that may be inadequate in dimension or poorly positioned to sufficiently cover the median nerve. The outcomes of a procedure using the hypothenar fat pad flap (HTFPF), which interposes tissue from the hypothenar eminence between the median nerve and overlying transverse carpal ligament and surgical scar, were reported.

Methods.—Fifty-eight patients with recurrent symptoms after failed open carpal tunnel release were included. Revision carpal tunnel decompression with an HTFPF flap was performed on 62 affected hands. The mean follow-up time was 33 months.

Findings.—At the final follow-up assessment, 95% of the patients said they were satisfied. The mean time to return to work was 12 weeks for the patients without workers' compensation and 37 weeks for those with workers' compensation. The outcomes of the HTFPF procedure were equal to or better than those of other soft-tissue flaps used for revision decompression in patients with recurrent symptoms after failed open carpel tunnel release.

Conclusion.—The HTFPF yields excellent outcomes in patients with recalcitrant idiopathic carpal tunnel syndrome. A prospective study comparing HTFPF surgery with other surgical approaches in patients with recurrent carpal tunnel syndrome would be useful.

▶ This article addresses a difficult problem, that of the painful hand secondary to failure of carpal tunnel decompression through an open approach. This retrospective study reviews 62 procedures using an HTFPF for coverage of the median nerve with vascularized smooth-gliding tissue. The paper describes, in thorough fashion, the technique used to raise the flap, the anatomy of the flap, and the anatomical studies that confirm the rich vascularity present within the hypothenar fat pad. In addition, the follow-up of these patients was thoroughly assessed and appears to validate the use of this flap in the case of the problem median nerve after surgery.

This well-done article provides an excellent solution to a very difficult problem. The authors have contributed outstanding anatomical and clinical data to support their hypothesis that this flap gives excellent coverage for the problem median nerve. We have used the flap on several occasions and have had outstanding results in otherwise recalcitrant hand pain.

S.M. Shenaq, M.D.

Reverse Radial Artery Fascial Flap: A Treatment for the Chronically Scarred Median Nerve in Recurrent Carpal Tunnel Syndrome

Tham SKY, Ireland DCR, Riccio M, et al (St Vincents Hosp, Melbourne, Australia)

J Hand Surg (Am) 21A:849–854, 1996 7–5

Background.—Recurrent carpal tunnel syndrome (CTS) after surgical decompression of the median nerve is a difficult problem to manage. Several techniques have been proposed, with the goals of restoring a gliding bed for the median nerve after neurolysis, providing a barrier from the transverse carpal ligament and other structures, and improving nutrition to an area of chronic ischemia. A reverse-flow vascularized radial artery forearm fascial flap was used in 6 patients with recurrent CTS and chronic scarring of the median nerve.

Methods.—The experience included 6 patients (5 women) who had undergone at least 2 surgical decompressions for symptoms of median nerve compression at the wrist. The mean patient age was 56 years. In each patient, the symptoms were severe enough to interfere with activities of daily living. At surgery, all patients had chronic scarring of the median nerve with flattening and perineural fibrosis. Decompression was performed, with epineurotomy and interfascicular neurolysis, as indicated.

The decision to place a fascial flap was based on the finding of severe scarring and wasting of the median nerve. A 4-cm wide and 5-cm long vascularized fascial flap, pedicled distally on the radial artery, was created. This flap was then turned down and passed under the flexor carpi radialis to wrap around the median nerve, with the gliding surface of the flap in contact with the nerve. The patients were studied for a mean of 25 months.

Results.—Unrestricted use of the hand was restored in all patients. Two patients achieved excellent results, with complete symptomatic relief and normal 2-point discrimination. Four patients had good results, with mild intermittent pain or paresthesia. Persistent irritability over the nerve was noted in 2 patients with neuromas of the palmar cutaneous branch of the median nerve. Sensibility improved in all patients. There were no problems with cold intolerance or painful claudication.

Conclusions.—The reverse-flow radial forearm fascial flap gives good results in patients with recurrent CTS and chronic scarring of the median nerve. This technique provides a vascularized flap of size sufficient to cover the length and circumference of the median nerve, and provides a gliding bed for the nerve. The need to sacrifice the radial artery, with reverse flow through the ulnar artery, is a drawback.

► I see recurrent CTS much less frequently than I did a decade ago. This is because most surgeons no longer manipulate (or for that matter touch) the median nerve during a carpal tunnel release. As a result, there is less likelihood of fibrosis and nerve ischemia. Nevertheless, the problem still exists. Treatment can be frustrating, and many procedures have been described to alleviate debilitating symptoms; however, none are uniformly successful. The reverse radial artery fascial flap seems promising. As the authors note, it provides circumferential coverage over a good length, adds vascularity, and should allow the median nerve to glide free of fibrosis with range of motion of the wrist. On the other hand, there is potential morbidity with sacrifice of the radial artery. Also, this series is small, with only 2 of 6 patients having excellent results. I think the jury is still out as to which is the best surgical procedure for the management of recurrent carpal tunnel syndrome.

P.J. Stern, M.D.

Complete Endoscopic Carpal Canal Decompression

Okutsu I, Hamanaka I, Tanabe T, et al (Japanese Red Cross Med Ctr, Tokyo)

Am J Orthop 5:365–368, 1996 7–6

Objective.—Operative treatment of carpal tunnel syndrome involves decompression of the median nerve either with standard open surgery or endoscopic release. In some endoscopic procedures, when only the transverse carpal ligament is released, the sectioned ends of the ligament are separated only 1 to 2 mm. To determine whether release of the transverse carpal ligament alone is sufficient for decompression, carpal canal pressure

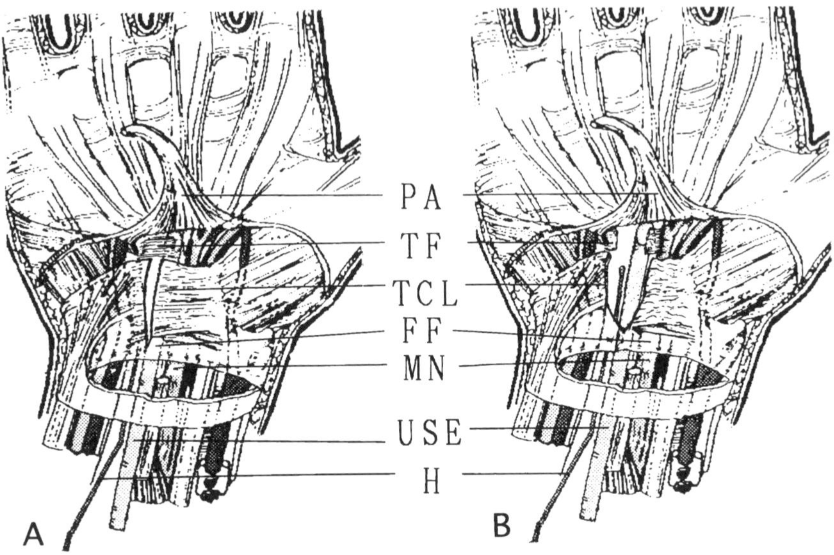

FIGURE 1.—Schematic drawing of carpal canal decompression. A, release of the transverse carpal ligament alone. B, release of the transverse carpal ligament and transverse fibers. *Abbreviations: PA*, palmar aponeurosis; *TF*, transverse fibers; *TCL*, transverse carpal ligament; *FF*, forearm fascia; *MN*, median nerve; *USE*, Universal Subcutaneous Endoscope system; *H*, hook knife. (Reprinted by permission of the publisher from Okutsu I, Hamanaka I, Tanabe T, et al: Complete endoscopic carpal canal decompression. *Am J Orthop* 5:365–368. Copyright 1996 by Quadrant Healthcom Inc.)

measurements and endoscopic observations were made using an operative model (Fig 1).

Methods.—Endoscopic release of the transverse carpal ligament, performed on 56 hands (43 patients, 2 men; ages, 31 to 87 years), was followed by release of the transverse fibers. Carpal canal pressure was measured with the hand in a resting position, and with power active grip, before surgery and immediately after each successive release. Data before and after release were compared statistically.

Results.—Mean resting preoperative carpal canal pressure was 50.1 mm Hg. Pressure after release of the transverse carpal ligament was 6.6 mm Hg, after release of the transverse fibers, it was 4.8 mm Hg, and after release of the forearm fascia, it was 4.5 mm Hg. The mean power active grip before and after release of the transverse carpal ligament was 125.5 mm Hg and 28.7 mm Hg, respectively; after release of the transverse fibers, it was 19.8 mm Hg, and after release of the forearm fascia, it was 16.3 mm Hg. All differences were significant except for release of the forearm fascia.

Conclusion.—Complete decompression requires release of the transverse fibers in addition to release of the transverse ligament.

▶ This article raises an interesting question: How much tissue requires release in carpal tunnel decompression? Uniform agreement would include the transverse carpal ligament, but what about the forearm fascia or the distal transverse fibers described here?

These authors state that complete decompression of the carpal tunnel should include the transverse fibers just distal to the transverse carpal ligament and the palmar aponeurosis. They support their comments by measuring carpal tunnel pressures at surgery and noting that only by releasing these distal fibers (as is currently done in open decompression) did the postoperative endoscopic canal pressure equal that of open decompression.

As most endoscopic techniques seemingly address only the transverse carpal ligament, are insufficient decompressions being done? Did the authors have a high recurrence rate in their initial series? Does release of these more distal fibers add to the complications with the superficial transverse arch or distal nerves? Does it create more "pillar pain"? These questions are not addressed by this article.

In my own endoscopic series using a 2-portal Chow technique, I expose the superficial transverse arch and distal nerves in the distal portal to ensure cannula placement. This alone would divide these transverse fibers. Secondly, the "open slot" on the cannula is 4 mm wide, and complete relief can be noted if only 1 cut leaf of the transverse carpal ligament is visible.

Lastly, I agree with the authors that from the scientific approach, surgical measurement of a carpal canal pressure is ideal. Several easy-to-use monitoring devices are currently being developed. Nay sayers will agree that this is just adding expense by making a simple successful procedure even more complex.

A.L. Osterman, M.D.

Avoidance of Transection of the Palmar Cutaneous Branch of the Median Nerve in Carpal Tunnel Release

Watchmaker GP, Weber D, Mackinnon SE (Washington Univ, St Louis)

J Hand Surg (Am) 21A:644–650, 1996 7–7

Introduction.—The palmar cutaneous branch of the median nerve (PCBMN) arises in the distal forearm. It travels distally in association with the flexor carpi radialis tendon to send sensory branches to the skin of the palm of the hand. This nerve can be injured in the distal forearm and palm, particularly during carpal tunnel release. Its relation to common surgical landmarks in the palm is not well described. To provide scientifically based guidelines for avoiding the PCBMN during carpal tunnel release, a cadaver study and clinical analysis were done.

Methods.—Dissections were done in 25 cadaver upper extremities to assess the relationship of the PCBMN to local structures and the incisions commonly used for carpal tunnel release. In addition, a clinical analysis of the palmar creases was done in 100 human volunteer hands.

Results.—In dissections, the PCBMN was found to be closely associated with the thenar crease (Fig 1). In the average hand, the nerve was located 0–2 mm radial to the thenar crease, although it could be found anywhere from 6 mm ulnar to 6 mm radial. It also crossed the axis of the ring finger, when this axis was determined with the finger flexed. The axis of the ring

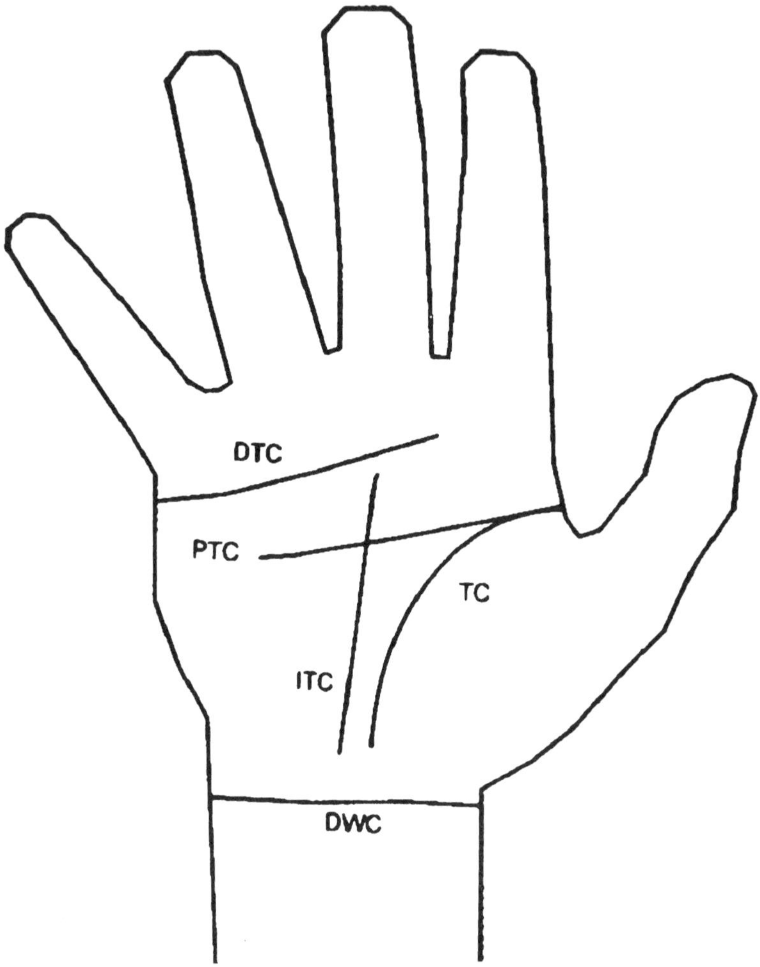

FIGURE 1.—The palmar creases. *Abbreviations: DWC,* distal wrist crease; *TC,* thenar crease (*life line*); *DTC,* distal transverse crease (*heart line*); *PTC,* proximal transverse crease (*head line*); *ITC,* interthenar crease (*destiny line*). (Courtesy of Watchmaker GP, Weber D, Mackinnon SE: Avoidance of transection of the palmar cutaneous branch of the median nerve in carpal tunnel release. *J Hand Surg [Am]* 21A:644–650, 1996.)

finger pointed in a more ulnar direction with the finger extended; in this projection, the PCBMN averaged 9 mm radial to the axis. In the clinical analysis, the interthenar depression—identified as the deepest point between the thenar and hypothenar eminences—was a constant finding. On average, the PCBMN was found 5 mm radial to the interthenar depression.

Conclusions.—The anatomy of the PCBMN in the human palm varies considerably. Because of this variation, the thenar crease and the axis of the ring finger are poor landmarks by which to plan incisions for carpal tunnel release. The best incision site to avoid injury to the PCBMN is about 5 mm ulnar to the interthenar depression, extending in the direction of the third web space.

► Although one applauds efforts at deriving the "safest" incision, the best way to avoid troublesome postoperative neuroma pain in the palmar cutaneous branch is to look for and recognize these structures and then avoid injuring them. This implies being aware of the variations in anatomy of this nerve and then performing a safe dissection both above and below the level of the palmar fascia, looking for any branches of the nerve crossing the path of the incision and sparing these. This also implies an incision through dermis and then basically blunt dissection through the fatty tissues superficial to the longitudinally oriented fibers of the most proximal element of the palmar fascia. One should not divide anything until satisfied that the crossing structure is a vessel and not a branch of the palmar cutaneous nerve. If I cannot decide which it is, a vessel or a nerve branch, then it goes undivided. Only then is the fascia split in line with its fibers, again while I am "looking" for these branches. The proper placement of the incision can only reduce the risk of encountering a sizable branch.

V.R. Hentz, M.D.

Carpal Tunnel Syndrome and Occupation in U.S. Navy Enlisted Personnel

Garland FC, Balazs LL, Garland CF, et al (Naval Health Research Ctr, San Diego, Calif; Univ of California, San Diego; Cornell Univ, Ithaca, NY)

Arch Environ Health 51:395–407, 1996 7–8

Background.—Carpal tunnel syndrome (CTS) and other nerve-entrapment disorders of the upper extremity are of increasing concern nationally and in the United States Navy. The Navy Occupational Safety and Health Program Manual contains a chapter on ergonomics, which focuses on cumulative trauma disorders amd nerve-entrapment syndromes. The demographic correlates of CTS, cubital tunnel syndrome, and other neuritis of the arm and hand were investigated, and high-risk occupations associated with these disorders in the Navy were identified.

Methods.—All cases of CTS, cubital tunnel syndrome, and other neuritis of the arm and hand found between 1980 and 1988 were identified in a search of all computerized records of first hospitalizations of all active-duty Navy-enlisted personnel. A total of 1,039 first hospitalizations, including 493 CTS cases, for all neuritis of the arm and hand occurred in 4,095,708 person-years among men, and 186 first hospitalizations, including 90 CTS cases, occurred in 365,668 person-years among women.

Findings.—For both sexes, the incidence rates of hospitalized patients with CTS increased with age. Rates in white women were about 3 times those in white men, although the rates did not differ significantly between black women and black men. Rates of cubital tunnel syndrome also rose with age in both sexes and were greater in white women than in white men. Significantly high standard incidence ratios for CTS among men were associated with the occupations of aviation-support equipment technician, engine man, hull-maintenance technician, boatswain's mate, and machinist's mate. Among women, high-risk occupations were boatswain's mate, engine man, hospital corpsman, ocean-systems technician, and personnel man. For each sex, several occupations had significantly high standardized incidence ratios for cubital tunnel syndrome. High rates occurred in male and female hospital corpsmen. Sex and racial differences did not explain the occupational differences.

Conclusion.—First-hospitalization rates for CTS and cubital tunnel syndrome in Navy-enlisted personnel were strongly associated with age, sex, and race. Additional studies are needed to determine the degree to which CTS and related disorders may be prevented by modifying the motions executed in occupations with high standardized incidence ratios.

▶ I find the study by Garland et al. to be interesting and useful. I would like the readers to consider several issues. In this study of active-duty enlisted Navy personnel, incidence rates for the diagnoses of CTS and cubital tunnel syndrome (CubTS) were obtained from hospital medical diagnosis codes. The authors do not indicate that the presence of underlying nerve pathology—a requisite component of the diagnosis of CTS and CubTS—was confirmed electrophysiologically. Estimating incidence rates by data extraction from files is prone to inaccuracy, as discussed by Franklin et al.[1] It is well known that estimates of incidence rates are sensitively dependent on the case definition used. The incidence rates were used to identify "high-risk occupations" by tallying the frequency of diagnoses per occupational category. In the absence of information on electrophysiologic confirmation of entrapment neuropathy, we must assume that the rates will tend toward overestimation of disease, which calls into question the magnitude of difference between "high-risk" and low-risk" categories.

I believe that calculation of occupational exposure by person-years degrades the potential for risk assessment. This method obviates the possibility of calculating the average length of employment for Navy personnel given a diagnosis of CTS or CubTS. This method of calculating exposure also does not allow for a determination of length of employment before symptom onset, a measurement that is helpful in determining whether the job caused the condition or the worker brought the condition to the job. We offer these examples to demonstrate that the attribution of cause must consider the progression of disease and the state of health of individuals before occupational exposure.

Despite these shortcomings, the study is useful, primarily because it shows trends in a segment of the United States population generally not affected by the potentially confounding factors of ill health and lack of physical fitness. This appears to be demonstrated by the authors' report of a markedly lower age-adjusted incidence of CTS among the naval subjects than that of Stevens et al.[2] in a general population or Franklin et al.[1] in a working population. This suggests that enlisted duty in the Navy is not, in itself, harmful to the upper extremities, and it could suggest that healthy, physically fit individuals in the general population are less prone to development of CTS or CubTS, despite occupation.

Additionally, the study confirms Stevens' findings[2] that incidence rates for CTS are strongly related to age and gender, as were incidence rates for CubTS. This, coupled with the fact that white Navy women were significantly more likely to have CTS or CubTS than were black Navy women, emphasizes the importance of considering factors such as age, gender, and race when studying the etiology of CTS or CubTS.

The authors' conclusion that CTS or CubTS in younger enlisted personnel was caused primarily by work factors, whereas the presence of these conditions in older personnel was age-related and not associated with work, was not substantiated by findings presented in the study. I wonder what the results would have been had the authors adjusted the CTS or CubTS incidence rates for personal factors that have been reported in the literature, and which were not considered. These include body mass index, wrist dimensions, avocational exercise, and use of legal drugs.[3, 4]

P.A. Nathan, M.D.

References

1. Franklin GM, Haug J, Heyer N, et al: Occupational carpal tunnel syndrome in Washington State, 1984–1988. *Am J Public Health* 81:741–746, 1991.
2. Stevens JC, Beard CM, O'Fallon WM, et al: Carpal tunnel syndrome in Rochester, Minnesota, 1961–1980. *Neurology* 38:134–138, 1988.
3. Nathan PA, Keniston RC, Lockwood RS, et al: Tobacco, caffeine, alcohol and carpal tunnel syndrome in American industry: A cross-sectional study of 1464 workers. *J Occup Environ Med* 38:290–298, 1996.
4. Stallings SP, Kasdan ML, Soergel TM, et al: A case-control study of obesity as a risk factor for carpal tunnel syndrome in a population of 600 patients presenting for independent medical examination. *J Hand Surg (Am)* 22A:211–215, 1997.

Steroid Injection for Carpal Tunnel Syndrome

Irwin LR, Beckett R, Suman RK (District Gen Hosp, Grimsby, England)
J Hand Surg (Br) 21B:355–357, 1996 7–9

Background.—Although steroid injections are commonly given for patients with carpal tunnel syndrome (CTS), their value is debated. Previous studies have attempted to identify factors associated with a good response to injection. A prospective study of steroid injection therapy for CTS is reported, including an assessment of the predictive factors.

Methods.—The study included all women with CTS referred to 1 of the authors during a 9-month period. All were initially treated with CTS injection with 100 mg hydrocortisone plus 4 mL lignocaine. The patients were reassessed at 1, 3, and 6 months. The response to treatment was determined by questioning of the patient. Previously reported predictive factors were evaluated for relevance.

Results.—The analysis included 45 wrists of 41 patients (average age, 48 years). The average duration of symptoms was 18 months. Eleven wrists had lasting symptomatic relief after steroid injection, 12 had initial relief followed by relapse, and 22 had no response to injection. Steroid injection tended to be more beneficial for patients with a longer duration of symptoms. Otherwise, none of the factors studied was significantly related to outcome.

Conclusions.—Only about one fourth of wrists treated with steroid injection for CTS have a lasting symptomatic response, according to this prospective study. Factors previously reported as predicting response to steroid injection did not correlate with outcome. Rather than performing carpal tunnel injections themselves, general practitioners should be encouraged not to delay referral of patients with CTS.

▶ Eleven of 45 patients with lasting relief is a result consistent with the various previous reports surveyed, but the number is higher than I would have suspected clinically. In my experience, less than 20% of those with mild CTS (defined as slightly prolonged sensory latency and no motor changes for latency or needle examination) have lasting relief, whereas any patients experiencing greater severity almost never did.

The 100-mg hydrocortisone dose is strong, and failure to relieve symptoms more often suggests that inflamed tenosynovium is not the problem.

A good response to injection, even an injection of plain lidocaine, still has diagnostic and prognostic value for a good response to surgery, but all bets are off when factors such as compensation and litigation prevail. Of course, the only true method to define the percentage of relief is to compare steroid injection with a placebo such as lidocaine in a controlled, blind, prospective way.

I do not understand why men were excluded from the study. Patients with rheumatoid arthritis are better excluded. Of course, a special case should be made for the injection of pregnant patients with severe symptoms that will likely abate with the birth of their children.

J.M. Failla, M.D.

Raynaud's Phenomenon in Idiopathic Carpal Tunnel Syndrome

Pal B, Keenan J, Misra HN, et al (Univ Hosp of South Manchester, England; Manchester Royal Infirmary, England; Wythenshawe Hosp, England)

Scand J Rheumatol 25:143–145, 1996 7–10

Background.—Carpal tunnel syndrome (CTS) and Raynaud's phenomenon, which both occur commonly in the general population, often cause similar symptoms, such as tingling, numbness, and a feeling of deadness in the fingers. These conditions also may coexist with scleroderma or rheumatoid arthritis. The association between Raynaud's phenomenon and idiopathic CTS was explored.

Methods and Findings.—Ninety-three patients with idiopathic CTS, confirmed by electrophysiologic testing, and 57 healthy individuals were included in the study. A previously validated questionnaire was administered to determine the presence of Raynaud's phenomenon in both groups. Raynaud's phenomenon occurred significantly more often in patients with idiopathic CTS than in controls. The prevalences were 36% vs. 12%.

Conclusions.—Idiopathic CTS and Raynaud's phenomenon appear to be associated. Although the precise mechanism underlying this association is not clear, sympathetic dysfunction may play a role. Clinicians need to be aware that these 2 conditions have similar symptoms and may coexist.

► This is a nice small study. It is interesting to know the increased prevalence of Raynaud's phenomenon in idiopathic CTS. Therefore, overuse of diagnostic tests for connective-tissue disease in patients with CTS needs to be cautioned, because Raynaud's phenomenon is so common (36%).

P. Wu, M.D.

Carpal Tunnel Release: Correlations With Preoperative Symptomatology

Wintman BI, Winters SC, Gelberman RH, et al (Harvard, Boston; Washington Univ, St Louis; Brigham & Women's Hosp, Boston; et al)

Clin Orthop 326:135–145, 1996 7–11

Introduction.—The objective diagnostic signs of carpal tunnel syndrome cannot predict the results of surgical carpal tunnel release. It has been suggested that the preoperative symptoms can help to predict the results of surgery, but no prospective outcome studies have addressed these correlations. The preoperative symptoms of carpal tunnel syndrome were correlated with the early subjective outcomes of carpal tunnel release.

Methods.—The prospective study included 54 hands of 50 patients undergoing surgery for carpal tunnel syndrome. Each patient had the clinical symptoms of carpal tunnel syndrome, and most had confirmatory electrodiagnostic studies. The patients were studied by questionnaire, physical examination, and Semmes-Weinstein monofilament pressure testing before, 3 weeks after, and 3 months after surgery. Pain of the hand, wrist, and forearm, night pain and paresthesias, intermittent paresthesias, clumsiness and weakness of the hand, constant numbness, and problems with work-related tasks were among the specific symptoms assessed. A subjective scale was designed to characterize the patients' symptoms along a continuum from "hot" (such as intermittent paresthesias and night symptoms) to "cold" (such as hand pain, constant numbness, and difficulty with work-related tasks). Objective outcomes were assessed as well. Correlations between specific symptoms and sets of symptoms and early subjective outcomes were evaluated.

Results.—Three months after surgery, all symptoms of carpal tunnel syndrome were significantly reduced. The mean symptom reduction at this time was 49%, and overall patient satisfaction was 7.8 on a scale of 0–10. There was a significant correlation between the severity of preoperative subjective hand weakness and reduced patient satisfaction with overall symptom relief at 3 months. Throughout the range from cold to hot preoperative symptoms, surgery brought marked improvement in the symptoms of carpal tunnel syndrome. However, satisfaction was greatest for patients with hot symptoms. The preoperative objective measurements were not correlated with the subjective outcomes, although some preoperative objective measures were related to the preoperative symptom severity scale.

Conclusions.—Carpal tunnel release significantly reduces the symptoms of carpal tunnel syndrome for most patients. Subjective outcomes tend to be better for patients with cold rather than hot preoperative symptoms, that is, more night symptoms and intermittent paresthesias and less hand and wrist pain, constant numbness, hand weakness and clumsiness, and problems with work-related tasks. The distinction between hot and cold symptoms may be useful in selecting patients for carpal tunnel release and in discussing the likely outcomes of surgery.

▶ This excellent article helps add some objectivity to a commonly held perception—that surgery for carpal tunnel syndrome (CTS) relieves symptoms of paresthesias better than it improves deficits in sensibility and strength. The use of an acuity rating (the hot–cold scale described here) proved helpful; patients with hotter CTS improved more and were better satisfied with the results of their surgery, at least in the first 3 months. The authors did not correlate the "heat" of CTS with duration of symptoms; one might assume that hotter CTS is also more recent CTS, but perhaps that is not the case.

P.C. Amadio, M.D.

Prognostic Value of a Hand Symptom Diagram in Surgery for Carpal Tunnel Syndrome

Bessette L, Keller RB, Lew RA, et al (Harvard Med School, Boston; Maine Med Assessment Found and the Maine Health Information Ctr, Augusta)

J Rheumatol 24:726–734, 1997 7–12

Introduction.—Patients receiving benefits for carpal tunnel syndrome (CTS) under Workers' Compensation have markedly worse outcomes than other patients. It would be helpful to have reliable, simple, and inexpensive tools for prognostic stratification so that selection of optimal treatment could be improved. A hand symptom diagram was prospectively evaluated for its ability to predict outcomes in patients undergoing surgery for CTS.

Methods.—Two-hundred two patients with CTS completed a hand symptom diagram before and 6 months after surgery. Three symptoms were evaluated separately for each of 6 regions: pain, numbness/tingling (NT), and "other" symptoms. At 6-month follow-up, outcome was expressed as the percentage of change on the Symptom Severity Scale and Function Status Scale of the Carpal Tunnel Syndrome Assessment Questionnaire and patient satisfaction with the result of surgery. Thirty-seven percent of patients were receiving Workers' Compensation.

Results.—Hand symptom drawing patterns significantly associated with greater symptom or functional improvement or more satisfaction with surgery were pain of 2 or more of the first 4 fingers; NT in fingers 2, 3, and 4; "other" symptoms involving the dorsal surface of the fingers; pain of the upper palm; and pain of the lower or upper arm. Hand symptoms drawings associated with less symptom or functional improvement or less satisfaction were NT involving the dorsum of the hand and/or wrist, and NT of the arm. Hand symptom variables accounted for total explained variance in 30% of satisfaction, 14% of symptom severity, and 24% of functional status. Patients who received Workers' Compensation had more wrist pain and NT of the arm, less pain involving the arm and upper palm, worse outcomes, and less satisfaction with surgery. Drawing expansion was correlated with a low score on the SF-36 mental health subscale. Psychological impairment was not associated with poorer outcome.

Conclusion.—Symptom drawing pattern variables in patients with CTS were able to predict symptom and functional improvement and satisfaction 6 months after surgery.

► It should come as no surprise that patients who complain of NT in the wrist or arm are less likely to experience improvement after CTS surgery than those whose sensory symptoms are confined to the median nerve distribution. I believe that hand diagrams are a useful adjunct to the evaluation of patients with CTS. As these authors also show, these nonmedian nerve symptom patterns may be more common in the Workers' Compensation group, and this explains much of the difference in outcome between compensation and noncompensation patients.

P.C. Amadio, M.D.

"Sympathy Pains" on Carpal Tunnel Syndrome

McLaughlin MR, Pizzi FJ (Univ of Pittsburgh, Pa; St Francis Med Ctr, Trenton, NJ)

Acta Neurochir (Wien) 138:1094–1098, 1996 7–13

Objective.—Although bilateral symptoms of carpal tunnel syndrome are common and are relieved with bilateral releases, a 10-year retrospective study suggests that not all patients with bilateral symptoms require bilateral surgery.

Methods.—After failure of conservative measures, carpal tunnel release was performed in 102 patients (26 men, average age, 52 years.) Of the 71 patients with bilateral symptoms, 26 had bilateral surgery, and 45 did not. The latter group was sent a follow-up questionnaire at a minimum of 14 months after surgery to evaluate symptoms in the contralateral hand. Patients were studied for an average of 5 years.

Results.—Twelve patients did not complete follow-up. Fifteen of the remaining 33 said their contralateral symptoms had disappeared, 4 said symptoms improved, 11 said symptoms were unchanged, and 3 had had carpal tunnel release on the second hand.

Conclusion.—A subgroup of patients with bilateral symptoms of carpal tunnel syndrome will have improvement of contralateral symptoms after surgery on the most seriously affected hand. This suggests that some patients experience sympathy pains.

▶ This is a 10-year retrospective study of 45 patients who were initially seen with symptoms of bilateral carpal tunnel syndrome and who, for various reasons, had only the most symptomatic side surgically treated. At an average of 5 years after their surgery, they were contacted to determine the status of the unoperated hand. Thirty-three of the 45 responded, and of these, more than 50% reported improved or absent symptoms.

This is a phenomenon recognized by most hand surgeons, bilateral symptoms with resolution of all symptoms after surgery on 1 hand. I attribute this to better utilization of the operated hand (usually the most symptomatic) and, therefore, less unilateral dependency on the less symptomatic hand, or to the presence of a condition characterized by a waxing and waning natural history. The authors suggest a third possibility, that of abnormal nociceptive processing by the CNS that alters perception of a unilateral pathology and turns it into bilaterally perceived symptoms. Perhaps "sympathetic" has more than 1 meaning.

V.R. Hentz, M.D.

Evaluation of Portable Nerve Conduction Testing in the Diagnosis of Carpal Tunnel Syndrome

Atroshi I, Johnsson R (Hassleholm and Kristianstad Hosps, Hassleholm, Sweden; Lund Univ, Sweden)

J Hand Surg (Am) 21A:651–654, 1996 7–14

Background.—In patients with a clinical diagnosis of carpal tunnel syndrome, electrodiagnostic studies may be done to confirm the diagnosis, evaluate the severity of median nerve compression, and exclude more proximal compression. Portable nerve conduction devices provide a simple and inexpensive tool for measuring the distal motor latency of the median nerve. Newer instruments can measure sensory latency as well. This new device was studied for its sensitivity and specificity in diagnosing carpal tunnel syndrome.

Methods.—Forty-three consecutive hands with clinical signs of carpal tunnel syndrome that did not respond to nonoperative treatment were included. The patients were 25 women and 11 men; mean age, 52 years. The Nervepace electroneurometer was used to measure distal motor and sensory latency of the median nerve. The patients then underwent endoscopic carpal tunnel release, which provided complete relief of their symptoms. Nerve conduction tests also were done in 2 groups of healthy controls.

Results.—In the patients with carpal tunnel syndrome, the mean distal motor latency was 5.86 msec, compared with an upper limit of normal of

4.40 msec. The mean distal sensory latency was 3.49 msec, similar to the upper limit of normal of 3.50 msec. The sensitivity of nerve conduction testing in the affected hands was 58% for distal motor latency and 65% for distal sensory latency. Specificity in the control hands was 87% for distal motor latency and 92% for sensory latency. Distal sensory latency was the better diagnostic test on receiver operating characteristic curve analysis. At an optimal upper limit of normal of 3.3 msec, sensitivity was 74% and specificity 87%.

Conclusions.—In many patients with clinical signs of carpal tunnel syndrome, portable nerve conduction testing can provide objective support for the diagnosis. Sensitivity and specificity are similar to the values reported for conventional electrodiagnostic studies. However, studies that use the electroneurometer are much simpler, less expensive, and quicker than formal nerve conduction studies.

► In some parts of this country, a neurologist who does an electromyogram and nerve conduction velocity testing for a patient referred by a hand surgeon for electrophysiologic confirmation of carpal tunnel syndrome is compensated more for the test than is the surgeon for the operative procedure. The neurologist argues that there is more to testing than reading the numbers. Temperature has a most important influence on nerve conduction velocity and must be rigidly controlled.

This study indicates that sensitivity and specificity using the device equals that of conventional nerve conduction velocity testing. The device cannot provide information about axonopathy, however.

V.R. Hentz, M.D.

Variability in the Median and Ulnar Nerve Latencies: Implications for Diagnosing Entrapment

Radecki P (Portland, Ore)

J Occup Environ Med 37:1293–1299, 1995 7–15

Objective.—Variations in nerve conduction testing suggest that determinants in addition to hand usage play a role in the development of arm pain in the workplace. The effects of personal characteristics, habits, occupational factors, and avocational hand activity on median and ulnar nerve latencies were presented.

Methods.—Electrodiagnostic and personal evaluations were performed on 1,472 patients aged 18 to 64 years with hand or forearm symptoms.

Results.—Regression analysis was performed on 427 women and 215 men, all right-handed. Pooled data on right- and left-handed patients yielded similar results. Age, body mass index, and wrist ratio were significantly related to longer median motor, sensory, and palmar latencies. Height, age, and body mass index were negatively associated with ulnar latencies. Alcohol was correlated with palmar latency variability in women, and smoking was correlated with ulnar palmar latency variability in men.

Conclusion.—When conduction tests of median and ulnar nerves are performed, age and anthropometric measures should be considered to avoid overdiagnosis of neuropathies such as carpal tunnel syndrome.

▶ This nicely done article reproduces and confirms the findings from previous studies. It seems clear that a study to establish the norm for median slowing (particularly median and ulnar palmar latency difference) in a large number of normal volunteers with different wrist ratios in different age strata would be useful for avoiding potential overdiagnosis of carpal tunnel syndrome.

P. Wu, M.D.

Ulnar Nerve Entrapment at the Elbow [Italian]

Lisanti M, Rosati M, Rossi B, et al (Dalla 2ª Clinica Ortopedica, Pisa, Italy)
Giornale Italiano di Ortopedia e Traumatologia 22:495–502, 1996 7–16

Background.—A revision of 41 cases of cubital tunnel syndrome is reported. According to McGowan 7 cases were rated as grade I, 19 as grade II, and 15 as grade III.

Methods.—Sixteen cases were treated with a simple nerve decompression according to the technique described by Osborne, and 25 with a medial epicondilectomy according to King and Morgan. An anterior transposition of the ulnar nerve was not performed for any case. Average follow up was 63.6 months.

Findings.—The results were evaluated according to Alnot and Frajman: 24 were excellent, 7 good, 6 fair, and 4 bad.

Conclusion.—Different surgical options must be considered when dealing with ulnar nerve entrapment at the elbow. A simple decompression is often effective. A medial epicondilectomy has no major drawbacks and must be performed whenever an impingement of the nerve is observed in maximal flexion at surgery. Anterior transposition of the nerve is seldom needed and must be performed only when a bony deformity of the cubital tunnel is observed.

▶ Here the authors describe very nicely the options of treatment of cubital tunnel syndrome. In particular I found very interesting the discussion of the inappropriate use of the anterior transposition of the ulnar nerve, which is still very often considered to be the first or unique choice of treatment for ulnar nerve entrapment at the elbow. Medial epicondilectomy is said to be preferred over anterior transposition because of the reduced morbidity following the operation, improved postoperative results, and earlier return of patients to work.

M. Ceruso, M.D.

Surgical Treatment of the Ulnar Nerve Entrapment Neuropathy: Submuscular Anterior Transposition or Simple Decompression of the Ulnar Nerve? Long-term Results in 79 Cases

Bimmler D, Meyer VE (Univ of Zurich, Switzerland)

Ann Chir Main 16:148–157, 1996 7–17

Objective.—Four different procedures have been recommended for the treatment of ulnar neuropathy of the elbow: simple decompression of the ulnar nerve, medial epicondylectomy, and subcutaneous or submuscular anterior transposition of the ulnar nerve. However, none of these procedures has consistently given optimal long-term results. The results of 2 of these procedures—simple decompression and submuscular anterior transposition of the ulnar nerve—were compared.

Methods.—The retrospective study included 79 patients operated on for cubital ulnar neuropathy from 1975 to 1988. Depending on the time of operation, 31 patients were treated by simple decompression and 48 by submuscular anterior transposition. The status of the patients was followed for a mean of 76 months. The McGowan classification was used to rate the preoperative and postoperative severity of ulnar neuropathy. A more detailed sensory and motor scoring system developed by the authors also was used.

Findings.—Before surgery, the distribution of patients in the 3 McGowan classes—mild, intermediate, and severe lesions—was similar between groups. After surgery, 29% of patients who underwent submuscular anterior transposition and 36% of those who underwent simple decompression improved to a better McGowan class. In the submuscular anterior transposition group, 8% got worse; 10% got worse in the simple decompression group. Thus, most patients in both groups stayed in the same McGowan class.

By the more detailed scoring system, the overall rate of improvement was 73% with transposition and 55% with decompression, a nonsignificant difference. Regardless of the results of the objective evaluation, 90% of patients rated their postoperative condition as improved. Complications occurred only after anterior transposition. The subgroup of patients with habitual ulnar luxation or subluxation of the ulnar nerve had better results with anterior transposition than with simple decompression.

Conclusions.—Submuscular anterior transposition and simple decompression of the ulnar nerve give similar results in patients with ulnar nerve entrapment neuropathy. Decompression is thus preferred, because it is the simpler procedure. The exception is patients with cubital dislocation of the ulnar nerve, who do better with anterior transposition. During surgery, a precaution taken was to always check after decompression to see whether the ulnar nerve dislocated during elbow flexion.

▶ Here is yet another study of the outcome of surgical treatment for ulnar nerve compression at the elbow. Interestingly, this study is not presented primarily to advocate 1 technique over another. It reports results based on 2 different procedures done at various times by the senior author on the basis of personal preference at the time. Early on, simple decompression was preferred, then for a number of years, anterior submuscular transposition, then simple decompression again. Therefore, to some degree, the effect of operator differences are minimized.

The authors conclude that there really is not much difference in the outcome, unless the nerve subluxes a lot, in which case it needs to be stabilized. Subjectively, patients were happy with the outcome, but objective measures did not necessarily agree. My belief is that pain and paresthesias diminish with all techniques and that if you avoid creating new problems, such as a subluxing nerve or a cutaneous neuroma, all the techniques will succeed in satisfying the patient.

V.R. Hentz, M.D.

Medial Epicondylectomy or Ulnar-nerve Transposition for Ulnar Neuropathy at the Elbow?

Geutjens GG, Langstaff RJ, Smith NJ, et al (Queen's Med Centre, Nottingham, England)

J Bone Joint Surg (Br) 78B:777–799, 1996 7–18

Background.—A variety of procedures have been recommended for the treatment of ulnar nerve lesions at the elbow. Medial epicondylectomy and anterior transposition for such lesions were compared in a prospective, randomized study.

Methods.—Fifty-two patients underwent surgery for ulnar neuropathy between 1985 and 1992. Forty-three were available for follow-up assessment. Patients were assessed neurologically and orthopedically. The mean follow-up time was 4.5 years.

Findings.—None of the patients reported spontaneous pain in the elbow. Hand pain was significantly more common after nerve transposition, but such pain was only mild. Considerably fewer patients who underwent medial epicondylectomy reported that they were no better or were worse postoperatively than those who underwent anterior transposition. Almost all the patients who underwent the former procedure said they would be willing to have the procedure again, compared with about half of those who underwent anterior transposition.

Conclusion.—The outcomes of medial epicondylectomy were better than those of anterior transposition, patient satisfaction being higher after the former than the latter. However, motor power and nerve conduction rates did not differ significantly. Sensory fibers appeared to be more vulnerable to devascularization after medial epicondylectomy. Neither procedure seemed to affect elbow function significantly.

► That there are at least 5 operations currently in vogue for managing cubital tunnel syndrome speaks to the need for studies such as this that compare results of various operative techniques. This report shows improved grip strength and less tenderness in the patients who underwent anterior transposition but greater patient satisfaction in patients who received a medial epicondylectomy. I have modified a subintramuscular anterior transposition as taught to me in 1981 by A.L. Dellon and continue to use this modification, with surgeon and patient satisfaction.[1, 2] I have also used this procedure to manage failed cubital tunnel surgery, including the classic anterior submuscular transposition.

It is my opinion that surgery for cubital tunnel syndrome is very operator dependent and that surgical technique is imperative for a successful outcome. Important details include the following: (1) protection of the medial antebrachial cutaneous nerves; (2) care to release the ulnar nerve proximally and, especially, distally; (3) neurolysis of posterior motor branches that can tether the ulnar nerve; (4) removal of tendinous bands within the flexor/pronator muscle origin that can compress the ulnar nerve; and (5) creation of a step-lengthened flap with the fascia of the flexor/pronator muscle; this prevents relocation of the ulnar nerve and does not compress it. Equally important is postoperative management, which includes early (48 hours) institution of range-of-motion exercises to allow the ulnar nerve to glide through the operative site, whether it is behind or in front of the medial epicondyle.

S.E. Mackinnon, M.D.

References

1. Watchmaker G, Lee G, Mackinnon SE: Intraneural topography of the ulnar nerve in the cubital tunnel facilitates anterior transposition. *J Hand Surg (Am)* 19A:915–922, 1994.
2. Mackinnon SE: Submuscular transposition of the ulnar nerve at the elbow, in Rengachary SS, Wilkins RH (eds): *Neurosurgical Operative Atlas*. Chicago, American Association of Neurological Surgeons, 1995, pp 225–233.

Diagnostic Value of EMG Studies and Advantages of a Cervical Approach for Thoracic Outlet Syndrome With a Neurologic Predominance [French]

Chardel P, Merle M, Petry D (Hôpital Jeanne-d'Arc, Toul, France; Centre de Réadaptation, Gondreville, France)
La Main 2:71–78, 1997 7–19

Introduction.—The thoracic outlet syndrome (TOS) is still a controversial subject, probably because it covers a number of different pathologies, often ones with a difficult diagnosis. This study emphasized the cervical approach and evaluated the diagnostic value of preoperative electromyography (EMG) studies.

Materials and Methods.—From 1988 to 1993, the authors performed 37 neurolyses for a neurologic dominant TOS in 31 patients (6 bilateral cases). All patients (29 women, 2 men; mean age, 34.5 years; range, 18–63 years) were operated on by the same surgeon. The topography was always

C8-D1; lower trunk; medial cord. In all cases, the patients had preoperative EMG studies and were operated on through a cervical approach (transverse cervicotomy). The patients were divided into 3 groups as follows: group 1 (6 cases), sensory and motor deficit with altered EMG; group 2 (14 cases), subjective symptomatology with normal EMG; and group 3 (17 cases), subjective symptomatology with altered EMG.

Results.—In 36 cases, the compression was located above the first rib, and in 1 case, at the costoclavicular passage. All surgeries with anatomic anomalies (including a complete cervical rib) led to satisfying results. The global series showed 20 good and very good results (54%), 11 improvements (30%), and 6 failures (16%). Group 1 had 1 very good result (16.5%), 4 improvements (67%), and 1 failure (16.5%). Group 2 had 4 good or very good results (30%), 5 improvements (35%), and 5 failures (35%). Group 3 had 15 good or very good results (88%), 2 improvements (12%), and no failures.

Discussion.—In case of a neurologic dominant TOS, the most frequent levels of compression are located at the suspended system of the pleura, the scalenic hiastus, or are correlated with these regions, and resection of a cervical rib is very easy. On the contrary, resection of the first rib is more difficult through this approach, but possible. Group 1 results suggest that patients with a clinical neurologic deficit have a poor prognosis. Group 2 and group 3 results clearly show the diagnostic value of preoperative EMG studies, which proved to be the only objective diagnostic tool currently available.

Conclusion.—Transverse cervicotomy seems to be the best approach to a neurologic dominant TOS because it gives direct access to the structures most frequently responsible for the compression. Diagnosing a TOS remains very difficult, and the diagnosis must be confirmed by EMG studies which currently are the only objective predictor of outcome after surgery and are, therefore, the best tool for patient selection.

▶ This paper deals with 2 problems related to TOS with a neurologic prevalence. The authors' choice of a transverse cervical approach is based upon 2 factors. From the 6 potential areas of compression defined by Poitevin,[1, 2] 3 are responsible for most neurological TOS: the suspending system of the pleura, the scalenic hiastus and the costoclavicular passage, along with the cervical ribs. All these areas are easily approached through a transverse cervical approach, with elevation of the scalenus anterior. The transaxillary approach described by Roos,[3] although more elegant, does not give easy access to cervical ribs and requires a well-trained and skillful surgeon. It has proven dangerous on many occasions. However, it is a better approach for first rib resection.

The diagnostic of TOS is based on a confluence of symptoms, most of which are subjective; signs, most of which have been questioned; and examinations, which have also been questioned, including EMG studies and somatosensory evoked potentials.[4, 5, 6] The authors have found the following alterations of EMG studies in 23 cases: fibrillation at rest, which is very rare (1 case), neurogenic alterations during voluntary contraction, slowing of sensory or motor conduction velocity at the subclavicular region, or altered evoked sensory or motor potentials.

Except for those 6 patients with associated clinical sensory and/or motor deficit, all patients with an altered EMG benefited from the operation (15 were rated very good, and 2 improved), whereas patients with no EMG alterations (N = 14) improved in 64% of cases (4 very good, 5 improved). From this experience, the authors advocate restricting surgery to cases in which the symptoms are associated with EMG alterations (including somatosensory evoked potentials when their alteration is significant) and those cases with a complete cervical rib.

C. LeClercq, M.D.

References

1. Poitevin LA: Thoracic outlet syndromes: Anatomical, dynamic and radiological study [French]. Paris, Thèse de Médecine, 1980.
2. Poitevin LA: Compressions at the thoracic outlet [French], in Tubiana R: *Traité de Chirurgie de la Main*. Paris, Masson, 4:362–378, 1991.
3. Roos DB: Transaxillary approach for first rib resection to relieve thoracic outlet syndrome. *Ann Surg* 163:354–358, 1996.
4. Komanetsky RM, Novak CB, Mackinnon SE, et al: Somatosensory evoked potentials fail to diagnose thoracic outlet syndrome. *J Hand Surg (Am)* 21A:662–666, 1996.
5. Roos DB: Diagnostic clinique des syndromes neurologiques de la traversée thoraco-brachiale, in Kieffer R: Les syndromes de la traversée thoraco-brachiale. Paris, Edition AERCV, 1989, pp 229–312.
6. Seror P: Somesthetic evoked potentials and serial motor evoked potentials in the study of proximal peripheral nerve conduction: Apropos of 7 cases [French]. *Ann Chir Main Memb Super* 14:182–191, 1995.

Suggested Reading

Ablove RH, Moy OJ, Peimer CA, et al: Pressure changes in Guyon's canal after carpal tunnel release. *J Hand Surg (Br)* 21B:664–665, 1996.

▶ While previous studies have suggested a decrease in pressure within Guyon's canal following a carpal tunnel release, this study reinforces this point and emphasizes that a separate release of Guyon's canal associated with a carpal tunnel release should be a rare surgical procedure.

S.E. Mackinnon, M.D.

Biyani A, Wolfe K, Simison AJM, et al: Distribution of nerve fibers in the standard incision for carpal tunnel decompression *J Hand Surg (Am)* 21A:855–857, 1996.

▶ The etiology of pillar pain still remains a mystery to most hand surgeons, although we are familiar with diagnosing it postoperatively in carpal tunnel syndrome patients. Those who perform endoscopic release have hoped that this would solve the problem, but all studies clearly show that it has not. The authors state that the postoperative scar is more frequently tender in the proximal half of the conventional incision for open carpal tunnel decompression, yet others claim that a transverse incision at the wrist crease, as performed with the Agee device, has less scar tenderness. Unfortunately, there is no internervous plane at the palm of the hand, and one cannot make an incision in the palm or at the wrist without cutting some small cutaneous nerves. This study has taught us that we cannot explain pillar pain or scar tenderness based on quantitative neural innervation of the skin in the base of the palm.

R.M. Szabo, M.D., M.P.H.

Chiou-Tan FY, Vennix MJ, Dinh T, et al: Comparison of techniques for detecting digital neuropathy. *Am J Phys Med Rehabil* 75:278–282, 1996.

▶ The authors introduce an electrodiagnostic test to evaluate potential injury to the third web space nerves following endoscopic carpal tunnel releases. However, the clinician will determine management based on the likelihood of an injury to the third web space that will not spontaneously recover (Sunderland 4th and 5th degree injury). Techniques of quantitative sensory testing will allow the surgeon to determine whether there has been significant injury to this nerve. An advancing Tinel's sign associated with decreased symptoms and improved sensibility in the third web space distribution will encourage the surgeon to follow this injury expectantly. By contrast, severe pain and a localized Tinel's sign at the level of the surgery which does not improve over time would indicate surgical intervention. The electrodiagnostic studies as suggested by these authors, in my opinion, would not be useful to the clinician trying to sort out whether secondary surgery would be necessary following this type of complication.

S.E. Mackinnon, M.D.

Lee H, Jackson TA: Carpal tunnel release through a limited skin incision under direct visualization using a new instrument, the carposcope. *Plast Reconstr Surg* 98:313–319, 1996.

▶ The authors have described one more innovative way of releasing the transverse carpal ligament. They recommend the transverse incision and have adapted a fiberoptic light retractor to help visualize in the dissection. The authors have actually demonstrated that their return to work data is more favorable in both compensation and noncompensation patients than the endoscopic carpal tunnel release data presented by Agee and others. There is a race out there for who can build a better mousetrap for carpal tunnel surgery since it is one of the most common operations performed by hand surgeons. We must not forget the important goals in this operation which is to release the entire transverse carpal ligament and to make sure no other offending pathology goes unrecognized. Complete visualization is the only way one can know if this goal has been accomplished and it can only happen with the open technique and a full incision, in my opinion.

R.M. Szabo, M.D., M.P.H.

Nouhan R, Kleinert JM: Ulnar nerve decompression by transposing the nerve and Z-lengthening the flexor–pronator mass: Clinical outcome. *J Hand Surg (Am)* 22A:127–131, 1997.

▶ This paper reports 31 patients in whom the Dellon technique of Z-lengthening of the flexor pronator origin was used with submuscular transposition of the ulnar nerve. Good results were noted in most patients. I believe this technique is a reasonable one; however, the bottom line is that the nerve must be moved to a wide, dry, gliding bed. Z-lengthening of the flexor pronator origin may help, but proximal and distal mobilization of the submuscular plane are still necessary and are still, for me, the keys to success with this procedure.

P.C. Amadio, M.D.

Pierre-Jerome C, Bekkelund SI, Mellgren SI, et al: Quantitative MRI and electrophysiology of preoperative carpal tunnel syndrome in a female population. *Ergonomics* 40:642–649, 1997.

▶ The authors have taken a major step forward in separating the theoretical causes of carpal tunnel from documented etiologies in a thorough MRI study of the volume and narrowest segments of carpal tunnel by comparing patients with clearly defined carpal with a matched population of normal controls. While it is not clear that patients with diabetes were excluded, nor is it clear how the sensory conduction studies were performed, the clinical and electrophysiologic criteria for patients with carpal tunnel syndrome are clear and appropriate. The absence of any measurable difference in the carpal tunnels of these patient populations suggest that carpal tunnel size is a less significant factor than had been thought. The results are an excellent reminder of the importance of looking for other etiologic factors contributing to the disorder. The absence of a clear relationship between the demonstrated increase in median nerve signal intensity and the electrophysiologic changes is intriguing, and it suggests the need for further characterization of the MRI changes in the nerve in search of those most directly related to the impaired function demonstrated on nerve conduction studies.

J.R. Daube, M.D.

Wheatley M: A simple technique for identification of the distal extent of the transverse carpal ligament during single-portal endoscopic carpal tunnel release. *J Hand Surg (Am)* 21A:1109–1110, 1996.

▶ The author describes a potentially useful technique, especially useful perhaps in the context of teaching the single-portal technique to residents and fellows. He describes palpating the tip of the synovial elevator at the point where it seems to become subcutaneous at the distal margin of the transverse carpal ligament, marking this point and inserting a small needle into the canal. The needle is then visualized via the scope as identifying the distal extent of the ligament.

V.R. Hentz, M.D.

8 Wrist

General

Anchorage of Wrist Joint Prostheses to Bone Using the Osseointegration Principle

Lundborg G, Brånemark PI (Lund Univ, Malmö, Switzerland; Inst for Applied Biotechnology, Göteborg, Sweden)

J Hand Surg (Br) 22B:84–89, 1997 8–1

Objective.—Problems with wrist joint arthroplasty can result in bone resorption and "subsidence," fractures, reactive synovitis, and bone destruction. An alternative technique for fixation of a wrist prosthesis to bone based on the osseointegration principle of Brånemark was described, and 5 cases were reported in which the technique was used.

Methods.—Individually designed joint mechanisms were used for wrist joint arthroplasty in 5 patients, aged 28–60 years, with rheumatoid arthritis. The silicone joint mechanism was used for the first 3 patients, and a second-generation mechanism containing a titanium ball within a high-density polyethylene socket was used for the last 2 patients.

> *Technique.*—The extensor retinaculum is raised, and a tenosynovectomy is performed if necessary. The ulnar head is removed, the distal ulna stabilized, and transverse osteotomies performed. Cancellous bone graft from the iliac crest are placed. The mechanism is screwed into the second and third metacarpal bones, the retinaculum is sutured to the extensor tendons, and the wrist is immobilized and elevated for 3 weeks. Patients were followed up for 4–6.5 years.

Results.—The silicone joint mechanism failed in the first 3 patients within 2 years and was replaced by the ball and socket mechanism. During the follow-up period, no bone resorption or screw loosening was observed in any patient. The screws integrated into the repair (Fig 4).

Conclusions.—Fixation of a second-generation prosthetic wrist joint to bone tissue with screws and without the use of cement, a technique known

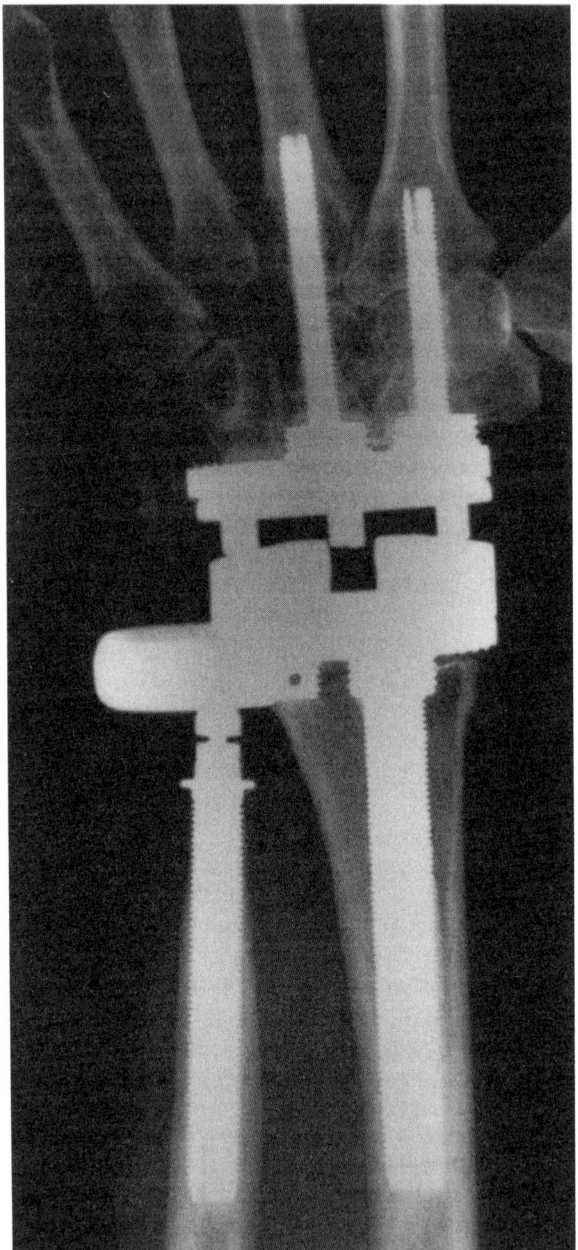

FIGURE 4.—Four years and 10 months follow-up after wrist arthroplasty (case 5). Note perfect osseointegration of screws in radius and ulna. (Courtesy of Lundborg G, Brånemark PI: Anchorage of wrist joint prostheses to bone using the osseointegration principle. *J Hand Surg [Br]* 22B:84–89, 1997).

as osseointegration, resulted in successful repair in all 5 patients with rheumatoid arthritis.

► The authors have sought to identify a technique of ensuring fixation in 9 total wrist joint prostheses. They have demonstrated an osseointegration fixation on the base plates of implants can be accomplished in the radius and the metacarpals, as evidenced in Fig 4 (note stress shielding of ulna in this photograph). There is quite a limited follow-up and a very small number of patients. The authors have commented that the design of the articular portion of the implant is not at this time ideal, but they are satisfied with the bony fixation aspect. The major problem with prosthetic replacement of the wrist with solid metal and polyethylene components has certainly been one of bone fixation and generally of the distal component. Menon has recently introduced a screw fixation system for the distal component of his wrist prosthesis similar to that used by the French Guepar prosthesis. The excellent results seen in the best total arthroplasties of the wrist warrant continued investigation into attempts to find a satisfactory functioning design and a satisfactory form of fixation and longevity. This concept has promise but is not yet convincing.

R.D. Beckenbaugh, M.D.

Biaxial Long-stemmed Multipronged Distal Components for Revision/ Bone Deficit Total-wrist Arthroplasty

Cobb TK, Beckenbaugh RD (Mayo Clinic and Found, Rochester, Minn)
J Hand Surg (Am) 21A:764–770, 1996 8–2

Background.—The incidence of complications associated with revision total-wrist arthroplasty is high. Distal implant loosening is a major problem. Because of the high failure rate of single-pronged distal implants after revision total-wrist arthroplasty, a custom multipronged distal component was designed for patients with deficient bone stock who were undergoing revision surgery.

Methods and Findings.—Ten patients underwent total-wrist arthroplasty with a custom long-stemmed, multipronged distal component between 1989 and 1992. Nine patients had a preoperative diagnosis of failed total-wrist arthroplasty. The average interval between previous total-wrist arthroplasty to revision was 5.6 years. By a mean follow-up of 3.8 years, 2 patients had had arthrodesis and 8 had functional total-wrist arthroplasties. All patients said that they were satisfied. Six patients reported no pain, and 2, mild pain. The average range of motion at follow-up was within the previously defined limits that enable patients to function in activities of daily living (Fig 3).

Conclusions.—Revision total-wrist arthroplasty with custom long-stemmed, multipronged distal components is an alternative for patients with deficient bone stock who decline arthrodesis. Preliminary findings

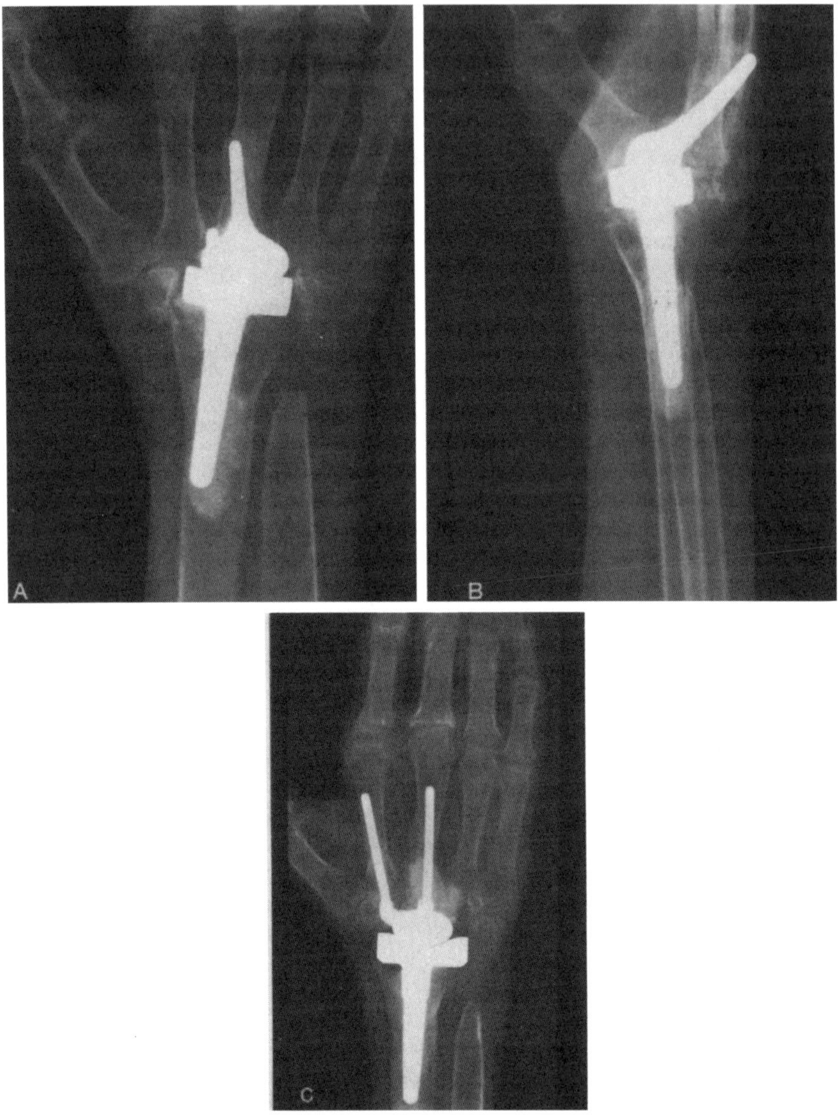

FIGURE 3.—A 70-year-old woman with severe rheumatoid arthritis. **A,** anteroposterior and **B,** lateral radiographs 4 years after primary total-wrist arthroplasty, with loosening and migration of distal component. **C,** anteroposterior radiograph after revision total-wrist arthroplasty using custom 2-pronged distal component. (Courtesy of Cobb TK, Beckenbaugh RD: Biaxial long-stemmed multipronged distal components for revision/bone deficit total-wrist arthroplasty. *J Hand Surg [Am]* 21A:764–770, 1996.)

show a greater longevity compared with single-pronged components for revision total-wrist arthroplasty.

► The material reported in this article represents a work in progress. The biaxial total-wrist prosthesis is, in my opinion, a good prosthesis and is my preference when the need arises. The prosthesis has been on the market for a number of years, and the developers apparently are continuing to work on improvements and modifications of the design. The track record for total-wrist prostheses, has not been very good, yet this particular design appears to have better survival and functional results than most of the others. Beckenbaugh previously reported results for total wrist revisions using the single-stemmed prosthesis and noted trouble in patients with poor bone stock.[1] He concluded that 1993 article by mentioning that he was already using the multipronged prosthesis presented here.

The results in this article are good, but failures still have occurred. Because 7 of the failed prostheses in this series were Biaxes, one wonders what the failure rate for primary Biax total-wrist prostheses has been. This information is not available. The authors honestly report their results treating an extremely vexing problem, and present a reasonable treatment option other than wrist arthrodesis for these unfortunate patients. This article shows, like others before it on the same subject, that even the best work of a talented team of developers and surgeons can't overcome the failings of biologically inadequate tissue.

L.B. Lane, M.D.

Reference

1. Rettig ME, Beckenbaugh RD: Revision total wrist arthroplasty. *J Hand Surg (Am)* 18A:798–804, 1993.

Anatomic and X-ray Film Studies of the Distal Articular Surface of the Radius

Mekhail AO, Ebraheim NA, McCreath WA, et al (Med College of Ohio, Toledo)

J Hand Surg (Am) 21A:567–573, 1996 8–3

Background.—Diagnostic and surgical procedures involving the distal radius require a knowledge of the operative and topographic anatomy of the distal articular surface of the radius. To help surgeons determine the location, displacement, and angulation of acute or healed distal radius articular fractures, the distal articular surface of the radius was evaluated in an anatomical and radiographic study.

Methods.—The distal articular surfaces of 50 dry radii were measured. In addition, in 12 adult cadaver radii, the margins and surfaces of the distal articular surfaces were marked by solder and radiopaque dye, respectively. Margins and bony landmarks then were delineated on radiographs.

Findings.—The area of the lunate facet surface was slightly greater than that of the scaphoid facet surface (53% vs. 47%, respectively). The marked radiographs showed both the palmar tilt and radial inclination. The 30-degree cephalad angled anteroposterior projection of the distal radius was useful for evaluating the dorsomedial fragment of the lunate fossa in a die-punch fracture (Figs 5 and 7).

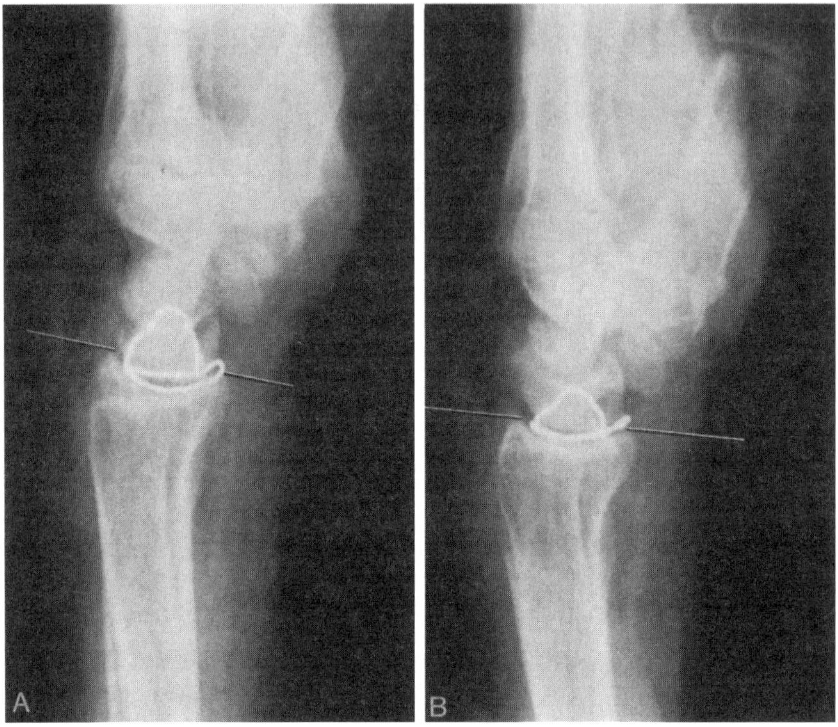

FIGURE 5.—Lateral x-ray films of the wrist. The labeling lines indicate the plane of palmar tilt. The wire marking the dorsal margin in this specimen is extended on the ulnar notch. **A**, true lateral projection. Note that the palmar margin of the articular surface is not well defined. **B**, lateral projection with cephalad angulation of the x-ray beam. The overlap of the wires and the clear joint line denote that the joint is seen tangentially. Note that with a clear joint line, the palmar and dorsal margins of the articular surface are well defined. (Courtesy of Mekhail AO, Ebraheim NA, McCreath WA, et al: Anatomic and x-ray film studies of the distal articular surface of the radius. *J Hand Surg [Am]* 21A:567–573, 1996.)

Conclusions.—Anatomical and radiographic findings may help clinicians assess and manage fractures and deformities of the distal radius. Additional imaging modalities may be of use in the interpretation and treatment of more complex wrist injuries. Fluoroscopy can be used to evaluate the radial inclination angle and palmar tilt by determining the cephalad angulation of the fluoroscopy tube at which a clear joint line is obtained in lateral and posteroanterior views, respectively.

▶ It often is difficult to evaluate the extent of intra-articular fractures of the distal radius on conventional posteroanterior and lateral views of the wrist. This article shows how modifications of these views can better reveal this pathology. First, anteroposterior (instead of the usual posteroanterior) view obtained with 30-degree cephalad angulation better shows a dorsomedial articular fracture fragment. Second, the lateral view obtained with 15-degree cephalad angulation shows a better tangential view of the articular surface than does a straight lateral view. The authors also found that the "palmar

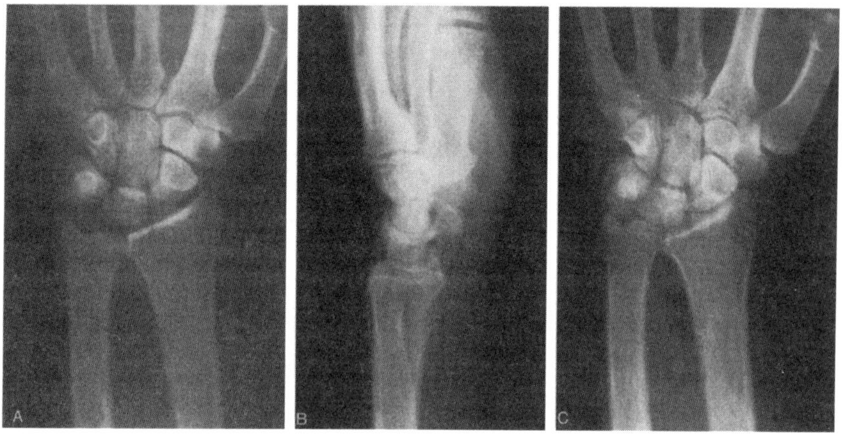

FIGURE 7.—Dorsomedial fracture of the distal articular surface of the radius. **A**, posteroanterior view. **B**, lateral view does not show the coronal extent of the fracture line. **C**, anteroposterior view with the x-ray beam directed 30 degrees cephalad, showing the configuration of the dorsomedial fragment on the articular surface. (Courtesy of Mekhail AO, Ebraheim NA, McCreath WA, et al: Anatomic and x-ray film studies of the distal articular surface of the radius. *J Hand Surg [Am]* 21A:567–573, 1996.)

prominence," often seen between the scaphoid and lunate fossae on posteroanterior radiographs of the wrist, divides the articular surface into 2 nearly equal halves. The location of this ridge, therefore, can be used to determine which fossa is involved by a fracture line, and to estimate what percentage of the articular surface of the radius is displaced by an injury.

G. Bergman, M.D.

Normal Disruption of Carpal Arcs

Peh WCG, Gilula LA (Univ of Hong Kong; Washington Univ, St Louis)
J Hand Surg (Am) 21:561–566, 1996 8–4

Background.—The concept of 3 normal smooth carpal arcs on the posteroanterior (PA) and anteroposterior (AP) radiographs of the wrist is widely accepted (Fig 1). However, no one has described the possible variations of carpal arcs simulating disruption in apparently normal wrists. In addition, the 3-arc concept has not been tested objectively in a large group of research subjects. Wrist instability series in asymptomatic wrists were reviewed to determine whether carpal arcs normally break in radial and ulnar deviation and remain intact in the neutral position.

Methods.—One hundred wrists were studied. Three carpal arcs were drawn on PA and AP radiographs in neutral and radial- and ulnar-deviated positions. Proximal-distal arc step-off was measured.

Findings.—On PA radial deviation at the lunotriquetral joint, arc I and II disruption was seen in 80 and 78 wrists, respectively. At the scapholunate joint, arc II was disrupted in 10 wrists. Findings on AP views were similar. In ulnar deviation, arc II was disrupted at the scapholunate joint posteroanteriorly in 30 wrists and anteroposteriorly in 12. Arcs I and II

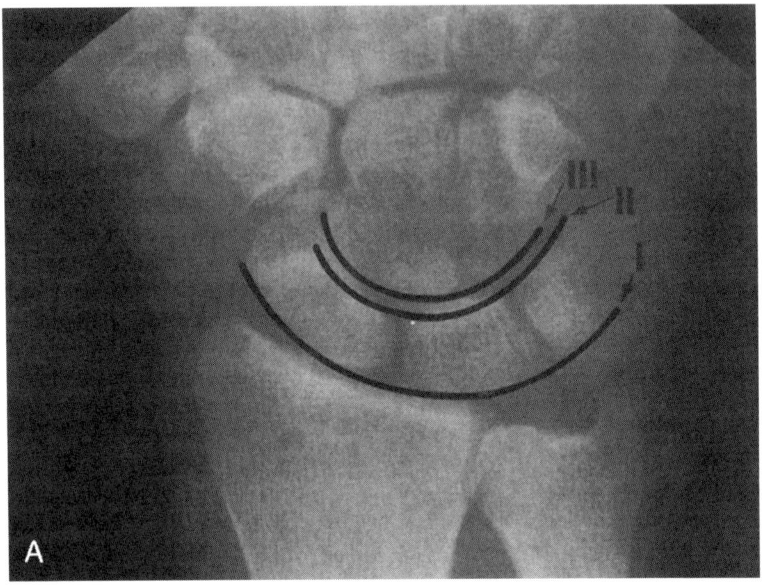

FIGURE 1.—A, the 3 normal carpal arcs are drawn on the neutral posteroanterior x-ray film. Arc I joins the proximal cortical convexities of the scaphoid, lunate, and triquetrum. Arc II links the distal concavities of the same 3 bones. Arc III connects the proximal convexities of the capitate and hamate. (Courtesy of Peh WCG, Gilula LA: Normal disruption of carpal arcs. *J Hand Surg [Am]* 21A:561–566, 1996.)

were normal in neutral AP and PA positions in all but 4 wrists. Of 20 wrists with a type II lunate, 6 had arc II disruption. Arc III was found to be intact in all positions (Figs 2, B and 3, C).

Conclusions.—Radiographic carpal arcs typically disrupt with radial and ulnar deviation. Clinicians must interpret arcs I and II and scapholunate joint width cautiously when the wrist is not strictly neutral in position.

▶ Posteroanterior views of the wrist during radial and ulnar deviation can be a noninvasive and inexpensive tool to detect a ligament tear in the proximal carpal row. A definite widening of the distance between the scaphoid and lunate bones, or the lunate and triquetral bones, usually indicates a ligament tear. It is important not to overdiagnose ligament tears of the wrist if there is a step-off in Gilula's carpal arcs I or II seen on deviation views but not on a PA view in neutral. This article concludes that step-offs in Gilula's arcs I or II occur on deviation views in a large proportion of asymptomatic and presumably normal wrists, and that these step-offs do not indicate ligamentous injury if the arcs show a return to a smooth contour without step-offs when PA views are obtained with the wrists in neutral position.

G. Bergman, M.D.

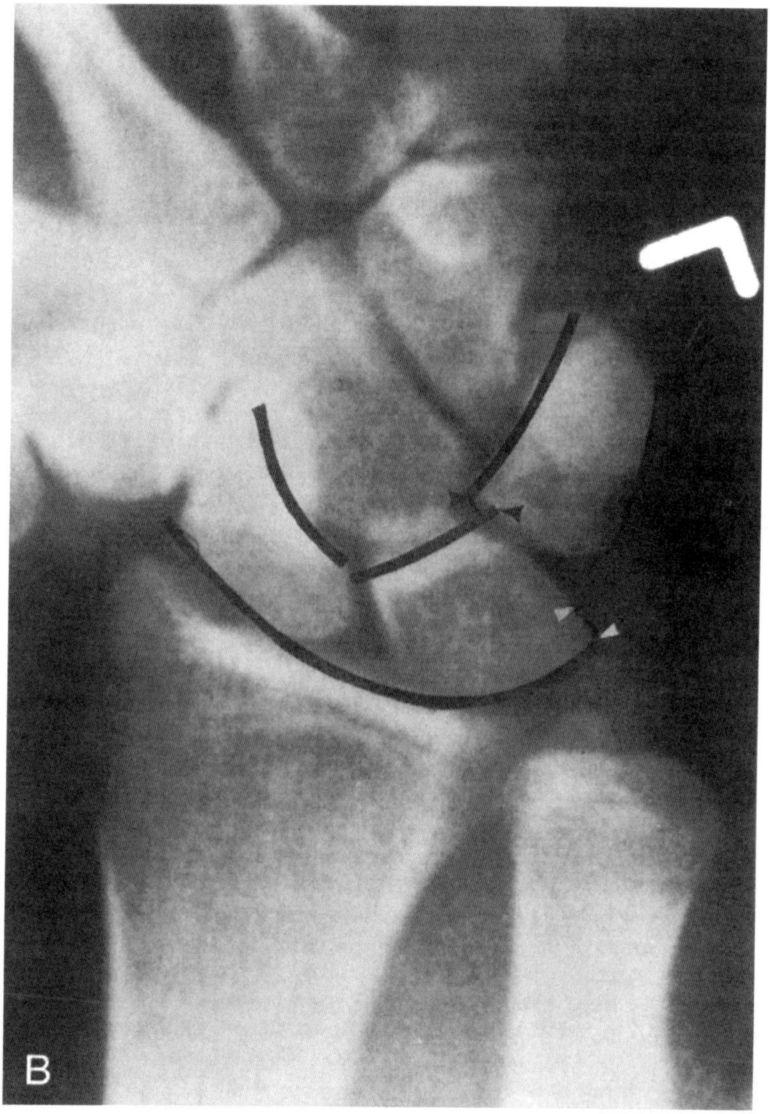

FIGURE 2, B.—Anteroposterior view of the left wrist in radial deviation. Arcs I and II are drawn to illustrate these disruptions. Proximal-distal step-off measurements of arcs I and II disruptions, at the lunotriquetral joint, are between *arrowheads.* (Courtesy of Peh WCG, Gilula LA: Normal disruption of carpal arcs. *J Hand Surg [Am]* 21A:561–566, 1996.)

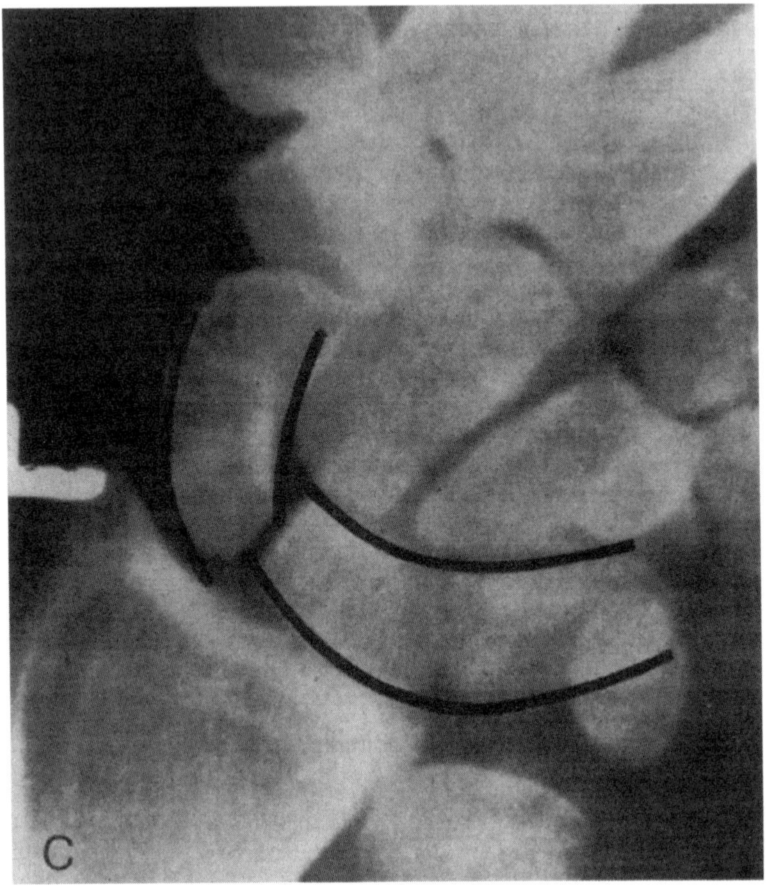

FIGURE 3, C.—Anteroposterior view of the left wrist. Arcs I and II are drawn to illustrate the disruptions. (Courtesy of Peh WCG, Gilula LA: Normal disruption of carpal arcs. *J Hand Surg [Am]* 21A:561–566, 1996.)

A New Radiographic Method of Measuring Carpal Collapse

Zdravkovic V, Sennwald GR (Univ of Zürich, Switzerland; Berit-Paracelsus Clinic, Teufen, Switzerland)
J Bone Joint Surg (Br) 79B:167–169, 1997 8–5

Objective.—It is important to assess the degree of carpal collapse in patients with rheumatoid arthritis, Kienböck disease, and other wrist disorders. The revised carpal height (RCH) ratio, based on the ratio between the carpal height and the length of the capitate, is an accurate measure of carpal collapse. The average normal value is 1.57, and a left–right RCH index can be calculated as well. However, the RCH method has some disadvantages. It is believed that direct measurement of the capitate–radius (CR) distance may provide a better estimate of carpal collapse (Fig 1). This measure was validated by comparison with the RCH method.

Methods.—The analysis included wrist radiographs from 16 normal research subjects and 11 patients with unilateral Kienböck disease. The radiographs were obtained by a standardized technique and read by 11 physicians. The CR and the RCH techniques were applied and compared for diagnostic accuracy using receiver operating characteristic curves. Subsequently, 40 normal wrists were studied to establish a norm for the CR index.

Results.—In the patients with Kienböck disease, both the CR distance and the RCH ratio were reduced in the affected wrist, and the difference for the CR distance was more significant. Across all readers, only the CR index was significantly lower in the patients vs. the controls. All readers found a significant reduction in CR in the Kienböck disease group, whereas only 8 found a highly significant difference in the RCH index. Diagnostic accuracy was much higher with the CR index on receiver operating characteristic curve analysis. The mean value in 40 normal wrists was 0.999 ± 0.034.

Conclusions.—The CR index appears to be a better measure of carpal collapse than the RCH ratio. The diagnostic accuracy is better with the CR index, which can be used for diagnostic purposes in patients with unilateral carpal collapse and for monitoring in patients with bilateral wrist

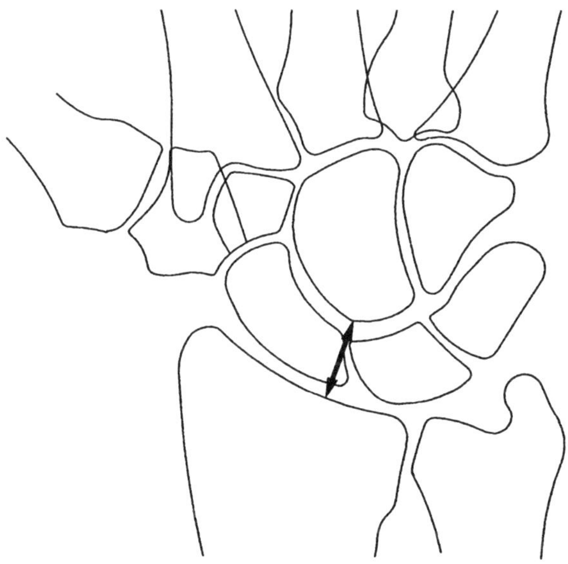

FIGURE 1.—Measurement of the capitate–radius distance. There is only 1 shortest line between 2 eccentric arches; the line is moved until the shortest distance is measured. (Courtesy of Zdravkovic V, Sennwald GR: A new radiographic method of measuring carpal collapse. *J Bone Joint Surg [Br]* 79-B:167–169, 1997.)

involvement. A CR index value of less than 0.92 can be considered abnormal.

▶ The desire to obtain objective information regarding the presence or absence of carpal collapse is highly clinically relevant, in both the staging of Kienböck disease and other disorders such as scapholunate dissociation. In the past, nondimensionalized indices based on either the length of the third metacarpal or the length of the capitate relative to the length of the entire carpus, which were based on measurements made from plain posteroanterior radiographs, have provided such objective information. The authors of this article have proposed a new means of defining carpal collapse based on a direct measurement, in centimeters, using the shortest distance between the subchondral cortices of the proximal capitate and the distal articular surface of the radius. The obvious advantages of this procedure are that it is simple, it requires no mathematics, and it is readily obtainable using a simple metric measuring system. The disadvantages of this system are that, by eliminating the nondimensionalization step, there may be some variations as a result of the size of the individual and a substantial error may be introduced with changes in the projection dimensions of the radiograph. This is particularly so with the increased use of the digitized format, which may substantially vary the size of the x-ray image on the film relative to the size of the individual undergoing radiography. Therefore, caution should be exercised when using this technique unless the enlargement or reduction factor of the image on the x-ray film has been determined. Until this information is available, I would advise the reader to continue using the nondimensionalizing techniques of determining either the carpal height index or the modified carpal height ratio.

R.A. Berger, M.D., Ph.D.

Bicompartmentalization of the Radiocarpal Joint

Ono H, Gilula LA, Marzke MW, et al (Washington Univ, St Louis; Arizona State Univ, Tempe; Univ Hosp Leiden, The Netherlands)

J Hand Surg (Am) 21A:788–793, 1996 8–6

Background.—Patients with bicompartmentalization of the radiocarpal joint can be diagnostically challenging for arthrographers and arthroscopists. Seven wrists with a septum connecting the lunotriquetral interosseous ligament and triangular fibrocartilage, resulting in radiocarpal joint bicompartmentalization, were described.

Patients and Findings.—None of the 7 wrists had been subjected to trauma; thus, the septa were thought to be congenital anomalies. In 1 wrist, obtained from a cadaver for dissection, histopathologic assessment of the septum indicated a fibrocartilaginous structure. Arthrographic findings demonstrated 2 types of radiocarpal joint biocompartmentalization. Two wrists were classified as type 1, characterized by a septum with a normal, intact lunotriquetral interosseous ligament. The remaining 5

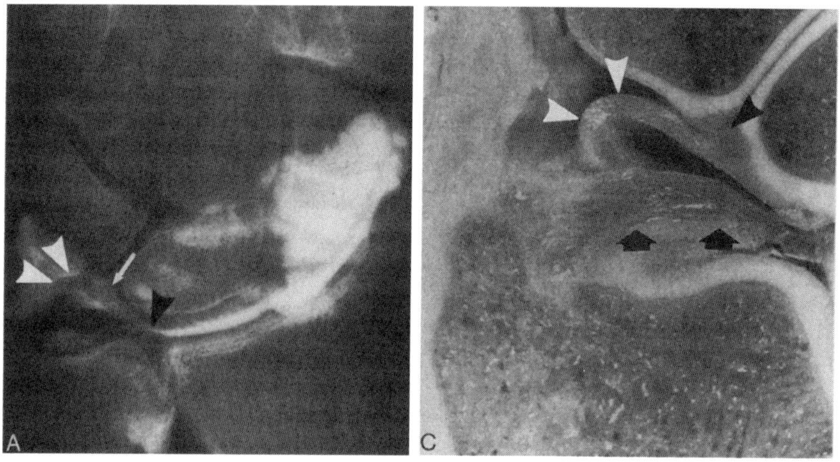

FIGURE 3.—Cadaveric specimen of patient. A posteroanterior view of the radiocarpal arthrogram (A) demonstrates an intact septum (*white arrowheads*) between the lunotriquetral interosseous ligament (*white arrow*) and triangular fibrocartilage. A radial-sided communicating defect of the triangular fibrocartilage (*black arrowheads*) is present. The photograph of a corresponding coronal cryosection of the same specimen (C) showed the fibrous connection or septum (*white arrowheads*) between the lunotriquetral interosseous ligament (*black arrowhead*) and triangular fibrocartilage (*black arrows*). (Courtesy of Ono H, Gilula LA, Marzke MW, et al: Biocompartmentalization of the radiocarpal joint. *J Hand Surg [Am]* 21A:788–793, 1996.)

wrists were type 2, characterized by a septum with a communicating defect of the lunotriquetral interosseous ligament (Fig 3).

Conclusions.—Septa probably are congenital malformations caused by a disturbance of the vacuolization of the mesenchymal mass between the forearm and carpus. No wrist abnormality other than the septa could be found in 2 patients—1 with ulnar-sided wrist pain and 1 with diffuse wrist pain. Hypothetically, the septa in these wrists may have been trapped between the lunate, triquetrum, and triangular fibrocartilage, causing the wrist pain.

▶ This article describes the features of a complete or perforated septum connecting the lunotriquetral ligament to the triangular fibrocartilage. Such a septum can be seen during wrist arthrography or arthroscopy and can present diagnostic challenges. A suspected connection between wrist pain and the presence of this septum was not proven in this study. The authors believe that these septa most likely represent incomplete resorption of fetal mesenchymal tissue, and are less likely to be related to prior trauma. This theory was supported by histologic findings in 1 cadaver wrist, and by similar septa found to be present at the dissection of wrist specimens of 2 nonhuman primates.

G. Bergman, M.D.

Extrinsic Radiocarpal Ligaments: Magnetic Resonance Imaging of Normal Wrists and Scapholunate Dissociation

Adler BD, Logan PM, Janzen DL, et al (Univ of British Columbia, Vancouver)

Can Assoc Radiol J 47:417–422, 1996 8–7

Objective.—Despite the major contribution to wrist stability made by the extrinsic radiocarpal ligaments, most radiologic studies of wrist pain have centered on the intrinsic wrist ligaments. Results of a study of oblique sagittal plane MRI, parallel to the course of the extrinsic wrist ligaments were presented, as were cases of scapholunate dissociation and rotatory subluxation of the scaphoid to determine the associated findings.

Methods.—Magnetic resonance imaging was performed on 1 cadaveric wrist, 23 normal wrists (8 women, aged 20–52 years), and 8 wrists (all men, aged 25–52 years), with scapholunate dissociation and rotatory scaphoid subluxation. The proton density and T2-weighted images ob-

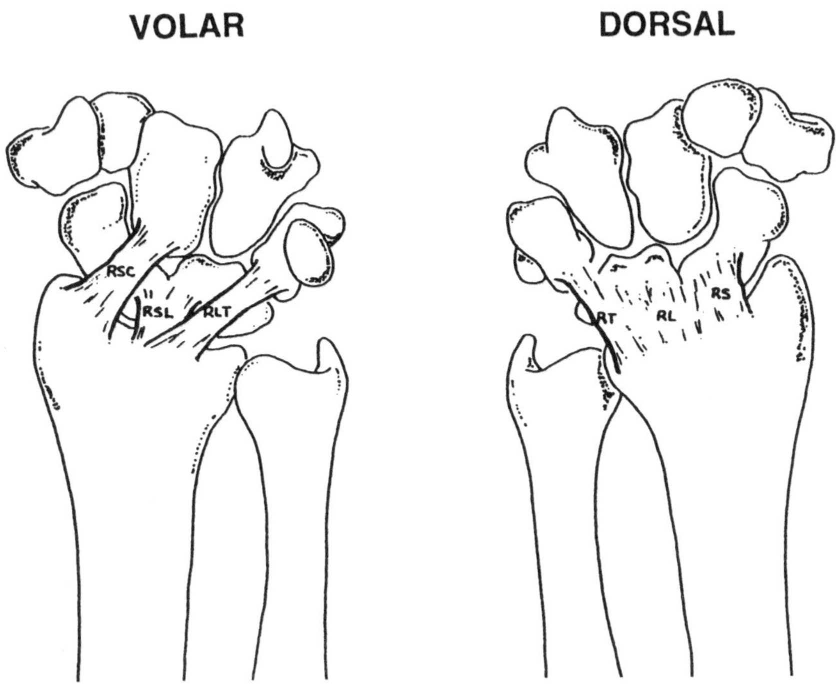

FIGURE 1.—**Left**, diagram of the radiocarpal ligaments from the volar and dorsal aspects. The volar ligaments consist of a deeper sagittal layer (the radioscapholunate ligament [*RSL*]), a superficial oblique layer (the radioscaphocapitate ligament [*RSC*], and the radiolunotriquetral ligament [*RLT*]). The dorsal ligaments consist of a single fanlike layer from the dorsal radius to the proximal carpal row (*RS*, radioscaphoid ligament; *RL*, radiolunate ligament; *RT*, radiotriquetral ligament). **Right**, coronal localizer image of the wrist shows the plane of acquisition for the oblique sagittal images. The plane is determined by a line passing from the midpole of the capitate through the waist of the scaphoid and the radial styloid process. (Reprinted by permission of the publisher from Adler BD, Logan PM, Janzen DL, et al: Extrinsic radiocarpal ligaments: Magnetic resonance imaging of normal wrists and scapholunate dissociation. *Can Assoc Radiol J* 47[6]:417–422, 1996.)

tained in the orthogonal sagittal plane and gradient recalled echo images in the oblique sagittal plane were assessed by 2 musculoskeletal radiologists. All ligaments were examined (Fig 1).

Results.—Extrinsic ligaments in cadaveric and normal wrists were best visualized by oblique sagittal imaging (Fig 3, A). Patients with scapholunate dissociation and rotatory scaphoid subluxation had abnormalities, and the dorsal radioscaphoid ligament was not consistently visualized (Fig 5).

Conclusion.—Magnetic resonance imaging in the sagittal and oblique sagittal plane is a reliable technique for visualizing extrinsic wrist liga-

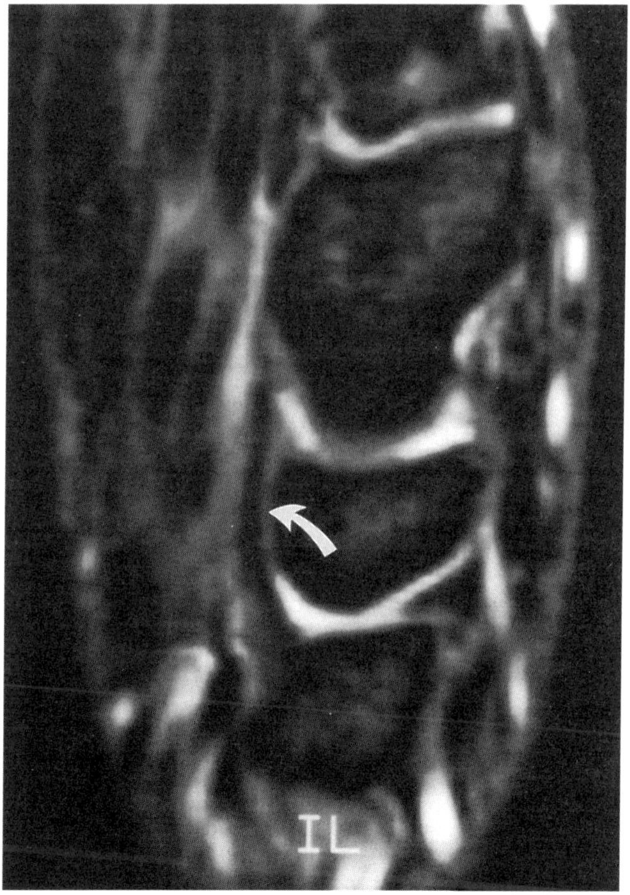

FIGURE 3, A.—Oblique sagittal gradient recalled echo image (repetition time, 700 ms; echo time, 16 ms; flip angle, 15 degrees) of a normal wrist shows the radioscaphocapitate ligament as a continuous, uniform, hypointense structure (*arrow*) extending from the radial styloid process to the midpole of the capitate. (Reprinted by permission of the publisher from Adler BD, Logan PM, Janzen DL, et al: Extrinsic radiocarpal ligaments: Magnetic resonance imaging of normal wrists and scapholunate dissociation. *Can Assoc Radiol J* 47[6]:417–422, 1996.)

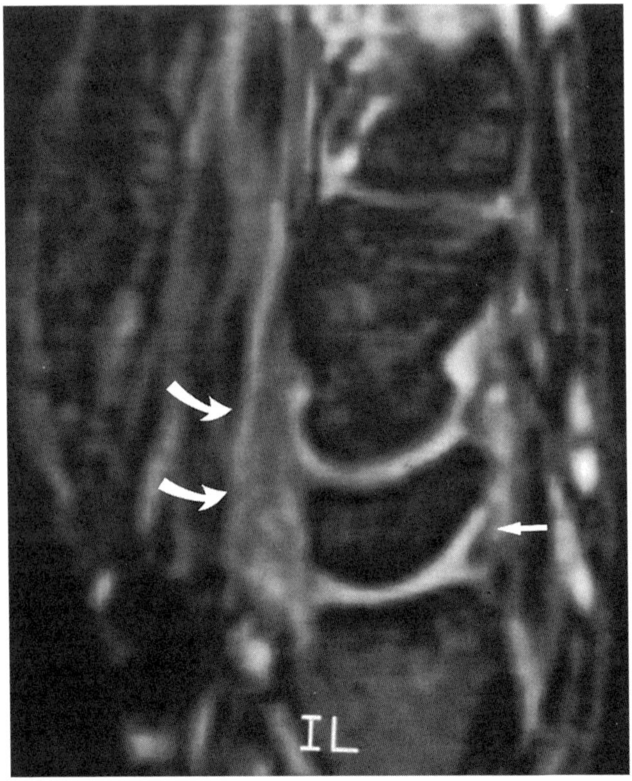

FIGURE 5.—Oblique sagittal image (repetition time, 700 ms; echo time, 16 ms; flip angle, 15 degrees) of the wrist in a case of scapholunate dissociation and rotatory scaphoid subluxation. The radioscaphocapitate ligament is thickened and of heterogeneously increased signal intensity (*curved arrows*). Thickening with fibrous scarring was confirmed at surgery. The dorsal radiolunate ligament is serpiginous (*straight arrow*), making it difficult to image in profile in the coronal plane. (Reprinted by permission of the publisher from Adler BD, Logan PM, Janzen DL, et al: Extrinsic radiocarpal ligaments: Magnetic resonance imaging of normal wrists and scapholunate dissociation. *Can Assoc Radiol J* 47[6]:417–422, 1996.)

ments and allowing evaluation of abnormalities in patients with scapholunate dissociation and rotatory scaphoid subluxation.

▶ The authors show how MRI in an oblique sagittal plane, parallell to both the superficial volar and the dorsal extrinsic carpal ligaments, improves demonstration of the full length of these ligaments. In normal wrists, when using this MR method, these ligaments are seen as continuous low-signal structures. In all 8 patients with a verified scapholunate ligament tear, the volar radioscaphocapitate ligament was shown to be abnormal on MRI of the oblique sagittal plane. The authors suggest that routine use of MRI in this oblique sagittal plane in patients with carpal injury may increase the specificity of MRI for detection of significant carpal ligament injuries with instability (e.g., with tears of both the intrinsic scapholunate and the extrinsic scapholunocapitate ligaments). This method deserves further evaluation in clinical use.

G. Bergman, M.D.

Radioscaphocapitate Ligament of the Wrist: Volar Filling Defect During Radiocarpal Arthrography

Rubin DA, Petropoulou KA, McIntosh JC, et al (Univ of Pittsburgh, Pa)

Radiology 201:501–506, 1996 8–8

Objective.—To confirm that the bandlike filling defect between the radial styloid and the capitate crossing the scaphoid waist appearing during arthrography is the extrinsic volar radioscaphocapitate (RSC) ligament, arthrography was performed in cadaveric wrists after labeling the RSC ligament. In addition, arthrograms in patients who were referred for evaluation of the intrinsic wrist ligaments were retrospectively reviewed to determine how frequently the RSC ligament is visualized.

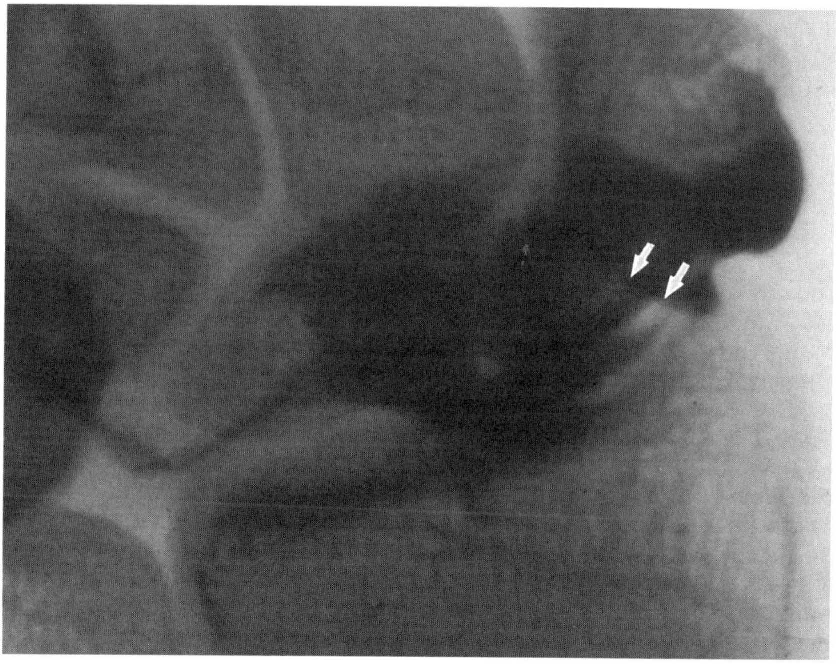

FIGURE 5, B.—Benefit of ulnar deviation in a 20-year-old man with a painful nonunion of the ulnar styloid. Radiograph obtained at the conclusion of the radiocarpal injection with the patient's wrist in ulnar deviation. With radial deviation, the radioscaphocapitate (RSC) ligament is not discernible, while its presence is unequivocal (*arrows*) when the wrist is in ulnar deviation. The radial aspect of the radiocarpal joint was not explored at surgery. (Courtesy of Rubin DA, Petropoulou KA, McIntosh JC, et al: Radioscaphocapitate ligament of the wrist: Volar filling defect during radiocarpal arthrography. *Radiology* 201:501–506. Copyright 1996, Radiological Society of North America.)

Methods.—Arthrograms were taken of marked RSC ligaments in 3 cadaveric wrists and forearms. Each wrist was examined. A total of 70 contrast-enhanced arthrograms were retrospectively reviewed to determine how frequently the RSC ligament was visualized. Scoring criteria were established. Pathologic findings were compared with the retrospective interpretations.

Results.—The cadaveric studies established that the filling defect seen on radiocarpal arthrograms is the RSC ligament. The RSC ligament was definitively identified in 55 of the 70 arthrograms, but was not observed in 15 arthrograms. Contrast enhanced visualization of the RSC ligament early on with the wrist in ulnar deviation (Fig 5, B).

Conclusions.—The RSC ligament was confirmed to be the volar filling defect seen during radiocarpal arthrography. It is best visualized soon after injection of contrast medium when the wrist is placed in ulnar deviation. Additional studies are necessary to determine the diagnostic capability of arthrography for detecting abnormalities of the RSC ligament.

▶ This article highlights the tremendous amount of information that can be gained, even with simple, straightforward, and commonly accepted imaging techniques such as arthrography. Our tendency is to utilize the arthrogram simply to determine the presence or absence of filling abnormalities, such as the triangular fibrocartilage complex (TFCC) tear or disruption of the proximal row interosseous ligaments. However, with diligence, the outlines of numerous features of the joint capsule, can be identified. Particularly, as highlighted by this manuscript, the RSC ligament may be seen as a filling defect, highlighted by the interligamentous sulcus, which separates it from the long radiolunate ligament. This information is very useful, particularly as we are identifying more conditions that involve the capsular ligaments, in addition to the more readily identifiable interosseous ligament disruptions. This information can then be used as a screening tool to determine whether further imaging, such as MRI or intervention such as arthroscopy is warranted.

R.A. Berger, M.D., Ph.D.

Surgeons' Decision Making in Patients With Chronic Wrist Pain: Role of Bilateral Three-compartment Wrist Arthrography—Prospective Study

Yin Y, Evanoff BA, Gilula LA, et al (Beijing Inst of Traumatology, People's Republic of China; Washington Univ, St. Louis)

Radiology 200:829–832, 1996 8–9

Introduction.—The value of a diagnostic procedure depends on how it affects the ordering physician's decision-making process. Wrist arthrography is generally regarded as an important tool in evaluation of chronic wrist pain, and it has become more accurate with the introduction of the 3-compartment injection procedure. However, there have been no studies of the impact of wrist arthrography on the surgeon's decision-making process. The influence of wrist arthrography on treatment in patients with chronic wrist pain was prospectively evaluated.

Methods.—Sixty-four patients undergoing bilateral, 3-compartment wrist arthrography were included. All were adults with unexplained unilateral wrist pain referred by 1 of 32 hand, orthopedic, or plastic surgeons. The surgeons were asked to state their diagnoses and management plans on 3 occasions: before arthrography, after arthrography of the symptomatic wrist, and after arthrography of the asymptomatic wrist. The effects of arthrography on the surgeon's management plan were evaluated.

Results.—The management plan tended to become more conservative after the surgeon had received the arthrographic results. The percentage of patients for whom surgery was planned decreased from 44% to 30%. The percentage of patients for whom any type of treatment was planned decreased from 86% to 77%. Overall, the treatment plan changed after arthrography in 45% of patients, becoming more conservative in 34% of patients and more aggressive in 11%. Most of the changes in treatment plan occurred in patients with no communicating defect on arthrography.

Conclusions.—In patients with chronic wrist pain, the results of bilateral 3-compartment wrist arthrography had a significant effect on the surgeon's decision-making process. Given the results of arthrography, surgeons tended to change their treatment plans in a more conservative direction. Because of protocol violations, it was not possible to evaluate the impact of the results in the asymptomatic and symptomatic wrist separately. This should be addressed in future studies.

► Recently, the value of wrist arthrography has been questioned when compared with arthroscopy for the evaluation of chronic wrist pain.[1, 2] On the other hand, Yin and coauthors make a strong argument in favor of arthrography. After arthrography, 45% of their patients had a change in treatment with a trend toward more conservative methods.

I believe that arthrography is of real value in the evaluation of chronic wrist pain, and I now recognize that an arthrographic communicating defect does not necessarily justify surgical intervention. First, the arthrographic abnormalities must directly correlate with the history and physical examination. Next, the treating physician must recognize that some arthrographic communications are merely ligamentous perforations that are clinically insignificant. Finally, the value of arthrography goes up considerably when the opposite asymptomatic wrist is studied, because when symmetric abnormalities (i.e., contrast communications) are found, the clinician tends to discount the findings in the symptomatic wrist. Unfortunately, the current study admittedly was unable to determine the value of bilateral studies because of a break in protocol.

P.J. Stern, M.D.

References

1. Cooney WP: Evaluation of chronic wrist pain by arthrography, arthroscopy, and arthrotomy. *J Hand Surg (Am)* 18A:815–822, 1993.
2. Weiss A-PC, Akelman E, Lambiase R: Comparison of the findings of triple-injection cinearthrography of the wrist with those of arthroscopy. *J Bone Joint Surg (Am)* 78-A:348–356, 1996.

Wrist Arthrography Versus Arthroscopy: A Comparative Study of 150 Cases

Chung KC, Zimmerman NB, Travis MT (Union Mem Hosp, Baltimore, Md)

J Hand Surg (Am) 21A:591–594, 1996 8–10

Background.—Wrist arthroscopy has been advocated as a procedure of choice for assessing ligamentous wrist injuries. However, there have been no large studies comparing wrist arthrography and arthroscopy. These modalities were compared in 150 patients with suspected wrist ligamentous injuries.

Methods.—All patients had received a clinical diagnosis of ligamentous wrist injury but had normal findings on radiographs. Triple injection wrist arthrography and arthroscopy were performed in all patients, and the diagnoses were compared.

Findings.—Arthrography detected intercarpal abnormalities in 71% of the patients and arthroscopy in 91%. Agreement between the 2 modalities was only 42%. Fifty-eight percent of the patients had their arthrographic diagnoses changed after arthroscopy. Eighty-eight percent of the 44 patients with normal arthrographic findings underwent arthroscopy because of the inadequate correlation between the findings on physical examination and on arthroscopy. Eighty percent of the 44 patients with normal arthrographic findings were found to have injuries by arthroscopy.

Conclusions.—Arthroscopy may be the most efficient way to definitively diagnose a patient with suspected ligamentous wrist injury. Cost analysis and outcome studies are now needed.

▶ The wrist arthrogram provides information regarding the presence or absence of a hole in the scapholunate ligament, the lunotriquetral ligament, or the triangular fibrocartilage complex. That's it! It does not tell us the size or significance of the hole. Neither does arthrography show us instability, chondromalacia, volar carpal ligament tears, or arthritis. Wrist arthroscopy gives us this information. Therefore, it is not suprising that the authors have found a significant discrepancy between arthrographic and arthroscopic data. Even 80% of patients in this study with normal arthrograms had injuries identified at arthroscopy. The question raised by this study is "why do wrist arthrography at all?"

Arthroscopy brings anesthetic risks and potential surgical complications and is a much more expensive procedure than arthrography. The decision to use arthroscopy diagnostically must be tempered by careful clinical judgement. At present, arthroscopy provides us with the most information, outside of clinical assessment, about the painful wrist.

E.R. North, M.D.

The Role of Arthroscopy in the Investigation of Wrist Disorders

Jones WA, Lovell ME (Broadgreen Hosp, Liverpool, England)

J Hand Surg (Br) 21B:442–445, 1996 8–11

Background.—A number of authors have described the utility of arthroscopy in the diagnostic evaluation of the wrist. Arthroscopy has also been recommended to confirm clinical diagnoses before surgery, suggesting that the findings may affect management decisions. However, this recommendation has been challenged because of its cost. The role of diagnostic wrist arthroscopy in the assessment of wrist disorders was further explored.

Methods and Findings.—Forty-eight consecutive wrist arthroscopies done in a 4.5-year period were reviewed retrospectively. When the clinical and arthroscopic findings were compared in 36 patients with wrist instability and triangular fibrocartilage injuries, concurrence was noted in 28. Arthroscopy was not helpful in the other 6 patients, in whom no provisional clinical diagnosis could be made. In 2 of the 6 patients in whom the articular surface was assessed, arthroscopy did prove useful in management decisions.

Conclusions.—Careful clinical assessment of the wrist is the cornerstone of diagnosis in patients with wrist disorders. Although arthroscopy is useful in certain patients, its role is limited and specialized, and it should continue to be provided at specialist centers.

▶ Through their retrospective study of 48 patients with various problems in 8 groups they made up, the authors conclude that wrist arthroscopy remains useful in selected cases but has a limited, specialized role that should continue to be provided from specialist centers. Unfortunately, the authors do not provide us with information how we can distinguish those selected cases without arthroscopy.

The authors emphasize the importance of clinical examination of the wrist in patients with wrist pain, and I wholeheartedly agree. I wish to add that a careful history taking—not only that of injury, but also of vocational and avocational history, pain characteristics, symptom duration and frequency, what makes it worse/better, and so on—is also most important in making a diagnosis of wrist pathology. I also believe that wrist arthroscopy should be considered when there is a possibility or a probability that arthroscopic findings may affect treatment course, and when a therapeutic arthroscopy is indicated.

J. Ryu, M.D.

Mechanoreceptors in the Palmar Wrist Ligaments
Petrie S, Collins J, Solomonow M, et al (Louisiana State Univ, New Orleans)
J Bone Joint Surg (Br) 79-B:494–496, 1997 8–12

Introduction.—Ligamentous mechanoreceptors are found in various joints. They play important roles in preserving mechanical stability, preventing degenerative joint disease, and permitting optimal control of movement. This study investigated the presence of mechanoreceptors in the palmar wrist ligaments.

Methods.—Palmar wrist ligaments from 6 fresh cadavers were dissected from the proximal to the distal insertions. A modified gold-chloride staining method was used to identify the mechanoreceptors.

Findings.—The radial collateral, radioscaphocapitate, and radiolunate ligaments all showed Golgi organs, Pacinian corpuscles, Ruffini endings, and free nerve endings. All 4 types of mechanoreceptors where found in the greatest density at the proximal and distal insertions in the radial collateral and radiolunate ligaments. They were distributed more uniformly in the radioscaphocapitate ligament.

Conclusions.—Mechanoreceptors are identified in the palmar wrist ligaments, suggesting the presence of a ligamentomuscular protective reflex in the wrist. Because mechanoreceptors are present, surgeons operating on the wrist should attempt to preserve the articular nerves of the ligaments. This may be technically difficult. In situations such as painful posttraumatic or degenerative conditions, wrist denervation may be desirable.

▶ In a number of joint systems, such as the knee, shoulder, and facet joints, investigators have identified mechanoreceptors that have been theoretically linked with proprioceptive feedback loops. It is therefore no surprise that the rich innervation of the carpal ligaments also contains such nerve endings. This is a very important study because it introduces the possibility of dynamic stabilization of the carpus, in addition to the static constraints of the wrist ligaments. With further consideration, disruption of the carpal ligaments may not only lead to a mechanical destabilization directly, but may interfere with appropriate equilibrium producing forces via the neurologic feedback loop. This may be particularly important with the dynamic nondissociative carpal instability patterns.

R.A. Berger, M.D., Ph.D.

The Effects of Exercise on Ligamentous Stiffness in the Wrist
Crisco JJ, Chelikani S, Brown RK, et al (Yale Univ, New Haven, Conn)
J Hand Surg (Am) 22A:44–48, 1997 8–13

Introduction.—The scaphoid helps to stabilize the carpus throughout a wide range of wrist motion and variations in external load via its stout ligamentous connections to the proximal and distal carpal rows. Sports involving extremes of wrist position, such as racquet sports, golf, hockey, and platform diving often result in injuries to the scaphoid ligaments. Before strenuous physical activity, warm-up and loosening-up exercise are overwhelmingly recommended to minimize these and other soft-tissue injuries. However, no studies have documented the efficacy of these exercises. The effects of exercise on the load-displacement behavior of the scaphoid bone were determined.

Methods.—In the palmar-dorsal direction of both wrists of 7 healthy volunteers, the load-displacement behavior of the scaphoid was studied before and after 2 grip and push-up exercise protocols. On 3 separate days, each wrist was tested with an initial test, a test that was repeated after 5 minutes, and again after 1 hour. The grip exercise was performed with a generic grip-strengthening device, consisting of 2 hard plastic handles connected by a torsional spring. The push-up protocol involved the subjects performing push-ups. A device that applied a dorsally directed load to the scaphoid bone of the wrist and measured the resulting displacement (Fig 1) was strapped to the wrist.

Results.—The displacement was significantly increased at 40 newtons by 47% with the grip exercise protocol and by 34% with the push-up protocol when compared to the rested values. There was a 36% decrease in stiffness with the grip protocol and a 32% decrease in stiffness with the push-up protocol. After 1 hour of rest, partial recovery was documented, and after 24 hours of rest, there were no differences between any of the groups.

Conclusion.—The ligament loads are reduced at comparable wrist positions with the increase in laxity documented during the exercise proto-

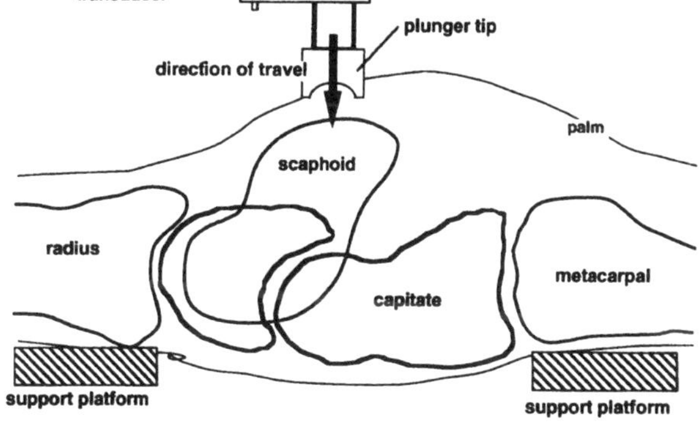

FIGURE 1.—A schematic of the testing apparatus and procedure for measuring the load-displacement behavior of the scaphoid in the dorsal direction. (Courtesy of Crisco JJ, Chelikani S, Brown RK, et al: The effects of exercise on ligamentous stiffness in the wrist. *J Hand Surg [Am]* 22:44–48, 1997.)

cols. The likelihood of traumatic ligamentous injury during participation in strenuous activity or sports may thereby be reduced.

► It is interesting how a general concept can be embraced and incorporated into our way of thinking and recommendations made without substantiation or validation in hard science. Although many believe in and recommend warm-up exercises before strenuous physical activity, feeling that it is beneficial in minimizing injuries, there has not been good, basic research to substantiate that belief. Although it has been shown that ligamentous laxity in the knee joint increases after exercise, we have generalized this information to other joints. The authors have utilized their testing apparatus for measuring load displacement of the scaphoid to address the question of whether or not exercise alters wrist joint laxity, based on the measured mechanical dorsal displacement of the scaphoid. This is a nicely designed study, which demonstrates in the wrist our beliefs that warm-up exercises do, in fact, result in increasing flexibility and transient ligamentous laxity of the joint that is being exercised. The fact that there is now information to demonstrate that exercising increases joint laxity, both in the knee and the wrist, further assists us in extrapolating this concept to other joints. Although the authors appropriately mention that the clinical effect of reducing ligament injury with exercise remains to be validated in the wrist, it is well demonstrated that preseason examinations can identify those individuals who are more likely to sustain injuries based on limited flexibility in joints such as the ankle. The authors are to be complimented on the design of this study and the addition they have made to the literature.

S.F. Viegas, M.D.

A Non-invasive Method for Studying In Vivo Carpal Kinematics

Wolfe SW, Crisco JJ, Katz LD (Yale Univ, New Haven, Conn)

J Hand Surg (Br) 22:147–152, 1997 8–14

Introduction.—In the workplace, wrist injuries account for a considerable and growing percentage of disability and dysfunction. Even though radiographs appear normal, patients may continue to be incapacitated by pain during stressful activities months after injury. Diagnostic modalities are not capable of determining the magnitude of the ligament injury. In vitro, there have been extensive studies of kinematics of the normal and abnormal wrist; however, little is known about in vivo injured and normal wrist kinematics. Carpal kinematics were quantified in vivo and it was determined whether abnormal carpal kinematics were present in patients with normal radiographic findings and carpal ligament injury.

Methods.—Using midsagittal CT images at 10-degree increments from full extension to full flexion, 7 uninjured and 3 injured patients were studied. Each patient had normal radiographic findings and a confirmed scapholunate ligament tear. Digitizations were made of CT bony contours, and using a specifically designed automated contour-matching algorithm, incremental motion was determined. Wrist motion was expressed as a ratio of lunocapitate (midcarpal) motion and radiolunate (radiocarpal) motion.

Results.—Motion occurred equally at the midcarpal and radiocarpal joints in normal wrists. Lunocapitate motion increased significantly throughout the arc of motion in wrists with scapholunate ligament disruption. The lunate-capitate and lunate-radius ratio of the normal volunteers was significantly different from the kinematic behavior of the injured patients.

Conclusion.—Despite radiographic intercarpal measurements that fall in the accepted normal range, there is a significant increase in the relative contribution of the midcarpal joint to flexion and extension after scapholunate ligament disruption. With a quantitative study of 3-dimensional kinematics of the normal and injured wrist in vivo, the technique of 2-dimensional feature registration of CT images lends itself well.

▶ The goal of measuring the kinematics of the normal and abnormal wrist in the in vivo setting has been an elusive one. The authors are to be commended on their attempt to obtain that goal with what the current technology has to offer. However, there are a number of issues regarding the limitation of this technique and its technology that raise some concerns. Even though only a single sagittal section was imaged, the image capture time is still sufficiently slow that true dynamic motion could not be obtained. Using a custom plexiglass device, a series of images of the wrist in static positions of 10-degree increments from flexion to extension were obtained. In our studies in the in vitro setting, in was noted that the kinematics differed between dynamic motion and that obtained by sequential static positioning of the wrist in different positions. There may be less difference in the in vivo situation between dynamic motion and a series of static positions. The greater concern is the fact that with the normal degree of translational motion of the carpal bones, and the fact that the normal flexion-extension motion is not a fixed axis or planar motion, the segment of the various carpal bones that are imaged from one position to another may, in fact, change. The authors have acknowledged this fact and further explained that 2 of the 7 scans showing no abnormality were discarded because of significant variations in the shape of the bone contours.

The relative contribution of the proximal and distal carpal rows to wrist motion, as the authors have mentioned, has been controversial, and a number of investigations using cadaveric wrists have been reported. In our own studies, we have found that the radiolunate joint contributed more than the lunocapitate joint in flexion, whereas the radiolunate joint contributed less motion than the lunocapitate joint in wrist extension. The authors made the assumption, and their results suggest, that the radiocarpal and midcarpal joints contributed equally to flexion-extension. Their findings in wrists with injuries of the scapholunate ligament are interesting and seem to be consistent with what is known about scaphoid instability and carpal kinematics in cases of scapholunate dissociation. They found that those injuries produced less motion at the radiolunate joint, which was compensated for by an increased motion at the lunocapitate joint. If the scaphoid is, in fact, unstable and assumes a flexed posture with the lunate assuming an extended position, this would diminish the overall range of the motion between the proximal carpal row and the radius.

I believe that the technology will continue to improve and increase our ability to obtain complete images of the carpus as we study both static and even dynamic carpal kinematics. At the present time, this study offers an interesting attempt to gain some insight into the carpal kinematics in the in vivo setting in both normal and abnormal conditions. Although the results are intriguing and offer additional information, it should be cautioned that it is still only a glimpse at a portion of the picture.

S.F. Viegas, M.D.

Study of the Transmission of Pronosupination Movements at the Wrist [French]

Roux JL, Micallef JP, Rabischong P, et al (Hôpital Lapeyronie, Montpellier, France; INSERM, Unité 103, Montpellier, France)

Ann Chir Main Memb Super 15:167–180, 1996 8–15

Purpose.—The wrist has an essential role in transmitting the movements of pronation and supination, which constitute the rotatory movement of the forearm around its longitudinal axis. Because the distal insertions of the 4 principal muscles responsible for these movements are proximal to the radiocarpal joint, the movements of pronation and supination are transmitted indirectly to the hand via the wrist. Radiometacarpal rotation (RMR) is defined as the displacement in pronation and supination of the carpal bones on the distal radius. An apparatus (designed by the author) was used to measure this passive intercarpal rotation.

Methods.—A 3-dimensional motion analysis device was used to measure RMR under 2 conditions: with the wrist relaxed and then during a grip of between 80 and 100 newtons. Radiometacarpal rotation measurements were obtained with the patient sitting on a chair, the upper arm hanging straight down along the torso, the elbow resting on the edge of the table, and the forearm bent at a 90-degree angle in relation to the upper arm. The measurements were taken in both wrists of 30 male and 20 female volunteers. Those with a history of wrist problems were excluded.

Findings.—The average RMR was 42 degrees. There was no significant difference between displacement measurements obtained with the wrist in pronation or in supination. Radiometacarpal rotation measurements between the dominant and nondominant sides also did not differ significantly. In contrast, the average RMR measured in the wrists of men was 37 degrees, whereas it was 49 degrees in women. The average rotation difference of 12 degrees between men and women is significant, as it is in agreement with the greater ligament laxity usually found in women. The results also showed that the center of RMR and the center of active pronation/supination are not concordant and that the average distance

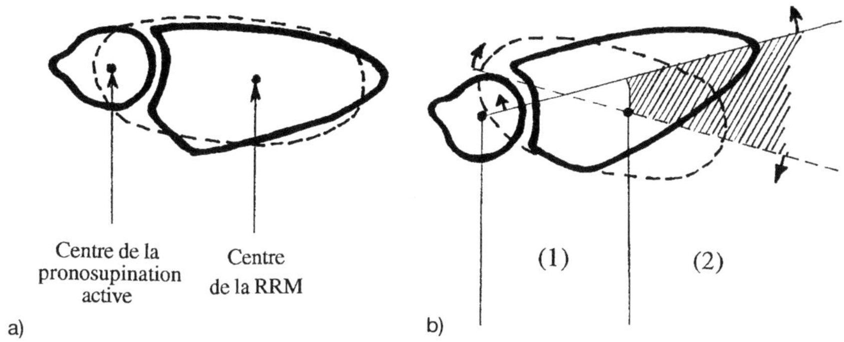

FIGURE 6.—Schematic representation of the rotation centers. The active pronosupination center and the radiometacarpal rotation (RMR) center are placed on horizontal superimposed sections of the carpal condyle and distal radial surface. The RMR center is always more lateral. **A,** neutral position; **B,** during pronosupination movement against resistance. Between the rotation centers, the carpal condyle and distal radial articular surface move in the same direction; displacements are concordant. Outside the RMR center, the carpal condyle and distal radial articular surface move in opposite directions; displacements are discordant. (Courtesy of Roux JL, Micallef JP, Rabischong P, et al: Study of the transmission of pronosupination movements at the wrist. *Ann Chir Main Memb Super* 15:167–180, 1996.)

between these 2 points is 24 mm (Fig 6). The maximal RMR occurs when the wrist is relaxed, and the range of rotation decreases as the fist is closed, because closing the fist increases tension on the ligaments.

Conclusion.—The transmission of pronation/supination movements is an essential function of the wrist. Active pronation/supination and RMR are interdependent.

► This is an excellent article to include in a study of wrist biomechanics. The authors define "radiometacarpal rotation" as pronation and supination of the carpal bones, and thus the hand, on the distal radius. They properly point out that this motion is separate from forearm rotation but is influenced by it via extrinsic wrist ligament pull on the scaphoid and also decreased by force of grip; they measured all 3 simultaneously with their device.

Most of the rotation took place on the radioscaphoid joint when the center of rotation was calculated (see Fig 6), with an average of 42 degrees when not gripping. This is an important concept biomechanically, because forced passive intercarpal rotation has been shown to cause perilunate dislocations. It is also important clinically, as physical measurement of forearm supination and pronation are often erroneously high if they include the hand rotating on the radius. For this reason, forearm rotation should be measured with the medial elbow against the straight trunk, with 1 limb of the goniometer on the flat dorsal surface and palmar surface of the distal one third of the forearm for pronation and supination, respectively; the other limb of the goniometer should be perpendicular to the floor.

The authors postulate that, in some cases, this movement may contribute to radiocarpal arthrosis, and may help in designing wrist prostheses. I wonder whether the diminution in RMR that occurs with grip may actually be protective and may be lacking in patients with ligamentous laxity and symptomatic midcarpal instability—for example, at the triquetro-hamate joint with dynamic, sudden, painful lunate snapping into extension in ulnar deviation.

J.M. Failla, M.D.

Total Wrist Fusion: A Functional Assessment

Field J, Herbert TJ, Prosser R (St Luke's Hosp, Sydney, Australia)
J Hand Surg (Br) 21B:429–433, 1996 8–16

Background.—Wrist fusion is indicated primarily by posttraumatic wrist problems and rheumatoid arthritis. The procedure appears to be effective in patients with rheumatoid wrist. These patients often have gross instability and a low functional demand. Wrist fusion is also performed in younger patients with high functional demand, especially for the scapholunate advanced collapse wrist after late scaphoid collapse and as a salvage procedure after limited carpal fusion. A functional assessment of total wrist fusion was reported.

Methods and Findings.—Twenty patients undergoing total wrist fusion for posttraumatic conditions were included. All reported good pain relief and were satisfied with the position of the fused wrist. All patients said they would have had the procedure sooner. Before fusion, a mean of 3 operations had been attempted. Forty-five percent of the patients had complications. Assessment using the Jebsen and Purdue tests indicated that hand function was poor, possibly because of decreased range of finger movements. Position of fusion, carpal height, and number of joints fused radiologically were uncorrelated with pain score, grip strength, or Buck-Gramcko score.

Conclusion.—Overall, patients are very satisfied with the outcomes of wrist function, although hand function is significantly decreased. A period of immobilization before surgery in an unremovable splint is recommended to determine the best fusion position and to allow patients to get used to the immobile wrist.

► Although this is not a large study, important information is presented. Half of the patients had some continued pain after surgery. Carpal tunnel syndrome occurred postoperatively in 25% of the patients. There was limitation of metaphalangeal joint motion in the fingers of the fused side, and certain activities of daily living were difficult. These findings concur with my observations of patients with wrist fusion. Although the authors found that 65% of their patients required plate removal, I have found that with use of the dynamic compression plate, a much higher percentage of patients eventually require plate removal. This study provides good information for surgeons to tell patients about the outcome of a contemplated wrist fusion.

E.R. North, M.D.

Suggested Reading

Cobb TK, Beckenbaugh RD: Biaxial total-wrist arthroplasty. *J Hand Surg (Am)* 21A:1011–1021, 1996.

▶ This report on 64 cases from the originator of the technique is worth a look, especially for its illustrations of the surgical technique. Rheumatoid arthritis was the diagnosis in each case. At a minimum 5 year's follow-up, 75% had no pain and 62% thought themselves much better. Eleven cases failed, primarily due to loosening of the distal component. Although total-wrist arthroplasty is still no panacea, it has clearly improved. This particular implant now has a track record going on 15 years, and I believe it is worth a look for patients with rheumatoid arthritis who have severe wrist arthritis, good bone stock, good tendons, and who are anxious to preserve wrist motion. Alternative motion sparing procedures, such as radiolunate arthrodesis, should, of course, also be considered in such circumstances. The number of patients satisfying all criteria will necessarily be small, as this series from a large medical center attests; the results in well-selected candidates can nonetheless be quite gratifying.

P.C. Amadio, M.D.

Werner FW, Palmer AK, Somerset JH, et al: Wrist joint motion simulator. *J Orthop Res* 14:639–646, 1996.

▶ This paper presents preliminary results for a computer controlled system to pull on the tendons of cadaver wrists to produce "natural" wrist motion. At this stage in the development of the system, I believe the results are not directly applicable to the clinical treatment of wrist pathologies, but the future studies of clinical problems proposed by the authors will surely yield important insights into the function of the wrist joint.

F.J. Valero-Cuevas, Ph.D.

Carpus

Corrective Osteotomy for Scaphoid Malunion: Technique and Long-term Follow-up Evaluation

Lynch NM, Linscheid RL (Mayo Clinic and Found, Rochester, Minn)
J Hand Surg (Am) 22A:35–43, 1997 8–17

Objective.—Little is known about malunion of scaphoid fractures, although 3 studies suggest that the condition can lead to premature radiocarpal arthrosis. A technique of corrective osteotomy for scaphoid malunion was discussed that corrects the intrascaphoid angles, restores palmar length to the scaphoid, and reduces the dorsal intercalated segment instability (DISI) deformity of the carpus, as well as assessing the long-term clinical and radiographic results. Three cases were presented.

Methods.—Five men, aged 19 to 25 years, underwent corrective osteotomy for scaphoid malunion resulting from a hyperextension injury to the wrist. Patients were followed for an average of 8 years and 9 months.

Technique.—The superficial branches of the radial nerve are accessed through a radial palmar zigzag incision and retracted.

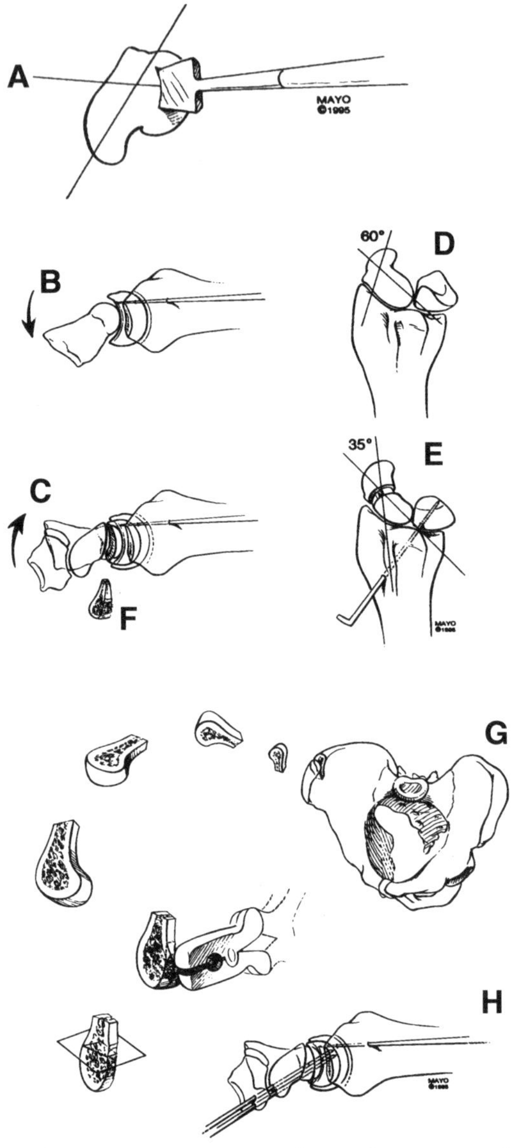

FIGURE 1.—Surgical exposure: **A**, osteotomy; **B**, flexion of wrist to align lunate, which then is transfixed with Kirschner wire; **C**, wrist extended to establish gap at osteotomy; **D** and **E**, anteroposterior schematic; **F**, a modest radial styloidectomy is performed after retracting the radial sensory nerves and radial artery and veins; **G**, tricortical iliac graft cut in trapezoidal fashion planned with the inner surface to reside next to capitate; **H**, graft, fixed and trimmed, is inserted. (Reprinted by permission of Mayo Foundation, from Lynch NM, Linscheid RL: Corrective osteotomy malunion: Technique for scaphoid and long-term follow-up evaluation. *J Hand Surg [Am]* 22A:35–43, 1997).

After retraction of the tendons, the scaphotrapezial joint is incised, and the osteotomy is performed (Fig 1). After the skin and capsule are closed, the arm is placed in a thumb splint and immobilized until radiographic union is demonstrated.

Results.—Wrist flexion improved from an average of 47 degrees preoperatively to 60 degrees postoperatively, extension from 35 to 46 degrees, ulnar deviation from 25 to 30 degrees, and total active range of motion from 127 to 156 degrees. Radial deviation was unchanged at 20 degrees. Mean grip strength improved from 16 kg to 32 kg and wrist score from 19 to 75. The mean lateral intrascaphoid angle was reduced from 39 to 23 degrees and scapholunate angle from 82 to 54 degrees. Three patients had no pain, 1 patient had mild pain and stiffness with athletic activity, and 1 patient with more symptoms is pursuing a workers' compensation claim.

Conclusion.—After the corrective procedure, all patients had improvements in symptoms and in flexion, extension, total active range of motion, and grip strength. Lateral intrascaphoid and scapholunate angles were reduced.

► Scaphoid malunion is now well recognized. Its treatment is not so clear. First, of course, is the question of what to do with the patient who has occasional symptoms. Should anything be done? For patients with more severe symptoms, it seems clear that treatment is indicated. But what treatment? Simple excision of the scaphoid hump? Will osteotomy provide lasting relief? Should a salvage procedure be done?

This article reviews the results of 5 cases of corrective osteotomy for scaphoid malunion. It helps, in that it reassures us that osteotomy can be done with a reasonable expectation of union and with at least short-term symptomatic improvement. The presence of posttraumatic arthritis in all 5 patients is, however, worrisome, but at a follow-up of up to 18 years, does not seem to have been so severe as to have required additional surgery.

I believe this technique of corrective osteotomy is a useful one. I would emphasize the importance of correction of secondary lunate malalignment—which has often been inadequately addressed—not only with malunion but also in cases of long-standing nonunion. I also agree that radial styloidectomy is helpful in eliminating a common site of posttraumatic arthritis. Personally, I would use this technique for significantly symptomatic patients with relatively early malunions and without evidence of posttraumatic arthritis. For patients with few symptoms, I would advise watchful waiting. For patients with arthritic changes and symptoms, scaphoid excision and midcarpal arthrodesis would be my procedure of choice.

P.C. Amadio, M.D.

Revision of Failed Bone Grafting for Nonunion of the Scaphoid: Treatment Options and Results

Smith BS, Cooney WP (Mayo Clinic, Rochester, Minn)
Clin Orthop 327:98–109, 1996 8–18

Background.—The best treatment for failure of bone grafting in scaphoid nonunion has not been established. One experience was reviewed to determine treatment options and outcomes.

Methods.—Twenty-five patients had a second nonunion after a failed initial bone grafting procedure at the Mayo Clinic in a 5-year period. Nineteen patients had a second grafting procedure. Four types of bone grafting procedures were performed based on preoperative assessment: conventional Russe procedures were done in 4 patients, Maltese cross bone graft procedures in 6 (Fig 3), interpositional wedge graft in 5, and vascularized pedicle bone graft in 4. Mean follow-up time was 57 months.

Outcomes.—Eighty-eight percent of the scaphoids united. Although the outcomes were satisfactory, the patients had varying degrees of pain. According to a modified Mayo Wrist Score, results were excellent in 3 patients, good in 5, fair in 10, and poor in 7. However, management involved many long periods of immobilization. There was often a delay in treatment, with a prolonged period of abnormal carpal mechanics.

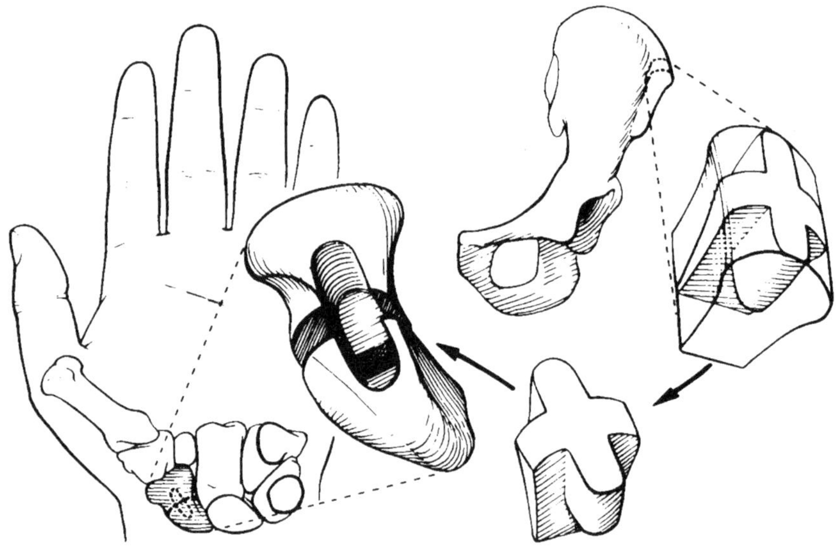

FIGURE 3.—Maltese cross bone graft. Large scaphoid cysts and mild-to-moderate humpback deformity with significant bone resorption is the best indication for this bone graft. A generous trough is created as in the conventional Russe graft. From a tricortical piece of iliac crest harvested at its widest point, a cross-shaped bone graft is carefully sculptured to fit precisely into the defect. The transverse portion will assist in reduction of the humpback deformity. Note, the transverse interpositional portion is slightly deeper than the longitudinal inlay portion. Kirschner wire fixation can be used if needed to supplement graft stabilization. (Courtesy of Smith BS, Cooney WP: Revision of failed bone grafting for nonunion of the scaphoid: Treatment options and results. *Clin Orthop* 327:98–109, 1996.)

Conclusions.—A second bone grafting attempt should be seriously considered for patients with failure of bone grafting in scaphoid nonunion. Success relies on matching the type of bone graft procedure to the specific unique characteristics of scaphoid shortening, carpal instability, and proximal pole vascularity.

► The authors present a logical and realistic approach to this vexing problem. They conclude that undertaking a second attempt at bone grafting the already failed scaphoid bone graft is reasonable. The biggest problem for the hand surgeon is deciding exactly which procedure to perform for one of these patients. The authors, using the combined experience of the Mayo Clinic during a 5-year period, have developed a realistic and practical treatment algorithm. A common problem with articles that describe unusually good results treating extremely difficult conditions is that they boast about their results yet give the reader a paucity of advice. In contrast, this article presents a number of constructive suggestions and is pleasantly self-effacing. The authors describe their Russe and Maltese cross techniques in a way that is quite helpful to the reader. The latter technique is particularly valuable for cases that need inherent bony stability and an opening volar wedge. Their explanation for the interpositional graft is also helpful. Although the authors discuss the dilemma of the avascular proximal pole for which they recommend the Zaidemberg technique,[1] their clinical tips are less helpful than for the other 3 methods. After reading this article, the hand surgeon should be better prepared to deal with the failed scaphoid bone graft. Although bony union is attainable and another surgery can be justified, it certainly is not an easy road, and patients should be warned that dissatisfaction can occur even when the scaphoid successfully unites.

L.B. Lane, M.D.

Reference

1. Zaidemberg C, Siebert JW, Angnigiani C: A new vascularized bone graft for scaphoid nonunion. *J Hand Surg (Am)* 16A:474–478, 1991.

Non-union of the Scaphoid: Treatment With Cannulated Screws Compared With Treatment With Herbert Screws

Trumble TE, Clarke T, Kreder HJ (Univ of Washington, Seattle)

J Bone Joint Surg (Am) 78A:1829–1837, 1996 8–19

Background.—Treating scaphoid nonunion is challenging. Whether screw placement, scaphoid alignment, and screw type are associated with time to scaphoid union and functional outcome were determined.

Methods.—The participants were 34 patients in whom scaphoid nonunion had been treated with bone grafting and internal fixation with 1 of 2 types of screws and with temporary placement of Kirschner wires parallel to the screw to prevent rotation. Sixteen patients (group 1), treated from 1986 through 1989, received a Herbert screw, and 18 patients (group

2), treated from 1990 through 1992, received a 3.5-mm cannulated AO/ASIF screw.

Findings.—Mean time to union, confirmed on tomography, was 7.6 months in group 1 and 3.6 months in group 2, a significant difference. In both groups, the alignment of the scaphoid was significantly improved, and carpal collapse was reduced. Time to union was significantly shorter when screw placement was in the central third of the scaphoid, regardless of screw type. Seventeen of the 18 cannulated screws and only 7 of the 16 Herbert screws had been placed centrally.

Conclusions.—Mean time to scaphoid union after fixation with the AO/ASIF cannulated screw was shorter than that after Herbert screw use. The rate of central placement in the proximal pole of the scaphoid was greater for the former type of screw. The postoperative improvement of scaphoid and carpal alignment was maintained at the latest follow-up assessment. Overall improvement of range of motion resulted from improved alignment of the lateral intrascaphoid angle.

▶ The authors compared 2 types of screws in the operative treatment of scaphoid nonunions. They found that central location of the screw in the proximal fragment leads to faster healing. To compare the effect of screw types, one should analyze the 7 centrally placed Herbert screws with the 17 centrally placed AO/ASIF cannulated screws. Unfortunately this comparison cannot be gleaned from presented data.

W. Engber, M.D.

Apparent and Partial Non-union of the Scaphoid

Barton NJ (Nottingham Univ, England)

J Hand Surg (Br) 21B:496–500, 1996 8–20

Background.—Sometimes during surgery for nonunion of the scaphoid, the scaphoid appears to be united. The outcomes of 1 group of such patients were reviewed.

Patients and Outcomes.—Surgical exploration was done in 10 patients with radiologic evidence of nonunion of the scaphoid and 4 with suspected nonunion. In 10 patients, there appeared to be complete union, although the supposed site of fracture could just be discerned in most patients, usually as a dark line on the articular cartilage. In the remaining 4 patients, part of the fracture site was visible at surgery, although no movement between the 2 halves of the scaphoid could be elicited. These findings suggested that the fractures had united across part of the surface. Five of the 10 scaphoids that appeared united at surgery went on to definite union and 5 to nonunion. All 4 thought to be partly united went on to union. The conclusion that no graft or screw was needed proved correct in less than half the cases.

Conclusion.—A fractured scaphoid may look nonunited on a radiograph and united at operation. Those appearing to be united at surgery may later prove to be nonunited. During surgery, the fracture site must be probed and preferably windowed. In doubtful cases, CT scanning is probably the most useful study technique.

▶ Barton describes his experience with 14 apparent nonunions of the scaphoid that were explored surgically by this very experienced hand surgeon. He found that even under direct vision, it was difficult to tell whether the scaphoid was healed. The surgeon in practice is therefore faced with 2 difficult questions: (1) to explore or not to explore a symptomatic patient who has a scaphoid that appears by x-ray studies to be healed and (2) if at surgery the scaphoid appears to be healed, what is the appropriate treatment. Barton concludes that long-axis CT of the scaphoid is probably the best method for determining union, and I agree. However, even this technique is not sufficient proof because internal fixation devices and other metal artifacts, such as screws, can obscure detail at the fracture site.

It is comforting to me, if not to the patients, to know that, even in experienced hands, this remains a conundrum. My approach has been to explore by CT patients who do not have at least 50% union. If the scaphoid appears healed at surgery, I try to find the nonunion site, with a Freer Elevator and fill any defects with cancellous bone, even if there is no clinical motion between the fragments.

L.K. Ruby, M.D.

Ununited Proximal Pole Scaphoid Fractures: Treatment With a Herbert Screw in 16 Cases Followed For 0.5–8 Years

Inoue G, Shionoya K, Kuwahata Y (Nagoya Univ, Japan; Kuwahata Orthopaedic Clinic, Hamaoka, Japan)

Acta Orthop Scand 68:124–127, 1997 8–21

Background.—Treatment of delayed unions and nonunions of the proximal third of the scaphoid has been debated. Recommended treatment includes bone grafting with or without internal fixation; pulsed electromagnetic fields and casting; vascularized bone grafting; excision of the proximal fragment and replacement with a prosthesis or allograft; and salvage procedures such as resection arthroplasty or partial or total arthrodesis of the wrist. Herbert introduced a headless compression screw in 1984 to obtain stable fixation. Herbert advocated its use in proximal pole nonunions of the scaphoid, with proximal-to-distal insertion through a dorsal approach.

Methods.—There were 16 patients with delayed unions and nonunions of the proximal third of the scaphoid. A bone graft and Herbert screw internal fixation were used with dorsal proximal-to-distal insertion. The patients were between 17 and 43 years of age. The median follow-up was 2 years.

Results.—Definite union was achieved in 13 patients. Compared with the uninvolved wrist, the average wrist flexion-extension range of motion was 83%, and the average grip strength was 90%. In the 13 patients with definite union, grip strength was 92% of that in the uninvolved wrist. Ten patients had no pain and 3 had mild pain with strenuous use of the wrist. The 3 patients in whom union was not achieved had moderate pain. Of the 16 patients, 15 returned to their previous occupation and 1 was able to do light work. Overall function was excellent in 5 patients, good in 5, fair in 5, and poor in 1. In 3 patients, misplacement of the screw occurred; 2 of these patients did not achieve bony union and had fair or poor outcome.

Discussion.—In these patients with nonunion of the proximal pole scaphoid, this technique offered a short period of immobilization and good function. Placement of the screw is easier in a distal-to-proximal direction, but a proximal pole fracture should also be treated by the retrograde insertion method. This technique can be used in cases of mild-to-moderate ischemic changes of the proximal fragment, but severe ischemic changes with sclerosis, fragmentation, or deformation of the proximal fragment are contraindications. Misplacement of the screw can result in union failure.

▶ This article confirms our own experience with the treatment of this most difficult fracture with a Herbert screw, inserted retrograde, and cancellous bone grafting. This is an elegant, quick, and reliable treatment. I also share the authors' experience with successful fracture surgery in spite of decreased signal intensity within the proximal fragment as shown on MRI. I was disappointed that reference was not made to a previous publication using this same technique[1] and to the Herbert[2] and Alnot et al.[3] papers advocating a similar approach to treating these fractures.

J. Taleisnik, M.D.

References

1. DeMaagd RL, Engberg WD: Retrograde Herbert screw fixation for treatment of proximal pole scaphoid nonunions. *J Hand Surg (Am)* 14A:996–1003, 1989.
2. Herbert TJ: Use of the Herbert bone screw in surgery of the wrist. *Clin Orthop* 202:79–92, 1986.
3. Alnot JY, Bellan N, Oberlin C, et al: Fractures and nonunions of the proximal pole of the carpal scaphoid bone: Internal fixation by a proximal to distal screw. *Ann Chir Main* 7:101–108, 1988.

Experience With Scaphoid Grafting

Barton NJ (Queen's Med Centre, Nottingham, England)
J Hand Surg (Br) 22B:153–160, 1997 8–22

Introduction.—Most studies have judged the success of bone grafting for nonunion of the scaphoid radiologically; few have based assessments on clinical results. One surgeon's experience over 24 years with varying types of bone grafting operations used in 150 ununited scaphoid fractures was reported.

Methods.—The following methods were used to graft nonunion of the scaphoid in just about equal numbers of patients during a 24-year period: original Russe graft, wedge graft and Herbert screw, modified Russe graft (in patients without dorsiflexed intercalated segment instability [DISI]) and modified Fisk's procedure (anterior wedge graft held by Kirshner wires instead of a Herbert screw). Patients in whom bony union could not be determined by radiography underwent CT scans. Radiologic categories evaluated at 12 months were union, uncertain, and nonunion. Clinical categories were based on range of movement, grip strength, activity level, and pain symptoms and were as follows: little or no pain (occasional pain on strenuous exertion or aching in cold weather, but no restriction of activities); less pain; same pain; or worse pain.

Results.—The wedge graft and Herbert screw yielded the best results radiologically (78% definite union). The worst results radiologically were observed with the original Russe operation. Clinical and radiologic outcomes frequently did not coincide. Pain was diminished by all 4 surgical approaches, but the modified Russe was most successful in achieving the rating of little or no pain. Patients regained the most movement with the modified Russe procedure. Recovery of grip strength and activity were best achieved with the Herbert screw and wedge graft.

Discussion/Conclusion.—One of the most striking findings in this series was the discrepancy between clinical and radiologic results. Explanations can only be speculative. Recommendations are as follows: treat nonunion of the wrist without DISI by modified Russe or dorsal approach, cancellous graft, and fixation by either Kirschner wires or Herbert screw; treat nonunion of the wrist with DISI with an anterior wedge graft held by a Herbert screw; and treat nonunion of the proximal pole with cancellous graft and freehand Herbert mini-screw from the proximal end.

▶ Dr. Barton's article is a benchmark in the treatment of scaphoid nonunion. Not only does it underline the inherent difficulties of confirming a scaphoid union, it highlights the discrepancy between clinical and radiologic results. Comparing the 4 techniques of scaphoid grafting for wrist nonunions, his data support Herbert screw fixation and volar wedge grafting as the superior approach compared with modified Russe grafting by the following measurements: the union rate (78% compared with 55%), symptom score (96% vs. 86%), grip strength loss (8% vs. 13%), and impairment of daily activities (9% vs. 15%). Some of these improved results may relate to the correction of the scaphoid collapse, which is easier with a volar intercolary wedge graft. Final wrist motion was not different between the grips, but this relates to the fact that even screwed scaphoids were immobilized an average of 8 weeks.

Dr. Barton raises concerns of late arthritis caused by scaphoid-trapezoidal joint mobilization necessary to insert the screw. No study has yet shown this to be a significant clinical problem—including a 10-year follow-up in 100 patients by yours truly. Such a problem may be more common in women and may require at least a 20-year follow-up to become clinically evident. An alternative to mobilizing the scapho-trapezial joint is to excise the tubercle of the trapezium with an osteotome. This allows a direct shot without joint mobilization.

Dr. Barton also questions a technical difficulty with the Herbert procedure. This may be particularly true if the scaphoid is cashew-shaped, (10% of scaphoids are). In that situation, Kirshner wire fixation may be a better option. Finally, the author addresses the problem of the proximal pole nonunion and admits that despite the Herbert screw or its miniaturized version (I certainly agree that this mini-version is more appropriate in this situation), did not solve this "problem." Perhaps this is because the problem relates even more specifically to the vascularity of the proximal fragment than to pure mechanical stability. The study did not address this. Currently, with proximal pole nonunions, I get an MR image. If the pole is avascular, a vascularized pedicle graft is used along with mini-screw fixation.

The ultimate take-home message from this article is that not all scaphoid nonunions are the same; thus, the surgeon should master not only volar Herbert screw/wedge grafting for collapsed nonunions with DISI, but also dorsal approaches for an undisplaced scaphoid nonunion, vascularized grafting for proximal pole nonunions, and Kirshner wire fixation for a comminuted or narrow-shaped scaphoid.

A.L. Osterman, M.D.

Radiographically Occult Scaphoid Fractures: Value of MR Imaging in Detection

Breitenseher MJ, Metz VM, Gilula LA, et al (Univ of Vienna; Washington Univ, St Louis)

Radiology 203:245–250, 1997 8–23

Background.—The diagnosis of scaphoid fracture is often delayed until 2 weeks after trauma, when follow-up radiography shows the "initially occult" scaphoid fracture because of resorption and better demarcation around the fracture line. The diagnostic value of MRI in 42 patients with clinically suspected scaphoid fractures and normal initial plain radiographs was assessed.

Methods.—The patients underwent MRI within 7 days of trauma. T1-weighted spin-echo. T2*-weighted gradient-echo, and short inversion time inversion-recovery (STIR) sequences were done. Radiographs were obtained again at 6 weeks.

Findings.—Magnetic resonance images showed occult fractures of the scaphoid bone in 33% of the patients, the capitate bone in 10%, the trapezium in 2%, and the distal radius in 5% (Fig 2). All wrist fractures were identified by combined STIR and T1-weighted spin-echo sequences.

The 2 radiologists examining the images were in almost perfect agreement, with sensitivities and specificities of 100% each for the first radiologist and 95% and 100%, respectively, for the second radiologist.

Conclusion.—Magnetic resonance imaging has a high sensitivity as the second diagnostic procedure in radiographically detecting occult fractures of the scaphoid and other wrist bones. This imaging modality may enable earlier diagnosis and treatment of scaphoid fractures.

► When a clinical suspicion of scaphoid fracture exists, but plain x-ray films are unrevealing, options include radionuclide scanning and tomography. Usually, trispiral or CT images are used—the former less often nowadays, as the equipment is no longer manufactured. These authors report success using MRI for the same purpose. It would be nice to know which method is most cost effective and has the greatest diagnostic sensitivity: radionuclide scanning, CT, or MRI.

P.C. Amadio, M.D.

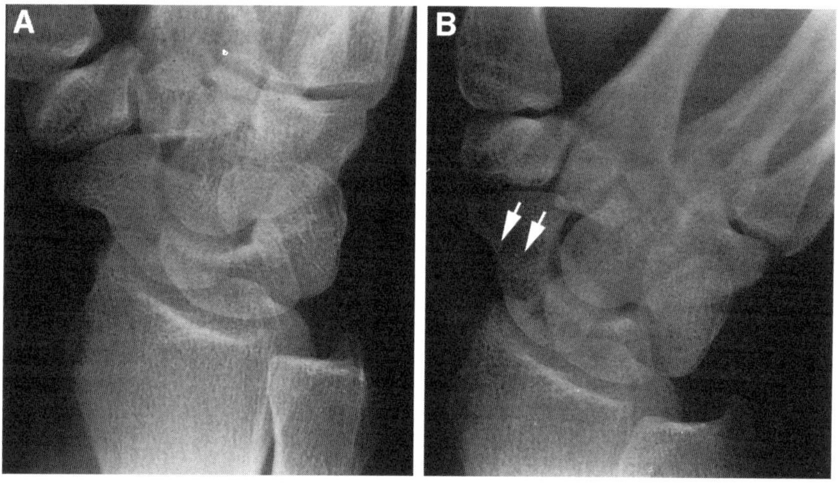

FIGURE 2.—Radiographically occult midthird scaphoid fracture in an 18-year-old man. **A,** initial radiograph of the scaphoid shows no fracture. **B,** radiograph of the scaphoid obtained at 6-week follow-up shows a midthird scaphoid fracture (*arrows*). **C,** coronal T1-weighted (500/20) image of the scaphoid obtained 3 days after trauma shows a hypointense trabecular fracture line in the midthird and proximal third of the scaphoid (*arrows*) with adjacent bone marrow abnormality (*arrowheads*). **D,** coronal T2*-weighted gradient-echo (60/17,20° flip angle) image demonstrates minimal increased signal intensity at this region, indicating bone marrow abnormality (*arrowheads*). The fracture line is not clearly depicted. **E,** coronal fast short inversion time inversion-recovery image (1,200/13/130) shows highly increased signal intensity of bone marrow abnormality (*arrowheads*). The trabecular fracture line (*straight arrow*) is less (*Continued*)

FIGURE 2 (cont.)

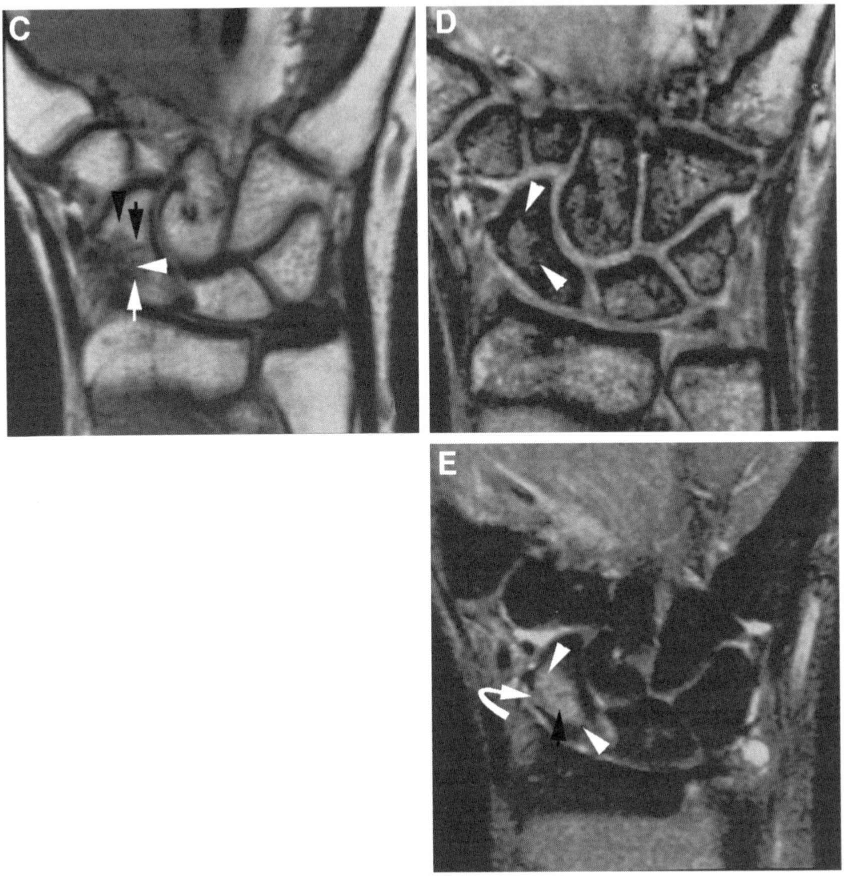

visible than in C; however, involvement of the cortex is clearly demonstrated (*curved arrow*). (Courtesy of Breitenseher MJ, Metz VM, Gilula LA, et al: Radiographically occult scaphoid fractures: Value of MR imaging in detection. *Radiology* 203:245–250. Copyright 1997, Radiological Society of North America.)

External Fixation and Cancellous Bone Grafting for Kienböck's Disease: A Preliminary Report

Zelouf DS, Ruby LK (Tufts Univ, Boston; Med College of Virginia, Richmond)
J Hand Surg (Am) 21A:746–753, 1996 8–24

Background.—The cause of Kienböck's disease is elusive, and its treatment is controversial. Lichtman stages I, II, and III Kienböck's disease have been treated with a combination of cancellous bone grafting and external fixation since 1985 at the study institution. The results of this procedure for the first 17 patients treated were assessed.

Patients.—Diagnosis in 16 patients was via clinical examination and plain radiography; 1 patient also required MRI. Lichtman stage I disease was present in 1 wrist, stage II disease in 9, stage IIIa in 5, and stage IIIb in 2. Preoperative carpal height ratio averaged 0.50, in contrast to the reported normal ratio of 0.54 ± 0.03.

Technique.—A longitudinal skin incision is made ulnar to Lister's tubercle; the extensor retinaculum over the third dorsal wrist compartment is incised, and Lister's tubercle is removed. The dorsal wrist capsule is exposed by radial and ulnar subperiosteal dissection. The wrist joint is opened longitudinally, exposing the proximal carpal row and dorsal pole of the lunate. A high-speed burr is used to make a small window in the lunate and then to curettage the avascular lunate. (Hand-held curettings of the lunate are first obtained for histologic examination.) Any possibly thermally damaged bone is removed after high-speed burring. When bleeding bone is visualized, the defect is filled with cancellous bone from the ipsilateral distal radius or the iliac crest. Curettage is carried to the subchondral bone if pink or red bone was not exposed. An external fixator is then placed across the wrist; distraction creating a 2-mm space between the lunate and the corresponding articular surface of the radius is produced and the fixator left in place for up to 12 weeks (Fig 1).

Results.—Duration of external fixation averaged 9.8 weeks. Kienböck's disease was confirmed in all 17 patients via histology. Follow-up was performed at an average of 4.7 years. The overall success rate was 71%. Fourteen patients were able to return to regular employment. Two patients showed poor results and underwent additional surgery: 1 underwent a proximal row carpectomy and 1 an arthrodesis of the scaphoid, capitate, and lunate articulations. A third patient with poor results has moderate pain but does not believe that his symptoms are severe enough (after 4.5 years) to warrant further surgery.

Conclusions.—This procedure is not technically demanding, does not significantly limit range of motion, and does not permanently alter carpal kinematics or the relationship between the radius and ulna. Furthermore, it "burns no bridges," yields results comparable with those of other modalities, and offers an alternative procedure in the ulnar-neutral or ulnar-positive variant. Disadvantages include lack of complete predictability and prolonged use of the external fixator. These workers no longer use this procedure in patients who have demonstrated collapse; the procedure is used only for stage I and II disease.

▶ Distraction external fixation and cancellous bone grafting of lunate is advocated for Kienböck's disease by the authors with not necessarily superior but commensurate results with other surgical treatment modalities such as joint-leveling procedures, intercarpal arthrodeses, and revascularization procedures. It has advantages, as noted by the authors, in that it is not technically demanding, it does not significantly limit motion, it does not alter carpal kinematics, it burns no bridges because other procedures can subsequently be performed, and it offers an alternative in the ulnar-neutral or ulnar-positive variants. But, also as noted by the authors, the results were unpredictable. I wonder how they could have a minimal follow-up length of

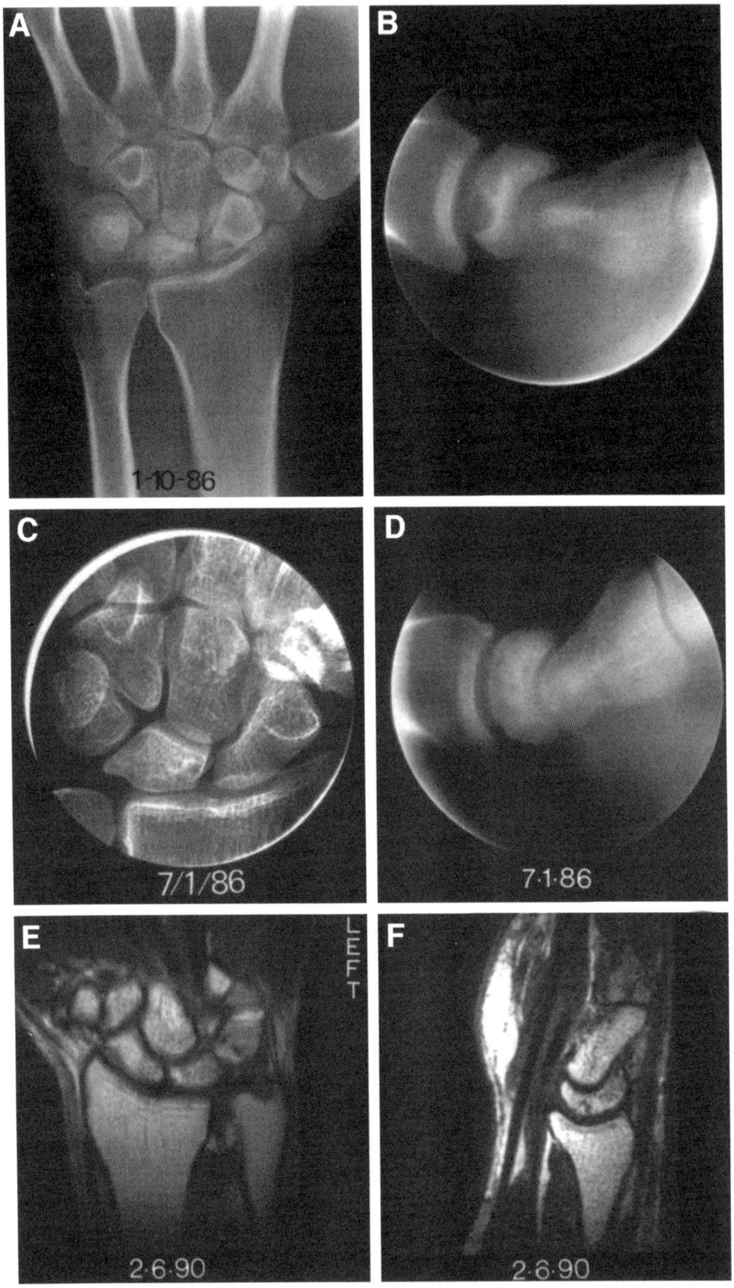

FIGURE 1.—**A**, posteroanterior radiograph shows stage II Kienböck's disease; **B**, lateral tomogram showing cyst and subchondral fracture of the lunate; **C**, posteroanterior radiograph showing healing of lunate 3 years and 3 months after surgery for application of external fixator and cancellous bone grafting; **D**, lateral tomogram showing healing of cyst and subchondral fracture of lunate; **E,F**, MR images at 4 years showing revascularization of lunate. (Courtesy of Zelouf DS, Ruby LK: External fixation and cancellous bone grafting for Kienböck's disease: A preliminary report. *J Hand Surg [Am]* 21A:746–753, 1996.)

2 years when at least 1 of the cases required a second procedure (scaphoid, capitate, and lunate fusion) at 13 months after the original procedure. Either the follow-up result was that of scaphoid, capitate, and lunate fusion, or there was a statistical error. I also wonder whether the diagnosis of the only case report presented with various imagings was a true Kienböck's disease or a simple bone cyst. Even though the authors claim the diagnosis was confirmed in all 17 patients by histology, how could one differentiate Kienböck's from regional sclerosis around a bone cyst histologically? I agree with the authors' final conclusion, however, that the procedure can be considered in the precollapsed lunate (not for stage III but for stage I and II disease only), especially in ulnar-neutral and ulnar-positive variants.

J. Ryu, M.D.

Kienböck's Disease in Children

Kim TY, Culp RW, Osterman AL, et al (Philadelphia)

1996 Jefferson Orthopaedic J 25:53–57, 1996 8–25

Objective.—Kienböck's disease in children is rare and appears to behave differently than in adults. Suggestions for treatment of Kienböck's disease in children were discussed.

Methods.—A retrospective review of medical records of 7 children (3 males), aged 9 to 15, with Kienböck's disease, revealed no specific injury leading to wrist pain in any of the patients. Five patients had a negative ulnar variance and 2 had a neutral variance. Two patients had stage II disease and 5 had stage IIIa disease. The average duration of symptoms was 7.3 months. The 3 younger patients were treated with a cast for 1 to 3 months followed by splint immobilization for up to 9 months. The 4 older patients failed immobilization. Two had capitate shortening osteotomies, and 2 with negative ulnar variance had radial shortening osteotomies with bone grafting to the lunate. Patients were followed for 12 to 96 months.

Results.—At last follow-up, the 3 younger patients were participating in full activities without wrist pain and had less than 1-mm loss of height at the radial aspect of the lunate; 2 of them had complete revascularization of the lunate. Grip strength was 71% to 100% of normal and an arc of wrist extension-flexion was within 15 degrees of the unaffected wrist. Three of the 4 older children had no wrist pain during full activities, an arc of wrist extension-flexion averaging 55 degrees, and a grip strength of 67% to 86% of the unaffected side. One older child had occasional wrist pain.

Conclusion.—Kienböck's disease in children younger than 12 years appears to resolve completely with immobilization. Kienböck's disease in older children tends to behave as in adults and requires surgical treatment.

► I agree with these authors that Kienböck's disease seen in children under age 12 years might call for a nonoperative approach. Those 12 years of age or older have pretty much completed the lunate growth, and I believe it is appropriate to treat them as one would an adult.

P.C. Amadio, M.D.

Treatment of Kienböck's Disease With Vascular Bundle Implantation and Temporary Triscaphe Arthrodesis: A Preliminary Report [Italian]

Ceruso M, Beltrami G, Marin E (Ospedale San Maria Nuova, Firenze, Italy)

Riv Chir Riab Mano Arto Sup 33:11–14, 1996 8–26

Background.—Six cases of grade III Kienböck's disease treated with curettage, cancellous bone grafting, and vascular bundle implantation into the lunate are discussed.

Methods.—A temporary triscaphe fixation was associated by means of K wires percutaneous pinning. K wires were removed 6 months after the operation. At subsequent controls all patients were evaluated with standard x-rays, tomography, and MRI.

Findings.—Lunate reconstruction was successful in five cases; in one case, lunate collapse was observed 2 months after the operation, following an untimely mobilization of the K wires.

Conclusion.—At the last follow-up (average, 16 months), 4 of the successful cases were rated as good and one as fair, according to Lichtman and Evans criteria.

▶ Revascularization of the lunate is one of the treatment options of grade III Kienböck's disease, according to the experimental studies of Saldana et al.[1] and Hory et al.[2] This procedure is associated with scapho-trapezio-trapezoid (STT) or scaphocapitate (SC) fusion or with an external skeletal fixation applied to reduce axial load on the soft revascularized bone. This article reports on the possibility of temporarily unloading the lunate using percutanous pinning of the STT or SC joint during the time needed for the revascularization to take place. The revascularization is obtained by implantation of the second dorsal metacarpal vascular bundle into the lunate. Satisfactory results are reported that confirm similar reports on two cases by Yajima et al.[3] The advantages of the procedure described here are to avoid a permanent alteration of scaphoid kinematics as it is produced by STT fusion or the discomfort caused by a long-lasting exernal fixation.

M. Ceruso, M.D.

References

1. Saldana MJ, Niebauer JJ, Brown R, et al: Microsurgical revascularization of ischemic rat femoral heads. *J Hand Surg (Am)* 15:309–315, 1990.
2. Hory Y, Tamai S, Okuda H, et al: Blood vessel transplantation to bone. *J Hand Surg (Am)* 4A:23–33, 1979.
3. Yajima H, Tamai S, Mizumoto S, et al: Treatment of Kienböck's disease with vascular bundle implantation and triscaphe arthrodesis, in Nakamura R, Linscheid RL, Miura T (eds): *Wrist Disorders*. Tokyo, Springer-Verlag, 1992, pp 101–109.

Shortening Osteotomy of the Radius for the Treatment of Kienböck's Disease: Review of 20 Cases [Spanish]

Botelheiro JC (Hospital Ortopédico "Santa Ana" Parede, Portugal)

Rev Esp Cir Mano 23:7–15, 1996 8–27

Introduction.—There are 4 radiologic stages of the lunate bone, including grade I as no radiographic changes; grade II as irregular condensation; grade IIIa as lunate collapse with carpal collapse and grade IIIb lunate collapse without carpal collapse; and grade IV as degenerative arthritis. Ulnar lengthening osteotomies were used to treat this, but in the majority of patients with Kienböck's disease, the ulna was shorter. Radial shortening osteotomies were performed on 20 patients, particularly those with neutral ulnar variance and carpal collapse. The procedure is based on the same principles as ulnar lengthening osteotomy to avoid the high complication rate of nonunions of the lengthened ulna.

Methods.—Radial shortening osteotomy was performed on 20 patients with Kienböck's disease and their charts and radiographs were reviewed. There were 13 patients with grade IIIa, 5 patients with grade IIIb, and 2 with grade IV. There was a shorter ulna in 11 patients. None of the patients had a longer ulna than the radius. Follow-up was conducted up to 7 years after the procedure.

Results.—In 18 patients, pain was improved, and in 2 patients, 1 with stage IV and 1 with a stage IIIa disease, it was unchanged. Six patients had radiographic progression of the disease, whereas no significant changes were seen in the other 8 patients. There was a slight improvement in the lunate morphological in the remaining 6 patients. Reoperations were performed on 9 patients. Three of those patients had delayed union in diaphyseal osteotomies and 6 had dorsal plate removal.

Conclusion.—There are fewer lower complication rates with distal metaphyseal osteotomies than with dorsal metaphyseal osteotomies. A distal metaphyseal osteotomy through an anterior approach and internally fixed with a T-plate will result in the lowest complication rate. Although radiographic appearance worsened in most patients, pain relief was evident in most patients. The natural course of the disease may not be influenced by osteotomy, and the pain may be relieved by denervating capsular structures and bone from the osteotomy.

▶ This is a well-detailed paper on the results of 20 radial shortening osteotomies for the treatment of Kienböck's disease. Although it is difficult to draw statistical conclusions from a review of just 20 cases, many conclusions can be made after reading this detailed and accurate review. The first conclusion is that distal metaphyseal osteotomies give lower complication rates than distal diaphyseal osteotomies. Of the 11 patients with dorsal metaphyseal osteotomies, 6 had to have their plates removed because of discomfort, and 1 had a delayed extensor pollicis longus tendon rupture. It can be concluded that the lowest complication rate will be obtained by doing a distal metaphyseal osteotomy through an anterior approach and internally fixed with a T-plate.

It is very interesting to observe that most of the patients experienced pain relief, while the radiographic appearance was unchanged or even worsened in the majority. This makes us think that the osteotomy may not influence the natural course of the disease, but rather relieve pain after denervation of capsular structures and bone from the osteotomy. Similar results are observed after proximal tibial osteotomies for the treatment of medial compartment degenerative arthritis of the knee, in which good clinical results can be obtained in spite of further deterioration of the joint. Another observation in favor of this hypothesis is that radial closing wedge osteotomies have proved to provide good clinical results, in spite of the fact that some studies have shown that this procedure has no effect on lunate stress reduction. A radial open wedge osteotomy is probably more effective in decreasing the load on the lunate, as the radius is brought into closer contact with the scaphoid. However, the compressive forces to the lunate will be transferred from the radius to the distal end of the ulna, which will be detrimental in the presence of an ulnar plus situation. The good results reported after a closing wedge can also be explained from the fact that the carpus has to ulnar deviate for the patient to align the fingers with the longitudinal axis of the forearm. By ulnar deviating the carpal bones, a better coverage of the lunate will be obtained, as well as a partial correction of its flexed deformity, as the scaphoid extends when the wrist goes into ulnar deviation. Some confusion can be observed in the literature when referring to the inclination of the distal articular facet of the radius in the coronal plane (anteroposterior view on radiographs), as it is frequently called radial inclination, when it should be described as ulnar inclination.

A. Lluch, M.D., Ph.D.

Suggested Reading

DeCoulx P, Marchand M, Minét P, et al: La maladie de Kienböck chez le Mineur. Etude clinique et pathogenique (avec analyse de 1330 radios du poignet). *Lille Chir* 12:65–81, 1957.

García-Elías M: (letter). *J Bone Joint Surg (Am)* 74A:1431, 1992.

Litchman DM, Degman GG: Staging and its use in the determination of treatment modalities for Kienböck's disease. *Hand Clin* 9:409–416, 1993.

Miura H, Uchida Y, Sugioka Y: Radial closing wedge osteotomy for Kienböck's disease. *J Hand Surg (Am)* 21A:1029–1034, 1996.

Nakamura R, Tsuge S, Watanabe K, et al: Radial wedge osteotomy for Kienböck's disease. *J Bone Joint Surg (Am)* 73A:1391–1396, 1991.

Quenzer DE, Dobyns JH, Linscheid RL, et al: Radial recession osteotomy for Kienböck's disease. *J Hand Surg (Am)* 22A:386–395, 1997.

Watanabe K, Nakamura R, Horii E, et al: Biomechanical analysis of radial wedge osteotomy for the treatment of Kienböck's disease. *J Hand Surg (Am)* 18A:686–690, 1993.

A Critical Look at Intercarpal Arthrodesis: Review of the Literature

Siegel JM, Ruby LK (Tufts Univ, Boston; Southern Sports Medicine and Orthopaedic Ctr, Nashville, Tenn)

J Hand Surg (Am) 21A:717–723, 1996 8–28

Background.—Limited intercarpal arthrodesis can be performed in various combinations for painful conditions of selected carpal bones. The outcomes of each type of arthrodesis and their comparison in terms of nonunion, rate of complications, postoperative grip strength, range of motion, and pain relief were investigated through a review of the English language literature between 1924 and 1994.

Methods.—True meta-analysis could not be performed; most reports in the literature were retrospective reviews.

Results.—For scaphotrapezium-trapezoid arthrodesis (258 patients), the average follow-up was 38 months. Nonunion rate was 13%; the complication rate was not reported by all authors, but those reported averaged 43%. Lunotriquetal arthrodesis (143 patients) was associated with an average follow-up of 17 months, a 26% nonunion rate, and a 43% complication rate. Scapholunate arthrodesis was reported for 16 patients; follow-up averaged 45 months, nonunion occurred in 10 of 16, and complications were reported in 2 of 10. Scaphocapitolunate arthrodesis was reported for 33 patients; follow-up averaged 30 months, nonunion rate was 12%, and complications occurred in 3 of 24. Capitolunate arthrodesis was reported for 29 patients; follow-up averaged 55 months, nonunion rate was 35%, and complication rate was 62%. Scaphocapitate arthrodesis was reported for 17 patients; nonunion occurred in 2 of 17 and the complication rate was 11.8%. Capitohamate-lunotriquetal arthrodesis was reported for 138 patients; follow-up averaged 40 months, nonunion rate was 4.3%, and the complication rate was 26.5%.

Conclusions.—This method of data gathering has several inherent flaws. The manner in which objective data were reported varied widely. Complications were not always reported, and some included nonunion whereas others did not (these workers differentiated nonunion whenever possible). Subjective reporting of pain was considered a positive result regardless of reported degree. The lowest rates of nonunion occurred with the arthrodeses involving the greatest surface area. Complete relief of postoperative wrist pain occurred in only 47% of all patients. Postoperative function appears more dependent on pain relief than on objective measurements.

▶ The authors reviewed the previously reported data on various intercarpal arthrodeses to obtain a clearer understanding of the outcomes of each type of arthrodesis, focusing on complications. This type of literature review has inherent flaws, which are well described in the paper. Furthermore, such a study stands only with the assumption that the same surgical technique with the same level of surgical fluency has been used by all surgeons involved in all previous literature. Nonetheless, I agree with the several conclusions they made: (1) the arthrodeses that involve the greatest surface area have the lowest rates of nonunion; (2) arthrodeses that cross the midcarpal row limit range of motion more; and (3) only 47% of patients who underwent any type of intercarpal arthrodesis had complete relief of their preoperative wrist pain, which has a strong correlation with functional ability. I would like to mention, however, that I have many patients who have occasional, residual pain—much less than preoperatively—and are happy that they underwent limited arthrodesis because of the limited yet present motion of their wrists.

J. Ryu, M.D.

Nonunion Rates of Limited Carpal Arthrodesis: A Meta-analysis of the Literature

Larsen CF, Jacoby RA, McCabe SJ (Natl Univ Hosp, Copenhagen; Univ of Louisville, Ky)

J Hand Surg (Am) 22A:66–73, 1997 8–29

Background.—Limited intercarpal arthrodeses are performed to treat disorders of the carpus, but wide variability has been reported in the nonunion rate, both within and between types of arthrodeses. This may be caused, at least in part, by the small number of cases included in most studies. A review was performed of the English language medical literature on limited intercarpal arthrodeses. A 95% confidence interval (CI) was calculated for each article, and these results were combined with those of similar cases. An overall nonunion rate was calculated with a 95% CI.

Study Design.—Reported cases of limited intercarpal arthrodesis were collected by computerized search of the English language medical literature from 1966 to 1993, review of surgical textbooks, and review of reference lists from relevant articles and book chapters. From each article, data on carpal bones included in the arthrodesis, publication date, patient number, number of good results as defined by the author of the paper, number of nonunions, donor bone graft site, and indications for and length of follow-up were retrieved. There were an average of 10 patients described in each article.

Results.—Of the 385 scaphotrapezium-trapezoid arthrodeses analyzed, there was a 14% nonunion rate, with a 95% CI of 11% to 18%. Of the 104 lunotriquethral arthrodeses analyzed, there was a 27% nonunion rate, with a 95% CI of 19% to 36%. Of the 17 scapholunte arthrodeses analyzed, there was a 47% nonunion rate, with a 95% CI of 26% to 69%.

Conclusion.—The difficulty in diagnosing nonunion of the scaphoid, as well as the bias in the literature against reporting negative results, suggests that the reported rates of nonunion may be optimistic. Despite this potential positive bias, nonunion rates are high for many commonly used arthrodeses. However, nonunion does not necessarily imply poor outcome, as many nonunion patients had good results. This reemphasizes the importance of patient-oriented outcomes in clinical research.

▶ This very useful summary of the literature on intercarpal arthrodesis comes as close as we probably will ever get to a realistic portrait of union rates. Perhaps these authors will do the same for functional results and indications.

P.C. Amadio, M.D.

A Surgical Technique to Align the Wrist Central Column

Higgs PE, Gilula LA, Weeks PM (Washington Univ, St Louis)

J Hand Surg (Am) 21A:724–726, 1996 8–30

Background.—Alignment of the capitolunoradius or capitolunate axes is important in certain operative procedures of the wrist, especially when attempting to reduce or align the carpus with chronic carpal instabilities or when treating severe dislocations of the lunate or perilunate structures. Some authors have reported good results by performing scapholunate reduction and fixation first, followed by scaphocapitate fixation. However, this sequence can be technically frustrating. A practical approach to aligning the capitate, lunate, and radius was presented.

Technique.—Obtaining comparison views of the noninjured wrist before surgery can be useful for determining normal alignment configuration. General or block anesthesia is induced for the procedure. Because smaller wires may be broken by minor wrist movement, a 1.6-mm or greater Kirschner (K)-wire is used. The

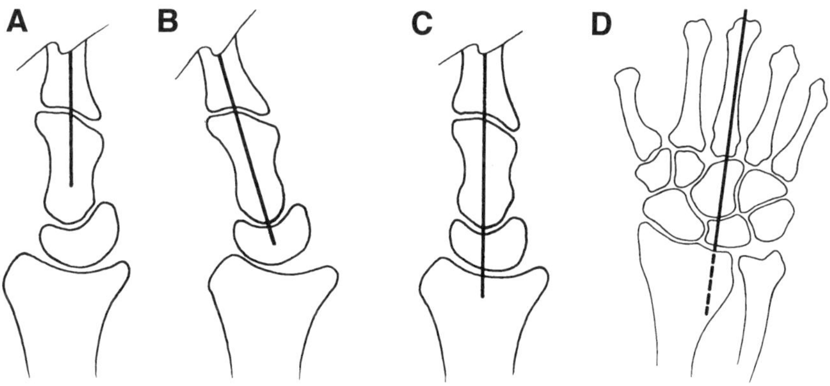

FIGURE 1.—Drawing of dorsal intercalated segment instability pattern. **A**, K-wire is passed down the axis of the metacarpal into the capitate. **B**, the metacarpocapitate unit is manipulated to align the axis of the capitate with the lunate. The wire is then advanced into the lunate. **C**, the metacarpocapitolunate unit is aligned with the radius and the wire is advanced into the radius. **D**, alternatively, the K-wire may be placed from radial or ulnar side of the metacarpal. (Courtesy of Higgs PE, Gilula LA, Weeks PM: A surgical technique to align the wrist central column. *J Hand Surg [Am]* 21A:724–726, 1996.)

surgeon passes the wire down the shaft of the long finger metacarpal into the capitate, then advances it to the proximal cortex of the capitate. Because the dorsal concavity of the capitate is exaggerated in some patients, the surgeon takes care to ensure that the pin remains in the axis of the capitate and has not exited through the dorsal concavity of the capitate waist. The capitate is reduced on the lunate under fluoroscopic control by manipulating the wrist to achieve neutral alignment, which may require extending, flexing, or deviating the wrist radially or ulnarly. After the capitate and lunate are aligned, the surgeon advances the K-wire in the capitate into the lunate. The K-wire can be passed into the metacarpal through the metacarpal head or from the radial or ulnar side of the metacarpal base. When the K-wire is passed through the metacarpal head, blocking metacarpophalangeal joint extension, the wire should be left in place for short durations, such as from 2 to 4 weeks (Fig 1).

Conclusions.—This method of completely reducing the central carpal axis can maintain rigid fixation of carpal bones initially and during healing. The procedure permits simple alignment and reduction and establishes an anatomically positioned central column around which other reconstructive efforts can be focused.

▶ This article presents a technical tip for alignment of the capitolunoradius axes after perilunate or lunate dislocations or for chronic carpal instabilities. The described technique uses a K-wire introduced through the long finger metacarpal, then into the capitate, lunate, and if desired, distal radius. It is a useful approach, especially in cases with significant instability in which control of multiple unstable carpals is necessary. By stabilizing this longitudinal axis first, other unstable carpals may subsequently be reduced to this axis.

E.R. North, M.D.

A New Surgical Technique for Carpal Instability With Scapho-Lunar Dislocation [Italian]

Brunelli GA, Brunelli GR (Università degli Studi—Brescia, Italia)
Minerva Ortop Traumatol 47:565–568, 1996 8–31

Background.—This report describes a new technique for correcting carpal instability with scapholunate dissociation. Rupture of the volar scapho-trapezo-trapezoid ligament seems to have an important role in the etiopathology of this instability.

Technique.—The scar between the scaphoid and lunate bones and the scar formed among scaphoid, trapezium, and trapezoid are removed. A slip of flexor carpi radialis is passed through a tunnel pierced in the distal pole of the scaphoid. This slip is sutured to the dorso-ulnar edge of the distal radius with correction of the dissociation and scaphoid flexion.

Discussion.—The cases of 13 patients with satisfactory results after a maximum follow up of 2 years were described. This technique is quick and easily performed.

▶ This method presents an interesting way of repairing scapholunate dissociation. The article is divided into 2 parts. In the first, the pathogenesis of the lesion is reevaluated: following cadaver studies it is said that the lesion of the scapholunate ligament cannot determine the flexion (per se) of the scaphoid associated to a scapho-lunate dissociation. It is said that a lesion of the scapho-trapezio-trapezoid ligament must be associated. This introduces a new concept in the evaluation of the sequence of ligamentous lesions needed to determine scapholunate dissociation.

In the second part of the study, the technique of reconstruction is described. It is particularly effective in keeping the scaphoid in the correct alignment as a double ligament reconstruction is obtained: the volar reconstruction which stabilizes the scaphoid at the scapho-trapezio-trapezoid level and the dorsal reconstruction which connects the distal pole of scaphoid to the radial rim. It is also demonstrated that an independent scaphoid mobility from the lunate is obtained.

M. Ceruso, M.D.

Scapho-Lunate Dissociation and Arthrodesis: An Experimental Study With Lesions of the Interosseous Ligament and Fusions With K-Wires

Hurkmans HLP, Kooloos JGM, Meijer RS (Univ of Nijmegen, The Netherlands)

Clin Biomech 11:220–226, 1996 8–32

Background.—Tearing of the ligament between the lunate and scaphoid is often seen during sectioning. Studies of experimental lesions of this ligament have yielded conflicting findings regarding their effects; some authors report significant changes, and others report little effect. Because understanding of the behavior of the scapholunate (SL) complex is essential for conceptualizing the wrist joint, sectioning experiments were performed.

Methods and Findings.—Sectioning experiments were done using roentgen stereophotogrammetry, and the kinematics of the carpal bones were examined. Very little effect was found. In addition, the scaphoid was fused to the lunate to determine the effects on the carpal mechanism when the ligament between the bones is stiffened. Fusion was achieved with K-wires. After fusion, the carpus began to behave unpredictably. The wire positions significantly influenced outcomes.

Conclusion.—A disruption of the SL ligament barely affects the carpal mechanism. However, over time, other ligaments may become overstretched, leading eventually to the pattern typically observed. K-wiring to restore the connection between the lunate and scaphoid results primarily in an unstable joint.

▶ This well-done in vitro study demonstrates, on 2 cadaver wrists, that no significant wrist instability developed with isolated section of the SL interosseous ligament under the circumstances of the experiment. This result agrees with Berger et al.[1] and Meade et al.[2] and is seemingly at odds with Ruby et al.[3] However, the latter study only demonstrated instability in 1 position, that is, flexion and ulnar deviation of the wrist under loaded conditions.

This combination was not tested in the study reported on here. Further, as the authors state, the clinical situation may be quite different from that in the laboratory in that complete SL interosseous ligament incompetence probably leads to clinical instability by overloading the secondary constraints of the scaphoid, causing gradual lengthening of those ligaments. The important clinical question as to how vital it is to restore the SL interosseous ligament remains unanswered by this in vitro work.

As a second part of the study, the scaphoid was pinned to the lunate, and the specimens were stressed and intercarpal motions measured. As expected, normal wrist mechanics were disturbed, suggesting that even if SL fusion could be easily obtained, it might have an undesirable outcome. Clinically, this is such a difficult fusion to obtain that the answer may be moot.

L.K. Ruby, M.D.

References

1. Berger RA, Blair WF, Crowninshield, et al: The scapholunate ligament. *J Hand Surg (Am)* 17A:87–91, 1982.
2. Meade TD, Schneider LH, Cherry K: Radiographic analysis of selective ligament sectioning at the carpal scaphoid: A cadaver study. *J Hand Surg (Am)* 15A: 855–862, 1990.
3. Ruby LK, An KN, Linscheid RL, et al: The effect of scapholunate ligament section on scapholunate motion. *J Hand Surg (Am)* 12A:767–771, 1987.

Carpal Instability in the Weight-bearing Upper Extremity

Schroer W, Lacey S, Frost FS, et al (Case Western Reserve Univ, Cleveland, Ohio; MetroHealth Med Ctr Rehabilitation Service, Cleveland, Ohio; Wade Park VA Med Ctr, Cleveland, Ohio)

J Bone Joint Surg (Am) 78A:1838–1843, 1996 8–33

Introduction.—Patients with spinal cord injury may experience impairment and disability of the upper extremities because of the weight-bearing stress placed on the shoulder, hand, and wrist. Some reports show an increased prevalence of shoulder impingement, tears of the rotator cuff, and carpal tunnel syndrome in these patients. A study of paraplegic patients sought to determine whether there is an association between chronic repetitive forces placed through their wrists and carpal instability.

Methods.—Eligible patients used a manual wheelchair and could transfer themselves independently; thus, they all had similar requirements for the upper extremities. Excluded were patients whose injury occurred less than 2 years before the start of the study, those with systemic disease, and those with a history of traumatic disease of the upper extremity. Sixty-two of 246 patients who completed an initial questionnaire met inclusion criteria, reported daily pain in the wrist or hand, and were available for evaluation. These patients underwent a complete physical examination of each upper extremity and radiographic examination of the wrists. Patients with a diagnosis of carpal instability were compared with patients in the entire paraplegic study population for potential risk factors for carpal instability.

Results.—Nine patients (16 wrists) had radiographic evidence of static carpal instability. None had a history of acute injury of the wrist. Nondissociative volar intercalated segmental instability, present in 6 patients (11 wrists), was the predominant pattern of instability. Flexion was substantially limited in these wrists, but extension was generally not limited. Patients with carpal instability had a significantly longer duration of spinal cord injury (average, 30 years) than patients in the entire study population (average, 16 years). The level of spinal cord injury varied in patients with carpal instability.

Conclusions.—Long-term survivors of traumatic spinal cord injury may subject the upper extremities to decades of increased demands. Static carpal instability was found in 6% of this paraplegic population; the rate was 18%, however, among patients who had the injury for more than 20 years. Chronic repetitive stress appears to be the etiology of carpal instability in such cases.

► The authors determined that the predominant pattern of instability in the wrists of these 162 paraplegic patients (most presumably male) was nondissociative volar intercalated segment instability. Having similar effects at the shoulder joint with longer and longer times in the wheelchair, these individuals experienced an increased incidence as they aged and continued to do weight-bearing activity. That the incidence was relatively low in comparison with the incidence of troubling shoulder pain or other problems of the hand and wrist (e.g., carpal tunnel syndrome) in this population is in itself interesting. In our own spinal cord unit population, scapholunate advanced collapse patterns were more usual, although still rare, as in this series of 9 patients of 162.

V.R. Hentz, M.D.

Chondral Lesions of the Midcarpal Joint

Dautel G, Merle M (Hôpital Jeanne d'Arc, Toul, France)

Arthroscopy 13:97–102, 1997 8–34

Introduction.—A retrospective study was based on the findings of midcarpal arthroscopy of 78 patients to confirm reported correlations between variations in the shape of the lunate and degenerative lesions of the midcarpal joints, to determine the frequency of chondral lesions of the midcarpal joints in a young adult population, and to compare chondral lesions detected during arthroscopy with clinical findings.

Methods.—Patients eligible for the study had wrist pain and underwent full exploration of the midcarpal joint through both the radial and ulnar midcarpal portal. The 56 men and 22 women included in the study had an average age of 32.8. Lunates were classified as type I (a single facet on the distal aspect) or type II (2 facets on the distal aspect, 1 medial and 1 lateral). The secondary facet of type II lunates was considered wide if larger than 3 mm. Chondral lesions were classified as stage 1 (isolated chondritis with no chondral defects), stage 2 (cartilage defect with no exposure of the underlying bone), or stage 3 (cartilage defect with exposure of underlying bone, arthritis).

Results.—Thirty-five cases (44.9%) were classified as type I and 43 (55.1%) as type II. Among the 14 type I chondral lesions, 6 were stage 1, 7 were stage 2, and 1 was stage 3. All chondral lesions were seen in association with other lesions. Among the 17 type II chondral lesions, 5 were stage 1, 7 were stage 2, and 5 were stage 3. Only 3 of the type II chondral lesions were not associated with any other cartilaginous or ligamentous lesions observed at arthroscopy. The secondary facet was larger than 3 mm in 14 of the 43 cases in which the lunate was classified as type II.

Discussion.—Degenerative chondral lesions can occur in midcarpal joints between the lunate, capitate, and hamate, and some authors report a correlation between the presence of a type II lunate and the onset of degenerative lesions. Unlike in previous anatomic studies, chondral lesions were found even in type I lunates (40% of cases in this series). Lesions involved the tip of the hamate in 25.7% of cases, the helicoidal slope of the hamate in 14.3%, and the distal facet of the lunate in 5.7%. Because of the frequency of associated lesions, painful syndromes cannot be attributed with certainty to chondral lesions.

▶ The authors have presented a fascinating series of 78 patients who underwent wrist arthroscopy for assessment and treatment of symptomatic wrist problems. Of these 78 cases, which were a subset of 130 consecutive wrist arthroscopies, they indexed whether the lunate was a type I, with 1 single facet on the distal aspect, or type II, with 2 facets on the distal aspect, 1 medial and 1 lateral, as had been categorized in our previous publications. Unlike in our previous series, in which almost all of the arthritic lesions with exposed subchondral bone at the proximal pole of the hamate were associated with type II lunates, in their series, they found these lesions to occur in wrists with a type I lunate and in wrists with a type II lunate.

There are differences between their study group and the previous studies we have reported. These differences include the fact that their population was younger and all individuals had wrist symptoms. The previous studies in which we reported and categorized the type I and type II lunates, as well as the incidence of ligament and joint pathology, were in a cadaver population whose average age was older; that population was random and most likely had a low incidence of symptomatic wrist pathology. In the cadaver population previously reported, there was a high incidence of ligament disruptions, but not of true carpal instability. However, in the patient population on which these authors are reporting, the history of trauma and symptomatic ligament disruptions may include or lead to carpal instabilities and further trauma. In the authors' patient population, they listed any lesions of the ulnar side of the midcarpal joint, both condromalacia and stage III changes with exposed subchondral bone associated with type I or type II lunates. In previous cadaver studies, it was specifically the lesions with exposed subchondral bone at the proximal pole of the hamate only that were dramatically correlated with the type II lunate. However, even looking just at the proximal pole of the hamate and the lesions that included exposed subchondral bone, the authors have still found a higher incidence of these lesions in the type I lunate than reported in previous cadaver populations.

A question can be raised with respect to the criteria for type I vs. type II lunates, and in those cases where the medial facet of the lunate is 1 millimeter or smaller whether these may inconsistently be categorized type I in some cases and type II in other cases. This may affect the reported incidence of type I vs. type II lunates; alternatively, it may simply reflect the random selection of samplings of the overall population of wrists. The authors found, as we have previously reported, that even in wrists with documented lesions with exposed subchondral bone at the proximal pole of the hamate, radiographs failed to demonstrate these lesions.

I find the authors' series to be quite provocative and stimulating. The information certainly raises questions, and I believe the whole issue warrants further study. I hope that there will be additional interest and work to assess the incidence of type I and type II lunates in populations and explore the possible correlations between lunate morphology and various types of pathology.

S.F. Viegas, M.D.

Suggested Reading

Feldman MD, Manske PR, Welch RL, et al: Evaluation of Herbert screw fixation for the treatment of displaced scaphoid nonunions. *Orthopedics* 20:325–328, 1997.

▶ Screw fixation alone resulted in union in 5 of 10 cases; addition of a K-wire to the construct resulted in union in 8 of 9 cases. Time to union was also less (5 months vs. 8 months) in the screw and K-wire group.

P.C. Amadio, M.D.

Miura H, Uchida Y, Sugioka Y: Radial closing wedge osteotomy for Kienböck's disease. *J Hand Surg (Am)* 21A:1029–1034, 1996.

▶ There has been considerable controversy as to whether a closing wedge osteotomy is helpful or harmful in the treatment of Kienböck's disease. Nakamura et al.[1] have argued for; Werner and Palmer[2] have argued against, citing experimental evidence of increased lunate fossa loading with a closing wedge. It is hard to argue, though, with a series like this of 26 patients followed for 4 years, with 80% good or excellent results in Kienböck's patients at Stage IIIA or less. Perhaps loading of the lunate fossa is not the be-all and end-all of Kienböck's disease; increased loading as an etiology is, after all, just a theory to explain clinical observations. When observations and theory do not jive, it is time to reconsider the theory, particularly when, as here, the observations have been reproducible among patients and in multiple centers.

P.C. Amadio, M.D.

References

1. Nakamura R, Tsuge S, Watanabe K, et al: Radial wedge osteotomy for Kienböck's disease. *J Bone Joint Surg (Am)* 73A:1391–1396, 1991.
2. Werner FW, Palmer AK: Biomechanical evaluation of operative procedures to treat Kienböck's disease. *Hand Clin* 9:431–443, 1993.

Quenzer DE, Linscheid RL, Vidal MA, et al: Trispiral tomographic staging of Kienböck's disease. *J Hand Surg (Am)* 22A:396–403, 1997.

▶ We commonly stage Kienböck's disease using Stahl's criteria, as modified by Lichtman: Stage I, lunate fracture; Stage II, density changes; Stage IIIA, lunate collapse; Stage IIIB, lunate and carpal collapse; Stage IV, arthritis. This paper shows that the stage applied to a given case depends upon the imaging modality used; tomograms see more than routine x-rays. This should come as no surprise, but it does remind us to be careful noting *how* the staging was done before comparing results between series. The authors, in my opinion, lost a golden opportunity, though, to study interobserver and intraobserver differences in staging x-rays and tomograms for Kienböck's disease. Such studies in other conditions have shown a distressing lack of consensus among observers. Thus, I should rephrase: this paper shows that one observer staged differently, depending on the imaging modality used. We must await another study to learn if this observation can be generalized, and to what extent.

P.C. Amadio, M.D.

Sotereanos DG, Mitsionis GJ, Giannakopoulos PN, et al: Perilunate dislocation and fracture dislocation: A critical analysis of the volar-dorsal approach. *J Hand Surg (Am)* 22A:49–56, 1997.

▶ Even with early, aggressive operative treatment, this series of 11 cases with short (30-month) follow-up showed significant sequelae. Only 5 patients were able to return to preinjury employment. Function, motion, and strength averaged 70% of normal. Perilunate dislocation is an injury best avoided. I agree with these authors that a combined dorsal and volar approach provides reason able anatomic results; unfortunately, it does not prevent long-term disability in most cases.

P.C. Amadio, M.D.

Wilhelm K, Hierner R, Brehl B: Callotaxis lengthening of the capitate after resection of the lunate for the treatment of Kienböck's disease Stage III: Operative technique and one year results. *Handchir Mikrochir Plast Chir* 29:10–19, 1997.

▶ The blood supply of the capitate enters distally, so I am not sure how this operation works; one would think that capitate lengthening would of necessity devascularize the proximal pole. Yet apparently it *does* work, at least some of the time, as the illustrated case attests. This is another option for the treatment of Kienböck's disease, when carpal collapse and lunate deformity suggest the need for lunate excision. Another option in such cases is proximal row carpectomy, a simpler, one-stage procedure which I prefer.

P.C. Amadio, M.D.

Zimmerman G, Heinisch W, Fischmeister MF: The fate of the calcium-dense proximal fragment in scaphoid fracture [German]. *Handchir Mikrochir Plast Chir* 29:20–26, 1997.

▶ The fate of proximal fragments with increased bone density is about the same as proximal fragments with normal density. Increased density may be a necessary, but not sufficient, criterion for osteonecrosis.

P.C. Amadio, M.D.

Distal Radius

Consistency of AO Fracture Classification for the Distal Radius

Kreder HJ, Hanel DP, McKee M, et al (Univ of Toronto)

J Bone Joint Surg (Br) 78B:726–731, 1996 8–35

Introduction.—The AO/ASIF classification system provides a measure of severity in patients with fractures of the long bones. This system is likely to be widely used in clinical research, so information on interobserver and intraobserver consistency is essential. Agreement in the use of the AO classification for distal radial fractures was assessed.

Methods.—Thirty patients were selected from a trauma database to represent a wide range of severe fractures. The fractures were classified by 36 assessors of varying clinical experience, from attending surgeons to nonclinical personnel. The assessors were briefly trained in AO classification, emphasizing the key points in grading a specific type, group, and subgroup. They were also asked to decide whether the articular surface was displaced. The same assessor reclassified the same injuries 2–4 weeks later.

Results.—Experienced assessors showed good agreement when grading AO type and the presence or absence of articular displacement. In contrast, assessors at all levels of experience did not always agree as to AO group or subgroup. Some cases were subject to more disagreement than others—no clear reasons for this variation could be identified. Intraobserver agreement was best for the more experienced assessors.

Conclusions.—The AO classification is a simple and reproducible tool for grading distal radial fractures according to joint displacement and type.

Subclassification into groups and subgroups is not as reliable. The authors suggest that severity could be graded by classifying the articular surface into displaced or undisplaced groups. The AO classification system remains to be validated as an outcome predictor.

▶ An ideal classification system for distal radius fractures has yet to be defined. Ideally, a classification system should be reproducible and simple to remember and should provide guidelines to treatment and help predict outcome. The AO classification system is a detailed anatomical classification system based on radiographic anatomy. The authors in this study statistically evaluate the interobserver and intraobserver reliability of this classification. It comes as no surprise that there was consistent agreement regarding fracture type (3 variables) and articular displacement (2 variables). However, there was much less consistency with subgroup classification (27 potential variables). Although it was not specifically stated, I assume that the hypothesis they wish to test is *the AO classification is a valid instrument for clinical research because of high intraobserver and interobserver reliability.* On the basis of their findings, one would reject, at least in part, this hypothesis. Furthermore, the authors accurately cite the literature supporting articular displacement as an important prognostic factor and suggest that the AO classification be supplemented with categories for joint displacement. Unfortunately, if one eliminates the "group" and "subgroup" categories and substitutes a description of joint displacement, the revised classification would not differ significantly from others already existing in the literature. The value of this study is that it points out some of the weaknesses of the AO classification and highlights the need for critical evaluation of any classification that is going to have widespread clinical use.

P.J. Stern, M.D.

Plaster Cast Versus Percutaneous Pin Fixation for Comminuted Fractures of the Distal Radius in Patients Between 46 and 65 Years of Age

Rodríguez-Merchán EC (La Paz Univ, Madrid)

J Orthop Trauma 11:212–217, 1997 8–36

Background.—Traditional management of distal radius fractures is by closed reduction and forearm plaster, but the instability of these comminuted fractures has prompted the design of methods to prevent redisplacement. This prospective, randomized study compared the results of treating unstable distal radius fractures by percutaneous pin fixation and plaster and by traditional closed reduction and plaster.

Study Design.—Between January 1992 and December 1994, 40 patients, aged 46 to 65 years, with unstable Frykmann III to VIII distal radius fractures sustained in falls entered this study. Twenty patients were randomly assigned to treatment with closed reduction followed by casting, and the remaining 20 were assigned to percutaneous fixation with K-wires followed by casting. Follow-up assessment occurred at 1, 3, and 7 weeks and again at 1 year. Outcome was assessed through initial displacement, carpal malalignment, articular step-off, range of motion, and grip strength.

Results.—Initial displacement and reduction were successful in both groups, but 7 days after surgery there was significant loss of position in the closed reduction group. The functional results in the fixation group were excellent in 12 cases, good in 8, and fair in 2. The functional results in the closed reduction group were excellent in 3 cases, good in 8, fair in 5, and poor in 4. Both functional and anatomical results were superior in the fixation group.

Conclusion.—The results of this prospective, randomized trial reveal that percutaneous fixation and casting is superior to traditional closed manipulation and casting in the treatment of unstable distal radius fractures. Although the cost of the fixation treatment is higher than the closed manipulation and casting treatment, the improvements in outcome justify this cost.

▶ This prospective, randomized study shows that percutaneous pin fixation combined with cast treatment improves the results of Colles' fractures in middle-aged adults, when compared with the results of cast treatment alone. Of course, no single treatment can be used for all cases of Colles' fracture; some will be amenable to casts, some to pins, some to external fixation, and some to open reduction and internal fixation. I believe this is a weakness of any study that randomly allocates all patients with a diagnosis of distal radius fracture to 1 treatment or another. Better preoperative stratification of cases before randomization would likely yield more striking results.

P.C. Amadio, M.D.

Intra-articular Fractures of the Distal End of the Radius Treated With an Adjustable Fixator System

Zanotti RM, Louis DS (Univ of Michigan, Ann Arbor)

J Hand Surg (Am) 22A:428–440, 1997 8–37

Introduction.—A wide range of complication rates (10% to 90%) has been reported for distal radius fractures treated by various methods. This prospective study was designed to evaluate the subjective, radiologic, and functional results of severely comminuted intra-articular distal radius fractures treated with an external fixator device (the Wrist Jack) alone or in combination with percutaneous pins.

Methods.—Study participants were 21 adults with 25 fractures; the mean age of the group was 34 years. All fractures were Frykmann type VII or VIII, involving both the radiocarpal and radioulnar joints. Five patients were lost to follow-up, leaving 16 patients (20 fractures) available for analysis. The average follow-up was 25 months after fixator removal. Eight fractures were isolated and 12 involved high-energy trauma with multiple injuries. Percutaneous pins were used to supplement fixation in 6

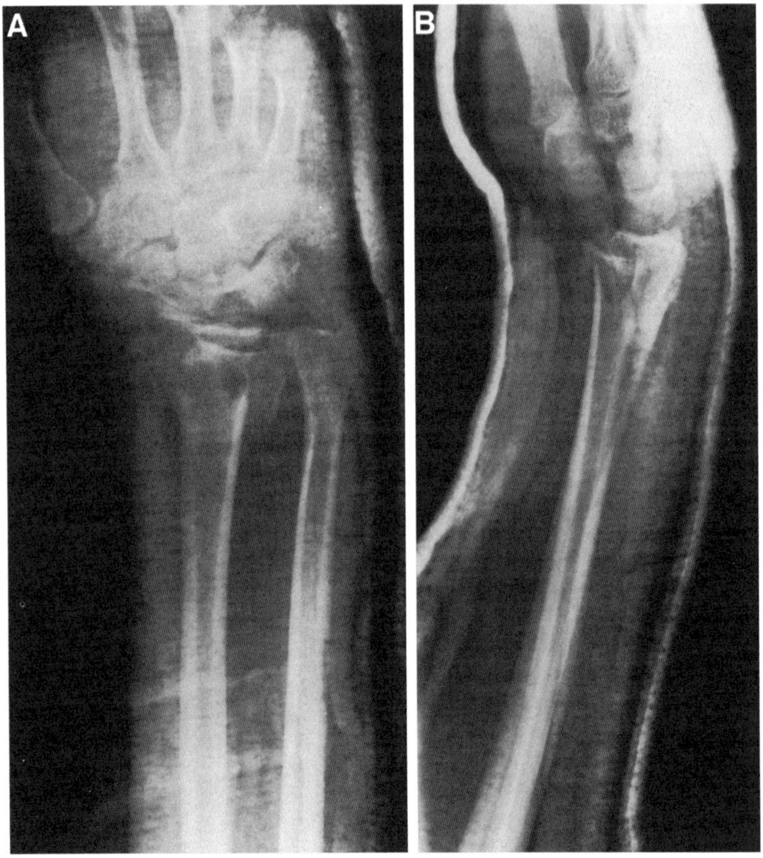

FIGURE 1.—A, anteroposterior and B, lateral radiographs of an injured distal radius show unacceptable alignment after closed reduction. (Courtesy of Zanotti RM, Louis DS: Intra-articular fractures of the distal end of the radius treated with an adjustable fixator system. *J Hand Surg [Am]* 22A:428–440, 1997.)

fractures. The goal of fixation was to restore articular congruity to within 1 mm. Radiographs obtained after closed reduction showed all fractures to have significant intra-articular incongruity, unstable fracture patterns, or a die-punch component (Fig 1). Intraoperative radiographs were taken to confirm joint alignment and articular congruity (Fig 2). Both anteroposterior and lateral radiographs (Fig 3) were obtained at follow-up.

Results.—Outcome at follow-up was judged good in 75% of patients, fair in 20%, and excellent in 5%; no patient had a poor result. The failure to achieve complete restoration of articular congruity, radial length, palmar tilt, and radial inclination in all cases indicates that the method used in some patients was insufficient. Seventeen of 20 fractures showed some evidence of articular incongruity, yet palmar tilt, radial inclination, radial length, and range of motion were acceptable. Grip strength averaged 80% of the unaffected limb. Most patients (85%) reported only occasional pain or none at all; 15% had some pain with weakness or limitation of motion.

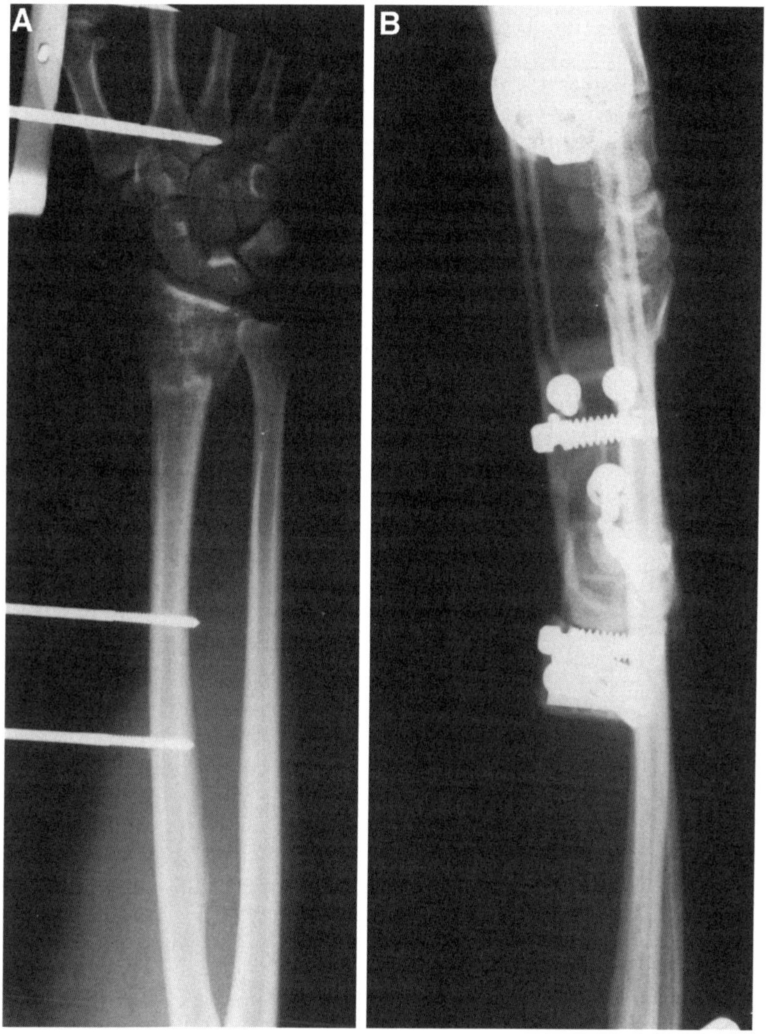

FIGURE 2.—A, anteroposterior and B, lateral radiographs of distal radius in Wrist Jack external fixation device after postoperative reduction in the same patient as in Figure 1. Note restoration of radial length, articular congruency, and palmar tilt. (Courtesy of Zanotti RM, Louis DS: Intra-articular fractures of the distal end of the radius treated with an adjustable fixator system. *J Hand Surg [Am]* 22A: 428–440, 1997.)

Patients with high-energy injuries had a poorer outcome than those with low-energy fractures. Although the rate of good/excellent results was higher in the fixator alone than in the fixator plus pins group, 5 of 6 fractures in the latter group were high-energy and substantially more severe.

Conclusion.—The outcome in this group of patients with severe, unstable distal radius fractures suggests that the external fixator, alone or in

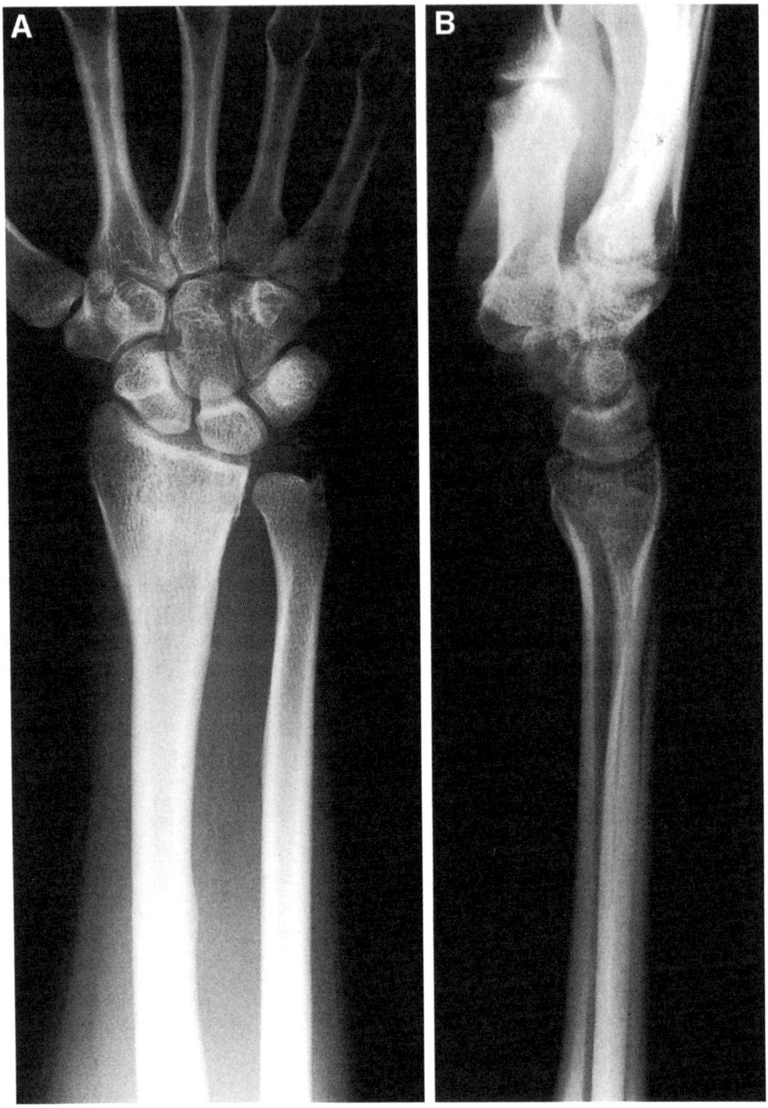

FIGURE 3.—A, anteroposterior and B, lateral radiographs of distal radius at follow-up evaluation over 2 years later (same patient as in Figures 1 and 2). (Courtesy of Zanotti RM, Louis DS: Intra-articular fractures of the distal end of the radius treated with an adjustable fixator system. *J Hand Surg [Am]* 22A:428–440, 1997.)

combination with multiple percutaneous pins, is an effective means of treating a difficult fracture fixation problem.

▶ The authors have shown significant benefits from the use of the Wrist Jack, an adjustable external fixator. Their patients had intra-articular fractures, and distraction fixation cannot produce reduction of all intra-articular fracture fragments. The operating surgeon needs to be aware of the occasional need to perform open reduction/internal fixation and/or closed reduction of the articular fragments with or without the use of an arthroscope. This provides for the best potential long-term result by restoration of the "nearest" to normal articular anatomy.

R.D. Beckenbaugh, M.D.

Open Reduction and Internal Fixation of Displaced Intraarticular Fractures of the Distal Radius: 31 Patients Followed for 3–7 Years

Hove LM, Nilsen PT, Furnes O, et al (Haukeland Univ, Bergen, Norway)

Acta Orthop Scand 68:59–63, 1997 8–38

Introduction.—In patients with fractures of the distal radius, open reduction may be indicated if there are problems achieving closed reduction of the articular surface. An experience with open reduction of displaced intra-articular fractures of the distal radius is reported, with internal fixation using a T-plate.

Methods.—The patients were 21 males and 10 females (mean age, 43 years). Each had a displaced fracture of the distal radius that was considered irreducible or in which attempts at closed reduction failed. Surgery was not performed on elderly patients and patients with severe osteoporosis who did not have a high demand for wrist function. There were 20 comminuted fractures, 4 multifragment chauffeur's fractures, 6 comminuted Smith's fractures, and 1 palmar articular lip fracture with a large fragment. Surgery was performed a mean of 5 days after the injuries. After open reduction through a dorsal, longitudinal incision, the fracture was fixed with a T-plate and small fragment screws. Additional fixation hardware was used as necessary. The patients were followed up for a mean of 4 years after their injuries.

Results.—The mean radial length increased from 2 to 11 mm, angulation increased from 18 degrees dorsal to 5 degrees palmar, articular step-off decreased from 2.4 to 0.3 mm, and the intra-articular gap decreased from 3.1 to 0.4 mm. One patient had a step-off at follow-up, and 2 had an intra-articular gap of 2 mm. There was no loss of correction during follow-up. Twenty-six patients had good-to-excellent function. Complications included 2 cases of median nerve paresthesia, 2 ruptures of the extensor pollicis longus, 1 postoperative wound infection, and 1 case of compartment syndrome.

Conclusions.—Good results are achieved with open reduction and T-plate fixation of displaced intra-articular fractures of the distal radius. The quality of reduction determines the functional outcome. The authors have had few major complications.

► The results of this retrospective clinical study by Hove and colleagues from Bergen, Norway support the impression by many that the treatment of intra-articular fractures of the distal end of the radius should follow principles similar to those that have evolved for articular fractures elsewhere involving the appendicular skeleton. Furthermore, these fractures more often than not involve 2 articulations, that is, the radiocarpal and radioulnar joints, and are not surprisingly associated with alterations in carpal kinematics as well as, in some cases, disruption of intracarpal ligament support. It has become quite evident that function follows form at the end of the radius as well as elsewhere.

As with the assessment of any management rationale, the results of this study must be subjected to a number of questions. In the first place, who are the patients that received this treatment? These were primarily younger patients, which suggests that these are more active individuals who may have been experiencing the sequelae of more energetic injuries. The reader should take heed in this that "elderly" patients and those with osteoporosis were not treated operatively. Given that this group of patients forms a large percentage of patients with fractures at the end of the radius, we must keep in mind that operative intervention at this stage in our collective experience is best reserved for a younger age group.

A second question lies in defining the problems associated with the fracture. It is quite evident that intra-articular fractures are wrist injuries that happen to involve the end of the radius. Although this study did not have a concurrent control that might illustrate whether these articular fractures could be treated by less invasive means, the authors support their management rationale sufficiently by previous studies in the literature to warrant acceptance of their more vigorous attitudes toward gaining anatomical restoration.

A third question involves the problems associated with the treatment. The reader should be mindful of the fact that there were some substantial complications in this study, including tendon rupture, acute carpal tunnel syndrome, and compartment syndrome. Additionally, it would appear that patients who had a dorsal plate applied had these plates removed, and this removal involved a second anesthetic and a second operative procedure. The authors may well have noted some disability associated with the need for this second operative procedure.

Yet another question involves what really influences the outcome in these injuries. The operative tactics strive to obtain a result that is as close as possible to realignment of the articular surface and that maintains the relationship between the end of the radius and the ulna and the end of the radius and the carpus. Although this study would not give us insight into problems with failure to regain the original anatomical positioning, this information is readily available in previous studies, and it would appear that, at least for these younger individuals, the ability to restore the original anatomical positioning, avoid the disabling effects of plaster immobilization, and allow a functional rehabilitation early on all have salutary effects on the outcome.

Finally, one has to ask, as with any rationale for fracture management, what are the costs? We do not learn any of this information from this study, but then neither was it intended to show this or the fact that costs in 1 health care system may be quite different than costs in another. The fact is that costs cannot be simply equated by a hospital stay or an operative procedure. Costs must take into effect issues such as the duration of follow-up, the need for occupational physical therapy, the time off work, and repeated office visits as a result of radiographs or cast changes, just to list a few. It is my impression that one could make a convincing argument that, in many instances, early restoration of function will prove to be cost-effective in the long run. Although this needs to be validated, as with every other area of musculoskeletal trauma, effective trauma care generally is cost-effective.

J.B. Jupiter, M.D.

Accelerated Healing of Distal Radial Fractures With the Use of Specific, Low-intensity Ultrasound: A Multicenter, Prospective, Randomized, Double-blind, Placebo-controlled Study

Kristiansen TK, Ryaby JP, McCabe J, et al (Community Health Care Plan, New Haven, Conn; Conway Hosp, SC; Emory Univ, Atlanta, Ga; et al)

J Bone Joint Surg (Am) 79-A:961–973, 1997 8–39

Background.—The application of a low-intensity ultrasound (US) stimulus may accelerate the healing of distal radial fractures after treatment with closed reduction and cast application. The efficacy of a specifically programmed, low-intensity, nonthermal, pulsed US medical device for reducing time to radiographic healing of dorsally angulated fractures of the distal aspect of the radius treated with manipulation and a cast was investigated prospectively.

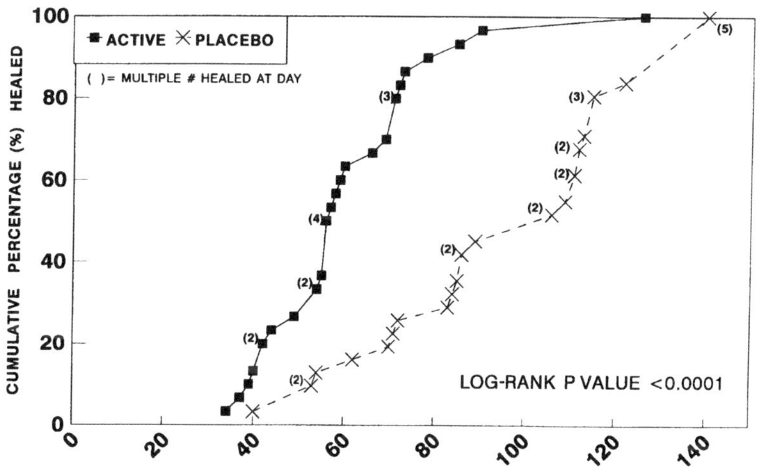

FIGURE 2.—Graph comparing the cumulative percentages of fractures that healed in the group treated with active ultrasound and the group treated with the placebo. (Courtesy of Kristiansen TK, Ryaby JP, McCabe J, et al: Accelerated healing of distal radial fractures with the use of specific, low-intensity ultrasound. *J Bone Joint Surg [Am]* 79-A:961–973, 1997.)

Methods.—Sixty patients with 61 fractures were included in the multicenter, randomized, double-blind, placebo-controlled clinical trial. The patients were enrolled within 7 days of the fracture. Thirty fractures were treated with an active US device and 31 with a placebo device every day for 20 minutes at home for 10 weeks. The placebo device emitted no US energy.

Findings.—Ultrasound-treated fractures had a significantly shorter mean time to union than placebo-treated fractures (61 and 98 days, respectively). The active treatment was also associated with accelerated healing at each radiographic stage; a significantly smaller loss of reduction, as determined by the degree of volar angulation; and a significant reduction in mean time until loss of reduction ceased (Fig 2).

Conclusion.—The US signal accelerates the healing of distal radial metaphysis fractures. The loss of reduction during fracture healing was also decreased with this treatment.

▶ This important article shows that US can stimulate fracture healing at the distal radius. This phenomenon is not unique to that site; US has been shown, in other studies, to stimulate fracture healing in both humans and experimental animals. In this study, faster healing (40 vs. 60 days to bridging the first cortex; 60 vs. 100 days for solid union) also resulted in fewer and less severe malunions, despite cast treatment. Although one could certainly never justify the use of US to the distal radius to avoid nonunion or even delayed union, it might be justified to accelerate healing and minimize external fixator time. It might also prove quite useful for scaphoid fractures and, perhaps, even for Kienböck's disease. Stay tuned.

P.C. Amadio, M.D.

Repair of Five Distal Radius Fractures With an Investigational Cancellous Bone Cement: A Preliminary Report

Jupiter JB, Winters S, Sigman S, et al (Massachusetts Gen Hosp, Boston; Stanford Univ, Calif; Norian Corp, Cupertino, Calif)

J Orthop Trauma 11:110–116, 1997 8–40

Background.—Fractures of the distal end of the radius with little displacement, impaction, or comminution of the supporting metaphyseal bone can be successfully treated with closed manipulative fracture reduction and plaster immobilization. Fractures characterized by wide displacement, comminution, or substance loss of the metaphyseal bone; impacted articular fragments; or instability of the distal radioulnar joint cannot be adequately treated with this method. Norian Skeletal Repair System (SRS) is a percutaneously injectable, fast-setting, high-strength calcium-phosphate cement for the treatment of compromised cancellous bone. Results were presented of a feasibility study of the clinical effectiveness and safety of Norian SRS injected percutaneously into the fracture site to prevent loss of distal radius fracture reduction.

Methods.—Patients seen at Massachusetts General Hospital from January 1994 to May 1994 who were between 45 and 80 and had a dorsally displaced extra-articular fracture of the distal radius occurring within 72 hours of presentation were eligible for inclusion in this study. Of the 20 patients whose radiographs fulfilled study criteria, only 5 agreed to participate. All 5 of these patients were women, aged 49 to 57, who had a fracture caused by a fall. Under anesthesia, the fracture was reduced by closed manipulation. Norian SRS paste was injected percutaneously to fill the defect, and the limb was immobilized for 10 minutes. A below elbow cast was applied, with the wrist in a neutral position. Active assisted range-of-motion exercises were prescribed for the digits, elbow, and shoul-

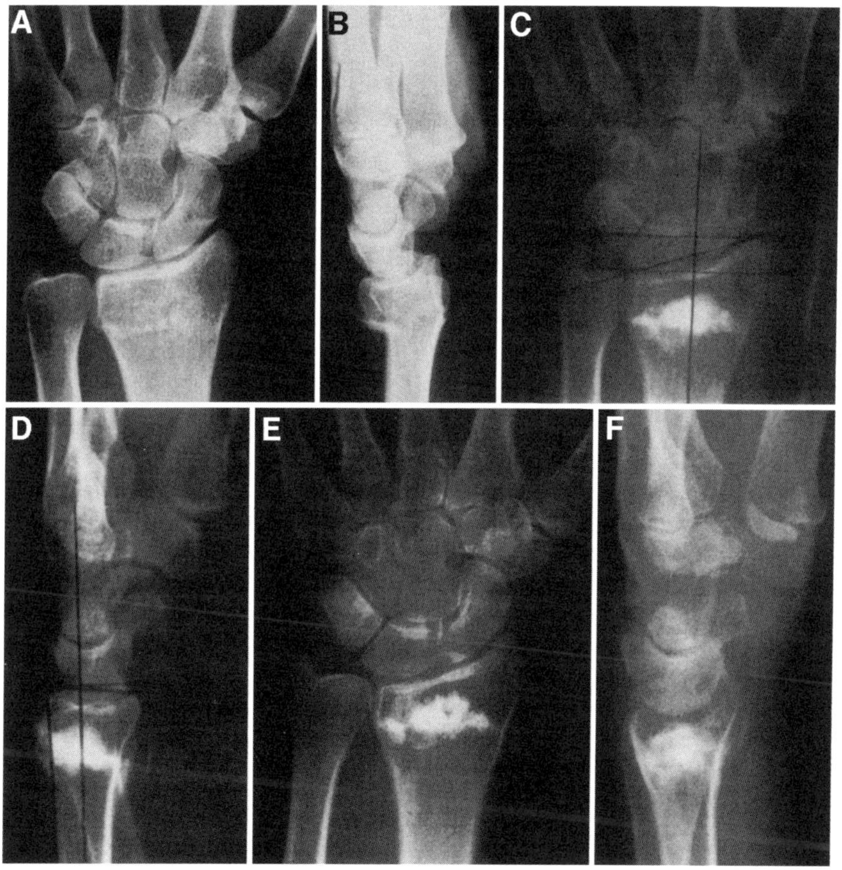

FIGURE 5.—Preoperative anterior (**A**) and lateral radiographs (**B**) of a 51-year-old woman who sustained a displaced extra-articular distal radius fracture after falling on ice. Immediate posttreatment posteroanterior (**C**) and lateral radiographs (**D**) show the radiopaque Norian SRS contained within the comminuted area. Fifteen months posttreatment, posteroanterior (**E**) and lateral radiographs (**F**) show reestablished cortices and subsequent remodeling of Norian SRS. (Courtesy of Jupiter JB, Winters S, Sigman S, et al: Repair of five distal radius fractures with an investigational cancellous bone cement: A preliminary report. *J Orthop Trauma* 11:110–116, 1997.)

der. The cast was removed after 6 weeks, and patients were then encouraged to use the affected wrist. Outcome was evaluated by prospective radiographic (Fig 5) and functional assessments performed during 1-year follow-up. The injured limb was compared with the contralateral limb.

Results.—At 1-year follow-up, the average loss of radial length was less than 1 mm. The radial angle was maintained at 25.4 degrees and the volar angle was within the normal range in 4 patients, whereas in 1 patient, the dorsal angle was 7 degrees. Wrist motion improved 50% between 6 weeks and 3 months. Further improvement occurred by 12 months, with grip strength an average of 88% of the contralateral side. Dorsal and volar extrusion of Norian SRS was resorbed over time. There were no clinically significant adverse effects or complications in this patient group.

Conclusion.—This small feasibility study demonstrated that Norian SRS was clinically safe and effective as a percutaneously delivered cancellous bone cement for maintaining reduction of unstable extra-articular metaphyseal fracture of the distal end of the radius. No significant complications were associated with its use in this setting.

► I believe that Norian SRS will prove to be useful as a replacement for cancellous bone grafting. However, the current protocol for the distal radius—in which the substance is used without adjuvants such as pins, plates, or fixators—is, I believe, unrealistic. In nearly all clinical cases in which bone graft is used in the distal radius, some additional fixation is necessary to ensure perfect articular alignment and to allow for soft-tissue and bony healing. This is true even if the graft provides immediate structural support, as the Norian substance does.

The Norian SRS substance is not a bone glue but rather a form of bone grout; fracture healing is still necessary around the substance, which is then replaced. Cast protection helps but cannot provide the fine tuning and additional support that is offered by internal fixation. I suspect that the use of Norian will increase once it comes off its new device protocol and is released for general use; I also believe that such use will commonly be coupled with various forms of internal and external fixation.

P.C. Amadio, M.D.

Injectable Calcium Phosphate in the Treatment of Distal Radial Fractures

Kopylov P, Jonsson K, Thorngren KG, et al (Univ Hosp, Lund, Sweden)

J Hand Surg (Br) 21B:768–771, 1996 8–41

Objective.—Secondary displacement after distal radial fracture and reduction is a common occurrence. Results of stabilizing the fracture during healing by using an injectable bone mineral substitute that hardens in situ to form a carbonated apatite were presented.

Methods.—Norian Skeletal Repair System (SRS) was used in 6 patients to repair distal radial fractures that had redisplaced after initial satisfactory reduction or for which primary reduction failed. Patients were operated on 8 days (range, 2–11 days) after the fracture. A short-arm dorsal splint was used to immobilize the wrist for 2 weeks. Patients received physiotherapy before and after surgery and after removal of the cast and were examined at 1 day, at 2, 5, and 7 weeks, and at 3, 6, and 12 months. Patients rated their pain, residual disability, and satisfaction on 3 visual analogue scales.

Results.—Two patients with Norian SRS in soft tissues appeared to have more postoperative pain than usual after wrist operations. One patient whose Norian SRS was manipulated too soon after introduction had a redisplacement of the fracture. Five of the 6 patients rated their satisfaction as good. They rapidly returned to activity, and their pain was minimal at 1 year. At 7 weeks, patients had regained 75% of their range of motion for pronation, 63% for supination, 55% for extension, and 50% for flexion. At 6 months, the results were 98%, 92%, 79%, and 64%, respectively. Compared with the contralateral side, grip strength was 75%. All patients showed radial angle changes at 1 year that resulted in measurements similar to preoperative values. The amount of Norian SRS diminished after 1 year in some patients (Fig 1, A and D).

Conclusions.—Patients had a shorter period of immobilization and an early return of motion. At 1 year, all but 1 were satisfied with their results. Norian SRS is a novel alternative for treatment of distal radial fractures.

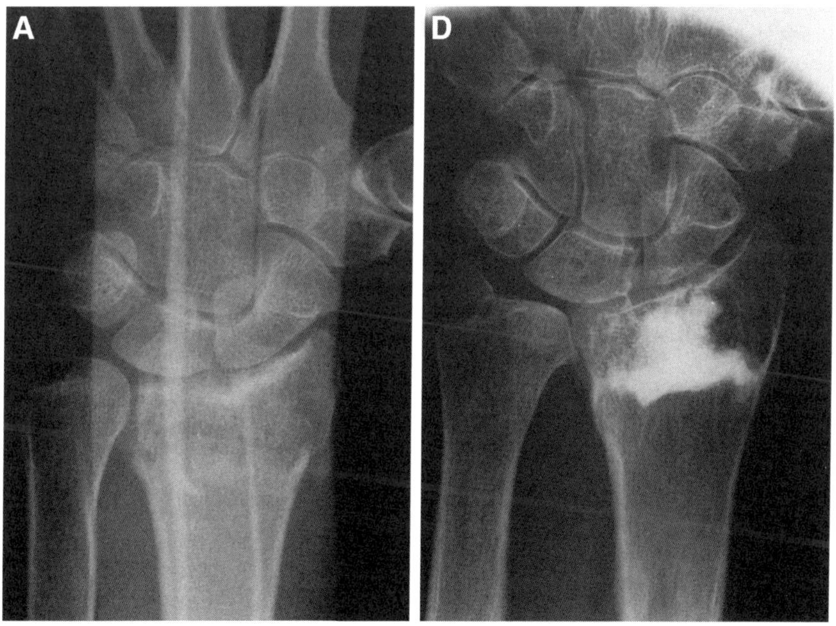

FIGURE 1.—**A**, this intraarticular fracture of the distal radius was treated by injection of Norian Skeletal Repair System (SRS). **D**, x-ray after 1 year shows healed fracture with remodeling of the bone. (Courtesy of Kopylov P, Jonsson K, Thorngren KG, et al: Injectable calcium phosphate in the treatment of distal radial fractures. *J Hand Surg [Br]* 21B:768–771, 1996.)

Additional studies are necessary to improve the technique and verify these preliminary results.

► This report of the Norian SRS bone mineral substitute shows promising results, as the figures attest. However, a review of Table 1 in the original article shows that only 1 patient had correction of palmar tilt to 0 degrees or better, and 4 patients lost 2–5 mm of length by final follow-up. These anatomical results, although perhaps better than what one would expect from 2 weeks of casting alone, are certainly not normal, and less than one should be able to achieve with other forms of operative treatment. I do not believe this is a problem of the SRS substance, but rather of the protocol used: SRS was used with 2 weeks of casting and no other form of fixation.

The SRS substance is designed to replace a bone graft. If one considers the circumstances when a metaphyseal bone graft is useful, in almost all cases one would likely wish to use some form of neutralization until the graft incorporates. In this case there is no graft to incorporate, but the fracture still needs to heal. I believe that, without some form of neutralization, it is reasonable to expect that the fracture fragments would collapse to some extent around the SRS (or any graft, including autogenous cancellous bone), due to the compressive load of the muscles crossing the wrist. It is that load which I believe should be neutralized until initial fracture healing has occurred. Neutralization can be by either internal or external fixation, as fracture anatomy and surgeon choice dictate. In the case of SRS, where the point is to remain minimally invasive, I would think that a minimum of 4–5 weeks of external fixation (just as one would do after cancellous grafting) should be included at least as an option in the SRS protocol.

P.C. Amadio, M.D.

Effects of Intra-articular Distal Radius Depression on Wrist Joint Contact Characteristics

Wagner WF Jr, Tencer AF, Kiser P, et al (Univ of Washington, Seattle)

J Hand Surg (Am) 21A:554–560, 1996 8–42

Background.—Intra-articular involvement is a common feature of many distal radial fractures, but the effect of disruption of the radial articular surface on joint contact properties is not known. The effects of scaphoid and lunate facet depressions on the contact characteristics of the radiocarpal joint were examined.

Methods.—One fracture type was examined: midsagittal with scaphoid or lunate whole-facet proximal depression. Using 12 cadaver extremities, pressure-sensitive film was loaded into the radiocarpal joints with varying degrees of depression. The specimens were loaded statically in 15 degrees of radial deviation, neutral position, and 15 degrees of ulnar deviation; the film was then removed and analyzed for contact area and pressure.

Results.—Lunate fossa depression caused a significant increase in scaphoid fossa pressure only with a 3-mm stepoff and the hand in neutral position. A 1-mm scaphoid fossa depression resulted in increases in lunate fossa pressures in the neutral position and with radial deviation. Lunate fossa contact areas increased over those of intact joints in all loading positions with 3-mm scaphoid fossa depression and in ulnar and radial deviation with 1-mm scaphoid fossa depressions.

Discussion.—Depression of the scaphoid side of the joint appears to have the most significant effect on radiocarpal joint contact characteristics. However, limitations of this study do exist. Intra-articular fractures of the radius are more complex than the model represents, and pressure-sensitive film can alter joint characteristics. The loading is quasistatic and does not account for the shear forces that occur during rotational wrist movement. These data do suggest, however, that even minimal depressions can lead to significant changes in joint contact characteristics; hence, the joint should ideally be restored to an anatomical position after intra-articular fracture of the distal radius. The advantage of surgical reduction of these fractures must be clarified by further research with long-term follow-up.

► The importance of the intra-articular nature of many fractures of the distal radius has long been ignored. A few clinical studies have warned us that anatomical reduction is necessary to expect a good outcome, but no biomechanical research work has been done until this limited but valuable report. The limitations are well described in the paper, and further studies need to be done to minimize them. In the meantime, I congratulate the authors for the good start and agree with their conclusion that we should not hesitate to restore the joint to an anatomical position after intra-articular fractures of the distal radius even with minimal depression.

J. Ryu, M.D.

Outcome After Colles Fracture: The Relative Responsiveness of Three Questionnaires and Physical Examination Measures

Amadio PC, Silverstein MD, Ilstrup DM, et al (Mayo Clinic and Found, Rochester, Minn)

J Hand Surg (Am) 21A:781–787, 1996 8–43

Introduction.—Patients with Colles' fracture often experience permanent impairment, but outcome has been difficult to assess accurately because of a lack of standard measures for symptoms and function. To assess the responsiveness of 3 questionnaires developed to measure outcome, 21 consecutive patients treated for Colles' fracture in a single hand-surgery practice were enrolled in a study.

Methods.—Each patient had a closed fracture of the distal radius metaphysis. The questionnaires used were the short form health survey (SF-36), the Arthritis Impact Measurement Scale, and the Brigham and Women's Hospital carpal tunnel instrument. In the 2 latter instruments, the word "fracture" was substituted for "arthritis" or "carpal tunnel syndrome." Patients underwent physical testing as part of the study and were asked to complete the surveys on the day fracture immobilization was discontinued and again 3 months later.

Results.—Patients ranged in age from 14 to 84 years; 18 of 21 were women. Thirteen fractures were treated by cast alone. Significant improvement occurred during the study period in 2 of the 9 SF-36 scales: physical role and mental health. Only the functional scale of the Brigham instrument showed significant improvement. The Arthritis Impact Measurement Scale included 37 components; significant improvement was recorded for 10, including mobility, hand and finger function, level of psychological function, and pain. Physical measures of outcome indicated improvements in grip, pinch, dexterity, and range of motion.

Discussion.—Patients with Colles' fractures completed questionnaires on 2 occasions 3 months apart. Significant improvements were observed between the day when fracture immobilization was discontinued and at 3-month follow-up. The changes observed during this period fit well with the spectrum of symptoms and impairments previously reported in Colles' fracture. Such standardized instruments should be a part of any study of clinical outcome after this injury. Consolidation of the most responsive items in the 3 questionnaires might provide a new, disease-specific Colles' fracture instrument.

▶ This excellent study once again shows that health survey instruments are important and capture an additional "outcome" besides the classic physical measurements.

B.P. Simmons, M.D.

Suggested Reading

Raimbeau G, for a roundtable study group: Fractures of the lower end of the radius: An appraisal of pinning techniques, based on 285 cases [French]. *Annales Orthopediques de L'ouest* 28:125–170, 1996.

▶ This publication (in French) is the report of a roundtable discussion on management of fractures of the distal radius by percutaneous pinning techniques. There are 10 chapters authored by different orthopedic surgeons, and these chapters include such topics as epidemiology, a classification system, clinical-radiologic correlations, extraosseous complications, and therapeutic indications. This technique of intrafocal closed pinning termed "l'embrochage" has been popularized by Kapandji and is rather widely used in many European Centers.

V.R. Hentz, M.D.

Distal Radioulnar Joint

Functional Anatomy of the Triangular Fibrocartilage Complex
Nakamura T, Yabe Y, Horiuchi Y (Keio Univ, Tokyo)
J Hand Surg (Br) 21B:581–586, 1996 8–44

Background.—The triangular fibrocartilage complex (TFCC) is a fibrocartilage–ligament complex that separates the radiocarpal from the distal radioulnar joint. The TFCC has been shown to stabilize the ulnocarpal and distal radioulnar joints, to transmit and distribute load from the carpus to the ulna, and to permit complex movements of the wrist. However, the TFCC structures that account for its function have not been adequately described.

Methods.—The functional anatomy of the TFCC was assessed in 20 fresh cadavers. Dynamic changes during rotation were assessed from the proximal and distal aspects.

Findings.—The TFCC was found to consist of 3 components: the proximal triangular ligament, the distal hammock structure, and the ulnar collateral ligament (UCL). The triangular ligament stabilizes the radius and ulna, and the hammock structure supports the carpus. The disk proper

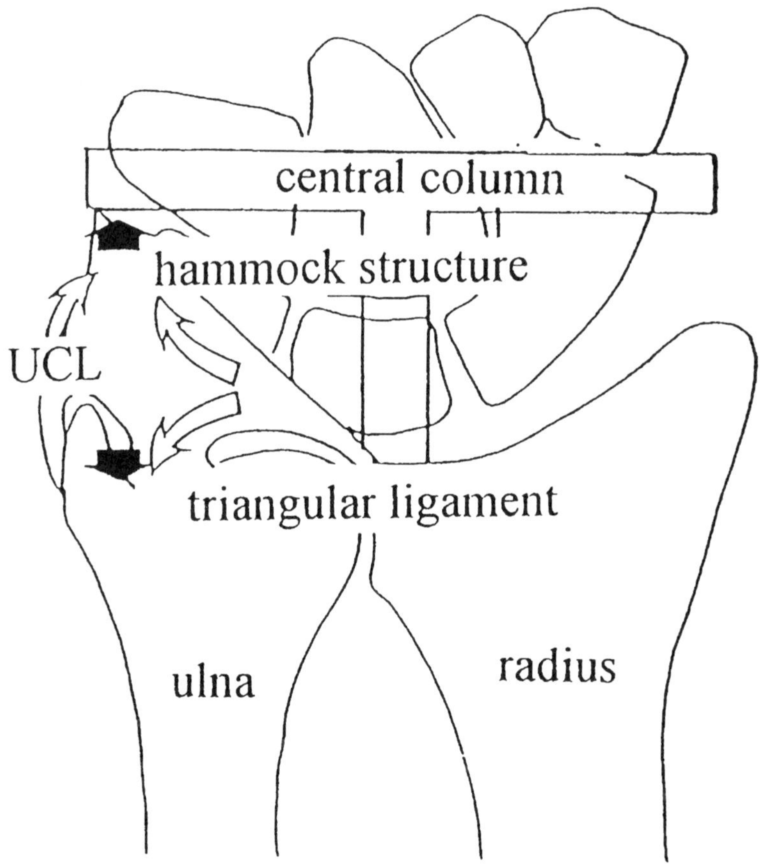

FIGURE 10.—Diagram of structure and function of the triangular fibrocartilage complex (TFCC). The TFCC is separated into 3 components: the proximal triangular ligament, the distal hammock structure, and the ulnar collateral ligament (*UCL*). These 3 components of the TFCC suspend each other, and the loose internal structure of the TFCC absorbs the strain so that both stability and mobility of the ulnar side of the wrist can be achieved. (Courtesy of Nakamura T, Yabe Y, Horiuchi Y: Functional anatomy of the triangular fibrocartilage complex. *J Hand Surg [Br]* 21B:581–586, 1996.)

corresponds to the floor, which is attached to the carpal bones. The suspended distal hammock structure vertically supports the origin of the triangular ligament. This can be deformed and twisted easily. Such twisting permits rotation with little deformity in the disk proper. During pronation and supination, the UCL is twisted. Local deformities at the triangular ligament and UCL are absorbed by the loose internal TFCC tissue. The 3 components' suspension of each other results in TFCC function and in stability and mobility in the ulnar side of the wrist.

Conclusions.—Three TFCC components were identified: the distal component, the proximal component, and the UCL (Fig 10). The first was stable and functioned like a hammock to suspend the ulnar carpus. The second was the fan-shaped triangular ligament, the true radioulnar ligament, which originated from the fovea of the ulna in a vertical fashion and twisted easily during rotation. The third component was the UCL, which also twisted during rotation.

▶ This is yet another attempt at elucidating the structure and function of the components of the TFCC. The authors propose 3 components to both the structure and the function of the TFCC.

The *proximal component*, called the *triangular ligament*, is a true ligamentous sheath spread from radius to ulna. It serves to support the distal radioulnar joint. The *distal component* is likened to a hammock. It represents a large, central, triangular piece of cartilage that is distal and ulnar to the ulnocarpal meniscus homologue. The third, or *ulnar component*, is called the *UCL*, although it represents the floor of the fibrous tunnel of the extensor carpi ulnaris.

Within this arrangement:

1. All 3 components relate to each other and help to stabilize each other.
2. Distal radioulnar joint support is provided by the proximal component or triangular ligament. This is unlike previous descriptions in which the distal radioulnar support was provided by the thickened margins of the triangular cartilage, which was referred to as dorsal and palmar distal radioulnar.
3. Therefore, the thickened margins of the triangular cartilage, the portion of the distal component or hammock of the TFCC, do not actually relate radius to ulna but instead relate radius to carpus. Therefore, these 2 thickened portions reinforce the function of the distal hammock and have no importance in stabilizing the radius to the ulna.
4. The distal component (hammock), unlike in previous descriptions, does not change shape during pronation and supination. All such changes or deformations occur within the insertion of the triangular ligament and the floor of the extensor carpi ulnaris and soft-tissue structures between them. I believe that this representation of the structure and function of the TFCC is quite valuable. To me, it is reminiscent of the soft-tissue structures surrounding the proximal interphalangeal joints of the fingers. The structure and function of the distal hammock are similar to the structure and function of the volar plate–checkrein ligaments complex. The structure and function of the trian-

gular ligament–UCL are reminiscent of the collateral and glenoid portions of the collateral ligament complex at the proximal interphalangeal joint level.

5. Finally, the deformation that occurs during pronation and supination at the triangular ligament and the UCL are absorbed by the loose internal tissues within the TFCC, as well as by the motions that occur between the hammock distally and the triangular ligament more proximally.

J. Taleisnik, M.D.

A Cadaveric Study of the Anatomy and Stability of the Distal Radioulnar Joint in the Coronal and Transverse Planes

Tolat AR, Stanley JK, Trail IA (Wrightington Hosp, Appley Bridge, England)

J Hand Surg (Br) 21B:587–594, 1996 8–45

Background.—Improved understanding of the anatomy of the distal radioulnar joint (DRUJ) would be useful for treatment. The detailed anatomy of the DRUJ was derived from study of 50 cadaverous wrist specimens.

Methods.—Fifty preserved cadaverous wrist specimens were obtained. The average age was 69 years and the male-to-female ratio was 33:17. There were 31 right and 19 left wrists. There was no known disease or injury of the DRUJ in any specimen. Dissection was performed to reveal the articular surface of the distal radius and the triangular fibrocartilaginous complex (TFCC) with the underlying ulna, without disturbing the DRUJ. Photographs were taken, and a midcoronal 5-mm section was removed from the distal articular surface of the radius and the adjoining ulna.

Findings.—There were 3 predominant types of DRUJ: type I, 55%; type II, 33%; and type III, 12%. The average DRUJ angle was 16 degrees. Type II angles were usually 10–15 degrees and type III were usually 15–20 degrees. In type I DRUJ, the apposing joint surfaces were parallel to the long axis of the radius and ulna. Positive ulnar variance was seen in 55%, negative ulnar variance in 33%, and neutral variance in 12%. There was a significant correlation between negative variance and DRUJ type II. The sigmoid notch articular seat was 8 mm, and the ulnar articular seat had an average of 7 mm. The average radius of the seat of the sigmoid notch was 19 mm and the ulnar seat was 10 mm. The sigmoid notch and the ulna were not congruous in the transverse plane. The sigmoid notch sector angle was an average of 60 degrees, whereas the ulna seat sector angle was an average of 100 degrees. There were 4 essential types of sigmoid notch: flat face, ski slope, C, and S (Fig 13). The most common type was the flat face, which was seen in 42%. The mean radioulnar ligament angle was 68 degrees. When only the flat-face sigmoid notch was analyzed, the average radioulnar ligament angle was 78 degrees. An extra-articular palmar osteocartilaginous lip was observed in 80% of the wrists. A smaller form was detected in an additional 18% of flat-face notches. The palmar radioulnar ligament and the palmar capsule were attached to this lip. Manual me-

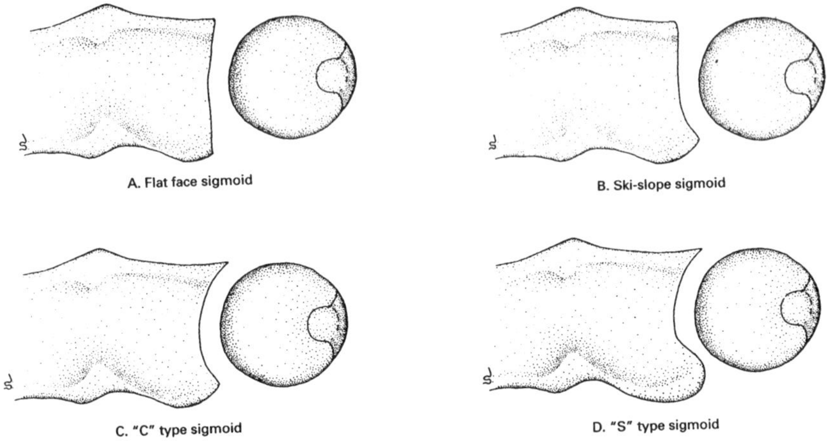

FIGURE 13.—Types of sigmoid notch: A, flat-face sigmoid; B, ski-slope sigmoid; C, "C"-type sigmoid; D, "S"-type sigmoid. (Courtesy of Tolat AR, Stanley JK, Trail IA: A cadaveric study of the anatomy and stability of the distal radioulnar joint in the coronal and transverse planes. *J Hand Surg [Br]* 21B:587–594, 1996).

chanical testing revealed that this palmar lip was a stable buttress to palmar dislocation of the ulna. There was an average of 9 mm of ulnar/triangular fibrocartilaginous complex articulation.

Conclusions.—The anatomy of the DRUJ is complex, with a variety of configurations in the transverse and midcoronal planes. A disparity in the radii of curvature of the sigmoid notch and the ulna-articular surface in the transverse plane results in articular incongruity. Motion of the DRUJ probably consists of sliding and rotation with a small area of true appositional contact. The palmar osteocartilaginous lip appears to be involved in DRUJ stability. Knowledge of the anatomy and stability of the DRUJ will have important clinical applications.

▶ Just as positive and negative ulnar variation in the axial plane has been shown to be important in a range of pathologic conditions affecting the ulnar wrist, so too might the variation in anatomy seen in the coronal and transverse planes, which is nicely explained in this paper, be found to have comparable importance in other wrist conditions. The study, potentially a landmark paper, defines the different shapes of the sigmoid notch in both the coronal and transverse planes and hypothesizes how the different shapes affect the stability of the DRUJ, especially on its volar side. The paper is, as titled, an anatomical study and, as such, gives little specific clinical instruction. However, it is packed with anatomical data that could lead to significant clinical advances. The serious hand surgeon would do well to become familiar with the authors' findings. Some of the information presented is either already known or intuitive, but the 4 transverse and 3 coronal shapes should be learned, and this knowledge could have clinical applicability on occasion. For example, although volar instability of the distal ulna is uncommon, learning the importance of the volar lip of the sigmoid notch might enlighten a hand surgeon treating a patient with such an instability. Ligamentous stability of the DRUJ is apparently more important in the "flat-face sigmoid" than the other types, and knowledge of this might help define when ligamentous reconstruction is needed. The paper is well-written and concise but requires careful reading because of the volume of data it presents.

L.B. Lane, M.D.

Isolated Tears of the Triangular Fibrocartilage: Management by Early Arthroscopic Repair

Trumble TE, Gilbert M, Vedder N (Univ of Washington, Seattle)
J Hand Surg (Am) 22A:57–65, 1997 8–46

Introduction.—The central region of the triangular fibrocartilage complex (TFCC) is limited in its ability to heal because of its hypovascularity. Multiple treatment options are available for repairing tears of the TFCC, but little is reported on repairing the TFCC. The efficacy of arthroscopic repair of the TFCC was retrospectively evaluated in 24 patients.

Methods.—Average patient age was 31 years, and average follow-up was 34 months. Thirteen patients had radial injuries, and 11 had ulnar injuries. All patients had a single traumatic injury with concurrent onset of symptoms. Preoperative arthrograms enabled identification of avulsion of the TFCC from the sigmoid notch in 12 patients. Ten of 11 patients with normal arthrograms had ulnar tears in capsular attachments of the TFCC. The TFCC was reattached to the radius in 9 patients. In 8 patients, the TFCC was attached to the peripheral capsule on the volar or ulnar side of the wrist.

Results.—Compared with the contralateral side, patients regained 89% of total range of motion (ROM) and 85% of grip strength. Compared with the contralateral side, patients with radial repairs had 87% total ROM and 89% grip strength, and patients with ulnar repairs had 91% total ROM and 83% grip strength. Pain was significantly relieved postoperatively, with no between-group differences in patients with radial or ulnar repairs. Fifteen of 20 patients returned to previous work or sports activities. Almost half reported changing the way they performed certain twisting and pushing activities at work. Thirteen of 20 patients submitted Worker's Compensation claims. Of patients with claims, 2 did not return to work. There were no infections. One patient had transient paresthesias in the region of the dorsal sensory branch that resolved in 3 months after an ulnar repair.

Conclusion.—Patients with TFCC repair (radial and ulnar) experienced improvements in ROM, grip strength, and pain relief. Fifteen of 20 patients returned to work in their original jobs.

▶ This manuscript reports a novel approach to increase the available space within the carpal tunnel. The management of carpal tunnel symptoms is based on the physiologic principle that increased pressure within the carpal canal, either from external compression (too small a space) or internal forces (excessive content), produces symptoms. Existing techniques for treating carpal tunnel syndrome decrease pressure within the carpal canal by reducing carpal canal content or increasing available space. Release of the flexor carpi radialis sheath increases the space in the carpal canal, thereby decreasing the pressure. This method should be considered one of many possible surgical approaches to the symptomatic patient with carpal tunnel syndrome.

L.A. Koman, M.D.

Arthroscopic Repair of Peripheral Avulsions of the Triangular Fibrocartilage Complex of the Wrist: A Multicenter Study

Corso SJ, Savoie FH, Geissler WB, et al (Tuckahoe Orthopaedic Assoc, Richmond, Va; Mississippi Sports and Orthopaedic Ctr, Jackson)

Arthroscopy 13:78–84, 1997 8–47

Objective.—Tears of the triangular fibrocartilage complex (TFCC) are now recognized as the major cause of ulnar-sided pain and instability of the distal radioulnar joint. Several different surgical options have been reported; treatment should emphasize the preservation of as much of the triangular fibrocartilage as possible. Excellent results are reported with arthroscopic repair of peripheral avulsions of the TFCC.

Methods.—The multicenter study included 45 wrists of 44 patients. Forty-one wrists had clinical instability after a traumatic event. Associated injuries were present in 27 wrists, including 4 fractures of the distal radius and partial or complete ligamentous ruptures (the scapholunate in 7 cases, lunotriquetral in 9, ulnocarpal in 2, and radiocarpal in 2). Two patients had fractures of the ulnar styloids, and 1 had scapholunate accelerated collapse wrist deformity. A zone-specific repair kit was used to repair the peripheral tears. Munster cast immobilization for 4 weeks permitted elbow flexion and extension but not pronation or supination. This was followed by 2–4 weeks in a short-arm cast or VersaWrist splint. All patients were followed up for 1–3 years, at which time they underwent independent medical examinations, physical therapy, and nursing assessments.

Results.—According to the Mayo modified wrist score, the results were graded as excellent in 29 wrists, good in 12, fair in 1, and poor in 3. Satisfactory results were achieved in 93% of patients, and normal activity was resumed. All wrists had normal motion, and the grip strength was at least 75% of that in the contralateral hand. Two patients had symptoms related to the ulnar nerve and 1 had chronic pain.

Conclusions.—Good results are achieved with arthroscopic repair of the TFCC. If performed with precision, this arthroscopic technique permits accurate approximation of peripheral TFCC avulsions with minimal soft-tissue trauma, good cosmetic results, and quick recoveries. The treatment and prognosis of these injuries depend on the type of tear present.

► As the technical capability of wrist arthroscopy improves, the ability to repair lesions of the wrist now exists as compared with simple débridement. This is particularly true of the peripheral portion of the triangular fibrocartilage.

In contrast to the central portion of the triangular fibrocartilage, the peripheral portion of the triangular fibrocartilage is well vascularized and therefore involves minimal repair. This multicenter study describes 45 patients who underwent arthroscopic repair of the peripheral portion of the triangular fibrocartilage. The repair described is an out–in repair using a mini-suture passer similar to its larger cousin in the shoulder. It should be noted that the procedure can be done equally well using any small cannulated needles, and that the purchase of a specific suture repair kit is not necessary.

Multiple sutures are placed and then tied at the capsular level. This is better than using a button as has been previously described. The preoperative diagnosis was believed to be positive on MRI in 17 cases and on arthrograms in 15 patients. In other patients, the tears were discovered incidentally during arthroscopies for other injuries. In fact, the study is clouded by the fact that 60% of the wrists had associated injuries, including distal radial fractures and ligamentous injuries. It would have been better to keep this study pure, that is, limiting it to the 18 isolated TFCC peripheral tears. A traumatic peripheral tear, the 1B lesion in Palmer's classification of a triangular fibrocartilage injury, is difficult to diagnose preoperatively. Ulnar wrist pain is a common symptom and not pathognomonic.

On physical examination the patients may show a tendency of the carpus to supinate relative to the ulna. The examiner should also test for subluxation of the extensor carpi ulnaris (ECU) tendon as we have found this to be a common co-injury associated with peripheral tears. Obviously, when ECU subluxation is present, not only is an arthroscopic repair of the peripheral portion of the triangular fibrocartilage required but also an open stabilization of the ECU sheath is necessary.

Magnetic resonance imaging and routine arthrography have not been helpful in my experience. I believe that the best indirect imaging technique is the distal radioulnar joint arthrogram because the dye flows out around the peripheral tear. Even so, it was only 65% sensitive in our series. The most accurate way of making a diagnosis is at surgery when the triangular fibrocartilage has lost its normal compliance. It is referred to in the paper as a loss of a trampoline effect. When this is present, particularly with peripheral synovitis, a tear should be suspected.

Despite the multiple associated diagnoses in this series, the overall results of peripheral repair using a Mayo modified wrist score were satisfactory (93%). Unfortunately, the series did not have a table comparing the preoperative values to the postoperative values. Our series has achieved good and excellent results using a similar wrist score in 88% of patients with peripheral repairs at 7½ years of follow-up.

In summary, it is important to classify and define the specific lesion of the triangular fibrocartilage. Relative to the peripheral tear of the triangular fibrocartilage, arthroscopic repair is a valid technique and offers results equal to, if not better than, open repair.

A.L. Osterman, M.D.

Sauvé-Kapandji Procedure for Disorders of the Distal Radioulnar Joint: A Simplified Technique

Rothwell AG, O'Neill L, Cragg K (Christchurch School of Medicine, New Zealand; Burwood Hosp, Christchurch, New Zealand)

J Hand Surg (Am) 21A:771–777, 1996 8–48

Background.—Many techniques have been described for the treatment of painful disorders of the distal radioulnar joint (DRUJ). A simplified version of the Sauvé-Kapandji (SK) procedure, which the authors have used for 10 years, was reported.

Methods.—The essential steps in the traditional SK technique are decortication with or without bone grafting, internal fixation of the DRUJ, removal of a 15-mm length of distal ulna and associated periosteum, and advancement of the pronator quadratus into the pseudarthrosis to be sutured to the sheath of the extensor carpi ulnaris (ECU). The modified procedure differs in several ways. The DRUJ is usually not exposed, nor is the periosteum of the distal ulna excised. In addition, the pronator quadratus is not advanced into the pseudarthrosis. Finally, the superficial and deep parts of the ECU and periosteum sheath are sutured firmly as a single layer over the ulnar stump and pseudarthrosis to stabilize the distal ulna.

Patients and Outcomes.—Of 28 operated wrists, pain relief was achieved in 27. Eighty degrees or greater of pronation and supination was achieved in 19 and 20 patients, respectively. In 18, the DRUJ was fused. Ulnar carpal shift was noted in 3. Equally good outcomes were achieved in rheumatoid and posttrauma patients. The main complications were associated with screw placement and length and prominence of the ECU tendon. The mean operating time was 20 minutes.

Conclusion.—The modified SK procedure reliably alleviates pain at the DRUJ, restores rotation, prevents carpal migration, and shortens operating time. In addition, rehabilitation can begin immediately. With careful attention to surgical technique. Complications are minimal.

▶ This is a retrospective clinical review of 28 wrists in 23 patients who underwent a modified SK procedure, which produced excellent pain-free motion in 17 patients. This is a 74% excellent rate. This result is consistent with those of other authors experienced with this procedure as well as that of ulnar head resection, that is, the Darrach procedure. Unfortunately, 19 wrists were in patients who had rheumatoid arthritis. Of the 9 nonrheumatoid wrists, 7 had distal radius malunion, 1 had osteoarthritis, and 1 had radial ulnar dissociation. This mixed cohort weakens the conclusions of the study.

To add light to the discussion as to which is the "better" procedure—ulnar head resection or ulnar pseudarthrosis creation—will require a randomized, prospective, comparative review of each technique, preferably by 1 surgeon. Until this study is done, the surgeon is faced with 2 apparently equally good alternatives for solving the problem of the painful DRUJ. I suspect that in rheumatoid patients, the choice makes less difference than in nonrheumatoid patients.

L.K. Ruby, M.D.

Arthroplasty of the Wrist by Island Transfer of the Distal Radioulnar Joint [French]

Roux JL, Mouzayek H, Allieu Y (Hôpital Lapeyronie, Montpellier, France; Hôpital Renaudot, Loudun, France)

Ann Chir Main Memb Super 15:121–131, 1996 8–49

Purpose.—The clinical experience with silastic wrist prostheses has been rather unsatisfactory because of their rapid degradation, even when placed in fairly inactive patients. The feasibility of transferring a vascularized distal radioulnar joint to reconstruct a radiocarpal joint damaged by advanced osteoarthritis was explored. The initial clinical experience with the selected procedure was also reported. The distal radioulnar joint was isolated on its anterior interosseous pedicle after its release over a distance of 7–8 cm. After 90-degree rotation, the distal radioulnar joint space was placed in the radiocarpal position with preservation of the pedicle. Bone remodeling was performed to enable correct positioning of the transferred pedicle.

Methods.—The blood supply to the distal radioulnar joint was examined in 40 fresh cadaver upper limbs. Tinted latex was injected into the anterior interosseous artery near its origin. The artery and its various branches were dissected via a dorsal approach. Based on the anatomical findings, surgical options were investigated.

Results.—The lower perforator of the anterior interosseous artery supplied the dorsal epiphyseal periosteal network in all 40 specimens, and the interosseous artery supplied 38 limbs. The anatomical study confirmed that the transfer under consideration was technically possible because the anterior interosseous pedicle was always long enough. Perioperative and postoperative dynamic radiographs confirmed that the reconstructed wrist was stable, with a mobility of approximately 100 degrees in the sagittal plane and 40 degrees in the frontal plane (Fig 9).

Conclusion.—An island transfer of the distal radioulnar joint provides a viable nonprosthetic alternative for patients with advanced osteoarthritis of the wrist who would otherwise undergo arthrodesis as their only therapeutic option.

► This is an ingenious use of the distal radioulnar joint (DRUJ) as a pedicle transfer to avoid wrist fusion. My concerns are (1) lack of long-term follow-up; (2) technical difficulty, specifically whether the rotation necessary would kink the pedicle; (3) inherent relative instability of the DRUJ, which the authors address by soft-tissue enchancement; and (4) ulnar stump impingement against the radius. Some authors from Europe prefer the Sauvé-Kapandji procedure, rather than the Darrach procedure, to avoid stump

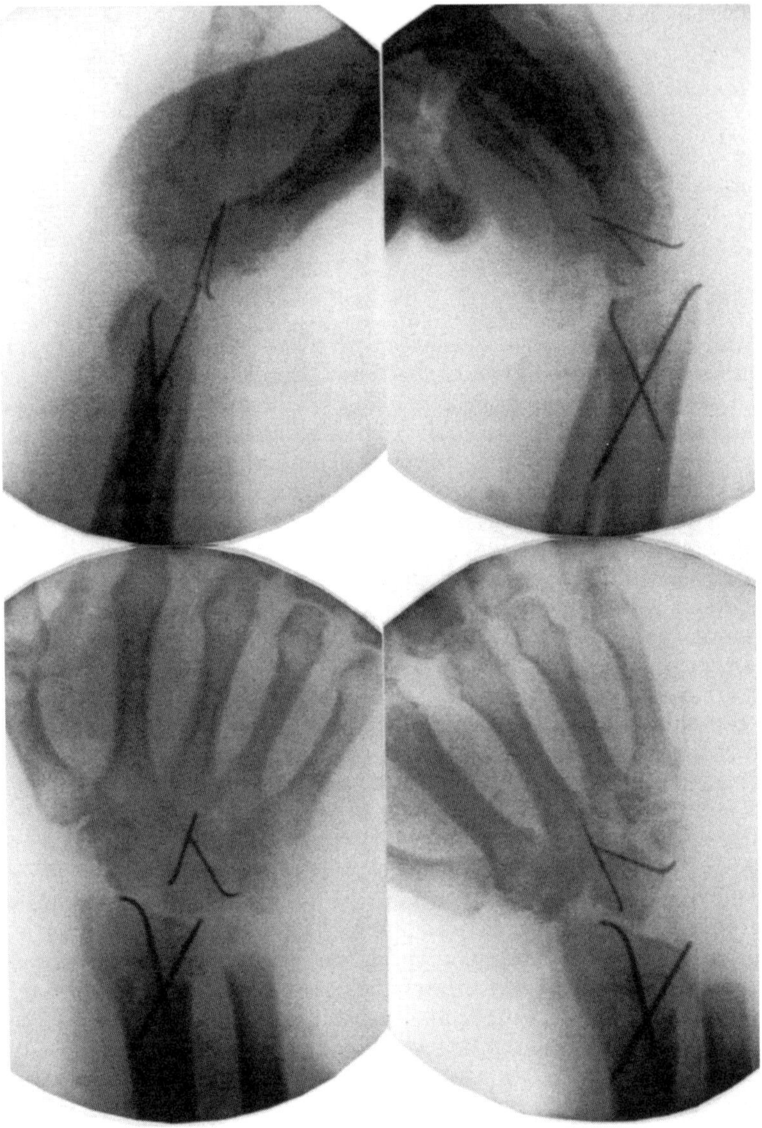

FIGURE 9.—Dynamic postoperative films, confirming the stability of the surgical repair and the range of movement of the reconstructed radiocarpal joint. (Courtesy of Roux JL, Mouzayek H, Allieu Y: Arthroplasty of the wrist by island transfer of the distal radioulnar joint. *Ann Chir Main Memb Super* 15:121–131, 1996.)

impingement, but it was interesting to note that this was not a concern here, in light of the very short ulna created. The authors do say that their indications are limited to a last resort to avoid wrist fusion, but I still could not recommend this procedure over wrist fusion for lack of long-term comparitive results. (Note that because of an editing error in the original article, the text referring to Figure 7 actually explains Figure 8, and that referring to Figure 8 actually explains Figure 9.)

What else will the DRUJ be called on to do in the future? There are rumblings from abroad that the Sauvé-Kapandji procedure might be used to unload the lunate for Kienböck's disease. We will have to wait and see.

J.M. Failla, M.D.

Ulnar Impaction Syndrome: MR Imaging Findings

Imaeda T, Nakamura R, Shionoya K, et al (Nagoya Univ, Aichi, Japan; Toyota Mem Hosp, Japan)

Radiology 201:495–500, 1996 8–50

Purpose.—Lesions of the triangular fibrocartilage complex are an important cause of ulnar wrist pain. It is important to differentiate ulnar impaction syndrome from the senescent changes that occur without clinical symptoms in this area. There have been few reports of the MRI appearance of the carpal bones in ulnar impaction syndrome. Such a study was performed and included arthroscopic confirmation and repeat MRI after ulnar recession or resection arthroplasty.

Methods.—The study included 30 wrists of 27 patients with clinical signs of ulnar impaction syndrome, that is, ulnar wrist pain, tenderness over the ulnar carpal bones or ulnar head or both, and a positive ulnocarpal stress test. All of these wrists underwent T1- and T2-weighted spin-echo MRI followed by arthroscopic ulnar-shortening osteotomy or partial distal ulnar resection (the arthroscopic "wafer" procedure). Eleven wrists had MRI before and after surgery. The MRI scans were analyzed for the signal intensity of the lunate triquetrum and the ulnar head.

Results.—Preoperative MRI showed focal abnormal signal intensity in the ulnar aspect of the lunate in 87% of wrists, in the radial aspects of the triquetrum in 43%, and in the radial aspects of the ulnar head in 10%. Postoperatively, the signal intensity abnormalities were reduced on T1-weighted images and increased on T2-weighted images. In the lunate, surgery shifted the signal intensity from low to slightly low to normal on T1-weighted scans and from low to high to normal on T2-weighted scans (Fig 2). Patients with changes on MRI tended to have greater symptomatic improvement. There was no significant difference in the MRI changes between the 2 types of arthroscopic surgery.

Conclusions.—Most wrists with ulnar impaction syndrome show a characteristic pattern of focal MRI signal intensity changes in the ulnar portion of the lunate. The syndrome is better appreciated on MRI than on plain radiography. With ulnar recession surgery, the signal intensity often returns to normal, and there is greater symptomatic improvement when the MRI picture does change.

▶ There are numerous articles in the literature on marrow abnormalities detected with MRI. Classic avascular necrosis of the hip, humeral head, and

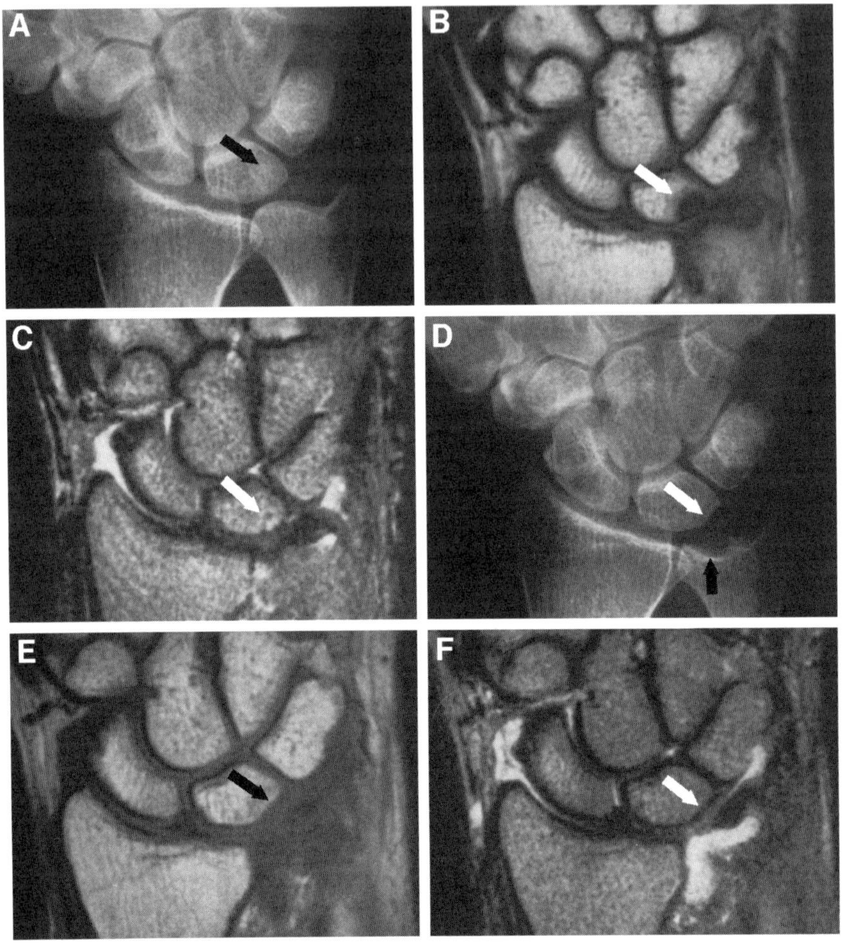

FIGURE 2.—Images obtained in the right hand of a 54-year-old woman (**A–C**) before and (**D–F**) after arthroscopic ulnar head resection arthroplasty. **A**, posteroanterior radiograph of the right wrist reveals a positive ulnar variance and a subtle lucent defect at the ulnar aspect of the proximal lunate (*arrow*). **B**, T1-weighted coronal MR image (500/20) demonstrates a focal area of low signal intensity in the lunate (*arrow*). **C**, corresponding T2-weighted image (2,000/80) demonstrates a focal subchondral area of increased signal intensity in the ulnar aspect of the lunate (*arrow*). **D**, posteroanterior radiograph demonstrates a collapse at the ulnar aspect of the proximal lunate (*white arrow*) and partial removal of the distal ulnar head (*black arrow*). **E**, T1-weighted image (500/20) and **F**, T2-weighted image (2,000/80) demonstrate that the signal intensity of the lunate (*arrow*) has changed to almost normal. (Courtesy of Imaeda T, Nakamura R, Shionoya K, et al: Ulnar impaction syndrome: MR imaging findings. *Radiology* 201:495–500, 1996. Copyright Radiological Society of North America.)

larger bones is seen with a well-defined geographic pattern. There is often associated marrow edema. Changes caused by ischemic disease in the carpal bones are more diffuse. Therefore, local changes, especially in the ulnar aspect of the lunate, are more often a result of ulnar impaction syndrome. The site and signal intensity changes seen with this condition are easily differentiated from osteonecrosis.

Ulnar impaction syndrome may be diagnosed clinically, and routine radiographs are often confirmatory. When indicated, MRI is the technique of choice to define this process, to follow the therapeutic response, and to exclude other causes for the patients' symptoms.

T.H. Berquist, M.D.

Suggested Reading

Nakamura R, Horii E, Imaeda T, et al: Criteria for diagnosing distal radioulnar joint subluxation by computed tomography. *Skeletal Radiol* 25:649–653, 1996.
▶ In this evaluation of criteria for axial CT measurements in DRUJ subluxation, modifications of the conventional methods are shown to markedly reduce the false positive rate.

G. Bergman, M.D.

Sagerman SD, Short W: Arthroscopic repair of radial-sided triangular fibrocartilage complex tears. *Arthroscopy* 12:339–342, 1996.
▶ The authors show us a technique of repair of TFCC tears from the avascular portion of the TFCC from the sigmoid notch (Palmer Class 1-D) tears. This is the type of tear that is frequently treated with arthroscopic débridement. About two thirds had good or excellent results. However, this technique requires 8 weeks of immobilization. Are their results enough superior to débridement of these lesions to justify 6 weeks of additional immobilization? The authors provide no information regarding pain relief, complication, and postoperative range of motion. This study does not provide enough information to justify the authors' recommendation that their direct suture technique should be used. A prospective study comparing arthroscopic débridement and the direct suture technique should answer these questions.

E.R. North, M.D.

Subscribe to the related journal in your field!

Yes! Begin my one-year subscription to ***Journal of Shoulder and Elbow Surgery*** (6 issues).

Name ______________________________

Institution ______________________________

Address ______________________________

City ____________________ State ________

ZIP/PC __________ Country ______________

Specialty ______________________________
(Students/residents, please list Institution)

Subscription prices (through 9/30/98)

		USA	Canada*	Int'l
Individuals	❑	$111.00	$147.66	$138.00
Institutions	❑	134.00	172.27	161.00
Students, residents	❑	55.00	87.74	82.00

Method of payment

Enclose payment (check or credit card number) and we'll send an extra issue FREE!

❑ Check (in U.S. dollars, drawn on a U.S. bank, and payable to ***Journal of Shoulder and Elbow Surgery***)

❑ VISA ❑ MasterCard ❑ Discover

❑ AmEx ❑ Bill me Exp. date__________

Card #______________________________

Signature ______________________________

*Includes Canadian GST

Individual/student subscriptions must be in the name of, billed to, and paid for by the individual.

Canada/Int'l prices include airmail postage.
Prices subject to change without notice.

J032983YA

Reservation Card for the Year Book

Yes! I would like my own copy of ***Year Book of Hand Surgery***® at the price of **$80.00** plus sales tax, postage, and handling. Please begin my subscription with the current edition according to the terms described below.* I understand that I will have 30 days to examine each annual edition.

Name ______________________________

Address ______________________________

City ______________________________ State __________ ZIP__________

Method of Payment

Check (in U.S. dollars, drawn on a U.S. bank, payable to ***Year Book of Hand Surgery***®)

❑ VISA ❑ MasterCard ❑ Discover ❑ AmEx ❑ Bill me

Card number ______________________________ Exp. date:__________

Signature ______________________________

Prices are subject to change without notice.

PMC-017

*Your Year Book service guarantee:

When you subscribe to the *Year Book*, you will receive advance notice of future annual volumes about two months before publication. To receive the new edition, you need do nothing—we'll send you the new volume as soon as it is available. If you want to discontinue, the advance notice allows you time to notify us of your decision. If you are not completely satisfied, you have 30 days to return any *Year Book*.

NO POSTAGE
NECESSARY
IF MAILED
IN THE
UNITED STATES

BUSINESS REPLY MAIL

FIRST-CLASS MAIL PERMIT NO 135 ST LOUIS MO

POSTAGE WILL BE PAID BY ADDRESSEE

SUBSCRIPTION SERVICES
MOSBY–YEAR BOOK, INC.
11830 WESTLINE INDUSTRIAL DRIVE
ST. LOUIS MO 63146-9988

NO POSTAGE
NECESSARY
IF MAILED
IN THE
UNITED STATES

BUSINESS REPLY MAIL

FIRST-CLASS MAIL PERMIT NO 135 ST LOUIS MO

POSTAGE WILL BE PAID BY ADDRESSEE

Mosby

PAT NEWMAN
11830 WESTLINE INDUSTRIAL DRIVE
PO BOX 46908
ST. LOUIS MO 63146-9934

Want to speed up the process?

**To order the *Year Book*,
you also may call 1-800-426-4545**

**To subscribe to the journal today,
call toll-free in the U.S.:
1-800-453-4351
or fax 314-432-1158
Outside the U.S., call: 314-453-4351**

Visit us at:
www.mosby.com/Mosby/Periodicals

Mosby–Year Book, Inc.
Subscription Services
11830 Westline Industrial Drive
St. Louis, MO 63146 U.S.A.

Mosby

9 Neuromuscular Disorders

Transposition of the Bicipital Tuberosity for Treatment of Fixed Supination Contracture in Obstetric Brachial Plexus Lesions

Eberhard D (Univ of Vienna)

J Hand Surg (Br) 22B:261–263, 1997 9–1

Background.—In many patients with obstetric brachial plexus lesions (Klumpke type), the forearm and hand are supinated by the action of the biceps muscle unopposed by the pronator teres, and the wrist is held in dorsiflexion. In other cases, supination is fixed. Supination contracture can result from contraction of the interosseous membrane or stiffness of the proximal or distal radioulnar joints. A surgical technique using reinsertion of the biceps tendon on the bicipital tuberosity was described.

Patients.—Of 23 patients with supination deformities from obstetric brachial plexus lesions, 9 could not achieve passive pronation in spite of mobilization of the radioulnar joint and longitudinal division of the interosseous membrane. In these 9 patients, impingement of the bicipital tuberosity on the ulna was the primary obstacle to achieving passive pronation. The mean patient age was 15 years.

> *Technique.*—A midlateral incision was made on the lateral aspect of the arm to the forearm. The muscle attachments to the proximal radius were divided, including the supinator muscle. The interosseous membrane was split longitudinally in 8 patients. The forearm was brought into supination after the bicipital tuberosity passed the ulna with a click. A chisel was used to remove the tuberosity and attached biceps tendon. The site of bicipital tuberosity reinsertion selected was the dorsoradial border of the radius to produce a neutral forearm position if no supinator muscle was available; reinsertion was more dorsal on the radius to produce a pronating effect in cases of a well-developed supinator muscle.

Results.—The hand achieved a more functional position in all patients at a mean of 29.4 months. In 5 patients, active pronation and supination were achieved. In 3 patients, active pronation only was achieved. In 1 patient, passive motion only was achieved. Seven patients were able to increase pronation by contraction of the biceps muscle.

Discussion.—In these 9 patients, the supinator muscle had lost its antagonists, and the pull of this muscle caused an approximation between the proximal radius and ulna. The short distance between the radius and ulna caused the bicipital tuberosity to impinge on the ulna. The bicipital tuberosity caused supination contracture in 9 of the 23 patients. This high percentage may be partly explained by the high average age of these patients.

▶ Eberhard's article describes a series of 9 patients with distal brachial plexus lesions (Klumpke type) in which chronic muscle imbalance has produced close approximation of the proximal radius and ulna, resulting in impingement of the bicipital tuberosity on the ulna as the primary cause of fixed forearm supination. Published reviews of obstetric brachial plexus lesions have reported that distal plexus palsies may occur in as few as 0.6% of all obstetric palsies.

Current literature recommends treatment of secondary obstetric plexus lesions within the first decade of life. Therefore, Eberhard's series of 9 patients treated at an average age of 15 years is quite unusual, and patients seen with this problem will be infrequently encountered. However, in the rarity of the problem is the usefulness of this paper. Eberhard's paper should alert the surgeon to possible bicipital tuberosity impingement when release of the interosseous membrane and mobilization of the proximal and distal radiounlar joints do not result in significant improvement in forearm pronation.

In addition to documentation of bicipital tuberosity impingement by direct visual inspection intraoperatively, the article describes a method of transferring the bicipital tuberosity and attached biceps tendon to the dorsoradial border of the radius, holding the forearm in a more functional position. Reattaching the tuberosity to the radius with a screw and washer provides excellent fixation and may be technically easier than rerouting the biceps tendon as described by Zancolli.[1] Although few objective results were reported, all patients had improvement of their fixed forearm supination. Eberhard alerts the surgeon to a potential cause of fixed supination deformity in the older child seen with a lower brachial plexus nerve palsy and describes a simple and effective reconstructive technique.

A.A. Stans, M.D.

Reference

1. Zancolli E: Paralytic supination contracture of the forearm. *J Bone Joint Surg (Am)* 49A:1275–1284, 1976.

Extensor Indicis Opposition Transfer in the Ulnar and Median Palsied Thumb in Leprosy

Mehta R, Malaviya GN, Husain S (Central Jalma Inst for Leprosy, Tajganj, India)

J Hand Surg (Br) 21B:617–621, 1996 9–2

Introduction.—Loss of thumb abduction and opposition is a serious disability that may result from peripheral nerve injuries, peripheral neuropathies, and poliomyelitis. In endemic areas, leprosy is the major cause of ulnar and median palsied thumb. Once the patient's leprosy has stabilized, early correction of the palsy is indicated to prevent secondary complications. A number of operative procedures have been proposed to restore thumb function, including transfer of the extensor indicis proprius (EIP), as originally described by Burkhalter et al. The results of EIP opponensplasty to correct ulnar and median palsied thumbs in patients with leprosy were reviewed.

Methods.—Transfer of the EIP as an abductor and opponens was done in 27 hands of 25 patients during 14 years. Most patients had borderline tuberculoid-type leprosy and were receiving adequate antileprosy therapy. Ulnar and median paralysis had been present for a mean of 3 years, 7 months. In each hand, EIP opponensplasty was done using Palande's modification of the technique of Burkhalter et al. Because of initial problems with tendon length, transinterosseous transfer was used in later cases. In this modification, the bulk of the flexor tendons was used as a pulley, and the transfer was routed medial to the flexor tendon mass up to the proximal crease, then along the abductor pollicis brevis to the level of the metacarpophalangeal joint. The metacarpophalangeal joint was stabilized by an additional transfer of the radial half of the flexor pollicis longus to the extensor pollicis longus. The patients were studied for a mean of 9 years, 7 months.

Results.—The thumb regained sufficient strength for activities by about 12 weeks, with stable results after 6 months. The results were rated as good in 13 hands, fair in 11, and poor in 3. The span of the hand increased after surgery in all hands but 1. Abduction was at least 41 degrees in 19 of the 27 hands. Improved ability and strength were reported by the patient in 25 of 27 hands. Complications included loss of full extension of the proximal interphalangeal joint of the index finger, recurrent thumb web contracture, and failure to learn how to use the transfer.

Conclusions.—Opponensplasty using the EIP gives good results in patients with ulnar and median palsied thumb as a result of leprosy. The problem of limited tendon length and excursion can be avoided by transinterosseous transfer. Adequate repair of the extensor hood of the index finger is essential. Also, the patient must receive training and encouragement in the use of transfer postoperatively.

▶ The authors describe a potentially useful modification of Burkhalter's extensor indicis transfer and provide a useful option in reconstructing pinch function in combined median and ulnar palsy. Passing the transfer transosseous instead of around the medial border of the ulna gains some length in a transfer that occasionally is a little short if passed in the typical manner. Attaching a distally detached slip of the flexor pollicis longus tendon to the extensor pollicis longus tendon over the proximal phalanx is useful in reducing the tendency of the interphalangeal joint to flex excessively (Froment's paper sign) and to stabilize the metacarpophalangeal joint against hyperextension. I have done this procedure many times in patients with tetraplegia who are undergoing brachioradialis to flexor pollicis longus transfer to restore pinch, and it has been a reliable performer.

V.R. Hentz, M.D.

Brachioradialis Transfer for Wrist Extension in Tetraplegic Patients Who Have Fifth-Cervical-Level Neurological Function

Johnson DL, Gellman H, Waters RL, et al (Univ of Kentucky, Lexington; Univ of Arkansas, Little Rock; Rancho Los Amigos Med Ctr, Downey, Calif)
J Bone Joint Surg (Am) 78A:1063–1067, 1996 9–3

Background.—Augmenting extension of the wrist in patients with high-level tetraplegia may be done by transferring the brachioradialis to the extensor carpi radialis longus and brevis. This procedure may also indirectly improve grasp and pinch, because active dorsiflexion of the wrist may bring about passive flexion of the fingers and thumb. The outcomes of this procedure in patients with traumatic tetraplegia and neurologic function classified at the fifth cervical level were reported.

Methods.—Nine patients were treated. The mean interval between injury and surgery was 6 years. Average follow-up time was 10 years. Patient assessment included range of wrist motion, manual muscle-testing of the strength of the brachioradialis and wrist extensors, functional assessment of the ability to perform activities of daily living, and evaluation of functional independence before and after surgery. Patients were also asked to assess their outcomes subjectively.

Findings.—Preoperatively, none of the patients had active extension of the wrist against gravity. Postoperatively, wrist extensor strength improved to a grade of good in 6 patients and to fair-plus in 3. Seven patients had a marked improvement in hand function. None of the patients had a loss of function. The patients' ability to pick up objects, feed and groom themselves, tend to personal hygiene, write and type, and use a telephone was improved.

Conclusions.—In these tetraplegic patients with fifth-cervical-level neurologic function, brachioradialis transfer improved the strength of the wrist extensors. Most patients also had improved function. Performing the brachioradialis and key-grip procedure in stages may have yielded better outcomes.

▶ Patients at the upper levels of spinal cord injury where reconstruction of voluntary function by voluntary tendon transfers is possible, benefit most from the addition of wrist extension. Johnson and colleagues highlight in this article the important increases in tenodesis function and functional ability that occur when wrist extension is replaced; even at Grade 3 (fair levels), more than simple wrist extension takes place. In addition to the movements afforded by tenodesis grip, a change in the balance of the hand, the addition of substitution patterns, and the usefulness of hand posture alone to position the fingers in space are small but significant improvements. Moreover, patients prefer the use of the voluntary powered wrist to the exclusion of static braces and tenodesis splints; this increases their satisfaction. In a time when diminished resources are available for severely disabled individuals, the most efficient combination of tendon transfers and other surgical procedures should be sought.

In this series, if brachioradialis did not achieve sufficient strength, then other adjunctive procedures were less successful. In tenodesis procedures, the balancing of the fingers is governed by the effectiveness of the outcome of the brachioradialis transfer. A substantial number of patients with C5 lesions will not have the strength, coordination, or wrist range of motion to provide sufficient finger function.

M. Keith, M.D.

Localizing Muscles for Botulinum Toxin Treatment of Focal Hand Dystonia

Geenen C, Consky E, Ashby P (Univ of Toronto)
Can J Neurol Sci 23:194–197, 1996 9–4

Background.—The best method for localizing muscles in the forearm for injection has not been established definitively. The value of electromyography (EMG) and stimulation for localizing muscles for botulinum toxin (BTX) injection and for predicting the risk of unwanted weakness in nontarget muscles was investigated.

Methods.—Twelve patients with focal hand dystonia were included. A single target muscle, clinically determined to contribute most to the dystonic hand posture, was selected for BTX injection. By random assignment, 8 patients had the target muscle localized by recording the EMG signals during voluntary contractions, and 4 had the muscle localized by local electrical stimulation. A standardized dose of BTX was then injected into the target muscle.

Findings.—The target muscle was weakened in 7 of the 12 patients 3 weeks after BTX injection. This was achieved in half the EMG group and in three fourths of the stimulation group. Noninjected muscles adjacent to the target muscle were weakened in 5 of the 7 patients, apparently because of toxin diffusion.

Conclusions.—Localization by stimulation appears to be as good or better than EMG, although each technique has advantages. Neither EMG nor stimulation consistently predicted nontarget muscles weakness, which suggests that BTX diffuses farther than the volume conduction of EMG signals or the spread of effective stimulus current.

▶ This article describes and compares 2 methods for localizing muscles within the forearm when injecting BTX. Accurate identification of the involved muscle(s), a prerequisite for treatment of focal hand dystonias, was not addressed. In 8 patients, EMG provided guidance while positioning the needle. In the remaining 4 patients, the injecting needle was repositioned until the target muscle was the first to contract with increasing levels of electric stimulation. In all but 1 muscle, a dose of 25 U of toxin was used. One patient received 10 U of toxin targeted for the index finger belly of the flexor digitorum superficialis. Outcomes were measured by subjectively assessing the strength of target and adjacent muscles and by the patients' reports of handwriting. Four of 8 patients injected using EMG guidance demonstrated at least 1 Medical Research Council grade strength decrease in the targeted muscle. Three of 4 patients injected using stimulation showed a similar result. Failure to cause weakness was attributed to technical factors, not to antibody formation. Half the patients reported handwriting improvement. The authors concluded that localization by stimulation is at least as good as localization by EMG and discussed clinical situations in which 1 technique may be superior to the other.

Some care should be taken when applying the results of this study. The authors fail to indicate whether the American or European formulation of BTX was used, and significant differences exist between the 2 in terms of potency. Current pulses, as described, stimulate peripheral nerves or terminal branches rather than muscle. It is possible, therefore, for muscle contraction to occur with the tip of the needle outside the fascia. Although stimulation for site localization appears to be a useful adjunct to EMG, it may not be sufficient alone.

C. Burgar, M.D.

Correction of Severe Spastic Flexion Contractures in the Nonfunctional Hand

Pomerance JF, Keenan MAE (Hand Surgery Associates, SC, Arlington Heights, Ill; Albert Einstein Med Ctr, Philadelphia)

J Hand Surg (Am) 21A:828–833, 1996 9–5

Background.—The main surgical treatment of spasticity in nonfunctional hands is directed at the extensor flexor of the hand and wrist; the major goal is improved hygiene. However, long-term follow-up of such patients has indicated that recurrence of the wrist deformity and incomplete digital correction from unaddressed intrinsic abnormalities can occur. The use of a single-stage procedure to provide comprehensive correction of the severely spastic hand was described.

Methods.—Fourteen patients underwent a total of 15 procedures during a 3-year period to alleviate severe flexion contractures of the hand and wrist. All patients had had unsuccessful nonsurgical treatment or had chronic skin problems. The single-stage, comprehensive procedure consisted of superficialis to profundus transfer, wrist flexor release, flexor pollicis longus lengthening, wrist arthrodesis, carpal tunnel release, and ulnar motor branch neurectomy or intrinsic release. The mean follow-up time was 1 year.

Findings.—Wrist fusion after the index procedure occurred in 13 patients. One patient needed replating, and another needed uniting after prolonged casting. In 2 patients, a residual claw hand resulted, with only partial correction of a thumb-in-palm deformity. All hygiene problems and infections seen before surgery resolved after surgery.

Conclusion.—The comprehensive protocol used in these patients enabled correction of severe hand and wrist contractures by a single operation. Improved care and appearance of the hand resulted. This protocol is recommended for all nonfunctional hands.

▶ The authors describe an aggressive approach to correcting the position of the spastic nonfunctional hand. Their goals were implied but not clearly stated: to alleviate or prevent skin breakdown, fixed contractures, and nerve compression. Although they successfully resolved hygiene problems and improved the position of the hand and wrist in all 15 treated hands, their complications were significant.

The authors recommend hospital admission for elevation for 24 hours (their tourniquet times averaged 160 minutes), but they did not stress this adequately. The patients selected for this surgical protocol will not have symptoms of compartment syndrome, and unless their home care is exemplary, they should be admitted for at least 48 hours of continuous elevation. The authors recommend this protocol for use in "all nonfunctional hands," but their argument for always doing a wrist arthrodesis is not convincing. They do not give the failure rate of soft-tissue procedures alone, although they imply that it is unacceptable.

This protocol will be useful for the surgeon treating a nonfunctional hand with severe fixed flexion contractures and intractable skin breakdown. The authors have not adequately identified other indications for this protocol. They have not provided convincing evidence that the benefits of the protocol outweight the risks for patients with asymptomatic fixed contractures or nerve compression in the absence of skin breakdown, although they have recommended it for these patients.

M.A. James, M.D.

Treatment of Spastic Thumb-in-palm Deformity: A Modified Extensor Pollicis Longus Tendon Rerouting

Rayan GM, Saccone PG (Univ of Oklahoma, Oklahoma City; Baptist Med Ctr, Oklahoma City, Okla)

J Hand Surg (Am) 21A:834–839, 1996 9–6

Background.—Thumb-in-palm deformity—a flexion adduction position of the thumb against the palm or between digits—occurs in patients with cerebral palsy or brain tumors or after head trauma or stroke. Releasing contractures and balancing the muscle forces by tendon transfers are effective. The vector of the extensor pollicis longus (EPL) muscle pull can be redirected by rerouting its tendon in line with the extensor pollicis brevis and abductor pollicis longus. The outcomes of EPL rerouting for thumb-in-palm deformity in a select group of patients using a modified surgical technique were reported.

Methods and Findings.—Fourteen patients with 15 hands affected by spastic thumb-in-palm deformities underwent modified EPL tendon rerouting. Deformities were corrected satisfactorily in 12 patients. Functional improvement, which was not anticipated in every hand, was achieved to some extent in 12. In severely affected hands, the best outcomes were achieved when rerouting was combined with metacarpophalangeal joint fusion and release of adductor pollicis and first dorsal interosseous muscles.

Conclusion.—Extensor pollicis longus tendon rerouting can provide satisfactory correction of severe thumb-in-palm deformity, particularly when combined with other procedures. This modified technique can be performed with 1 incision and permits easy adjustment of tension.

▶ The authors modified Manske's technique,[1] and expanded the indications for EPL rerouting to include severely involved patients with nonfunctional thumbs and skin problems, with good results. They cite the use of 1 rather than 2 incisions and easily adjusted tension on the tendon repair as the reasons for their modification.

Manske's technique works very nicely, and this article does not convince me that it requires modification. The authors have added metacarpophalangeal fusion in 7 of 15 procedures; this, rather than the tendon rerouting, is probably the reason they achieved respectable results in severely involved patients.

They performed metacarpophalangeal joint arthrodesis in 2 children under age 8 years; I would not recommend this procedure in this age group. As the authors acknowledge, arthrodesis is not necessary with Manske's technique.

They also added thumb intrinsic release in only 5 patients; in my experience, this is required more often. In addition, I disagree with their conclusion that sensory deficit has no bearing on functional outcome (which they did not prove, as they could only test sensibility in 2 patients). Sometimes the potential benefits of EPL rerouting outweigh the risks in a patient with poor sensibility, but this does not mean that sensibility has no effect on the outcome.

M.A. James, M.D.

Reference

1. Manske PR: Redirection of extensor pollicis longus in the treatment of spastic thumb-in-palm deformity. *J Hand Surg (Am)* 10A:553–560, 1985.

Suggested Reading

Faghri PD: The effects of neuromuscular stimulation-induced muscle contraction versus elevation on hand edema in CVA patients. *J Hand Ther* 10:29–34, 1997. ► Electrostimulation showed remarkable results. However, edema reduction was only temporary and only 8 subjects were tested.

K.A. Bengtson, M.D.

10 Repetitive Motion Disorders

Factors Prolonging Disability in Work-related Cumulative Trauma Disorders

Bonzani PJ, Millender L, Keelan B, et al (New England Baptist Hosp, Boston; Occupational Health & Rehabilitation, Waltham, Mass)

J Hand Surg (Am) 22A:30–34, 1997 10–1

Background.—Workers' compensation costs for the treatment of soft-tissue disorders are increasing. A classification system was developed to aid physicians in recognizing nonmedical issues that interfere with a rapid return to employment.

Classification System and Findings.—The charts of 50 patients with a diagnosis of a soft-tissue disorder associated with a repetitive motion or awkward posture were reviewed. After standard clinical and radiographic examinations, the patients' musculoskeletal disorders were classified into 3 groups: group 1, objective findings of swelling, limited joint passive range of motion, abnormal radiographic findings, or positive electrodiagnostic results; group 2, reasonable subjective symptoms, such as pain, tenderness, weakness, and/or sensory loss consistent with injury; and group 3, unreasonable subjective symptoms, including diffuse, vague, nonreproducible pain not corresponding to anatomical distribution or out of proportion to the injury.

Ergonomic factors were also classified into 3 groups: group 1, minor, easily correctable ergonomic issues; group 2, moderate issues, with minimal opportunity for job restructuring; and group 3, major ergonomic issues, with workstation designs and job demands that could not be modified in any substantial way. Psychosocial issues were classified as minor (group 1), consisting of administrative issues such as arranging modified duty, modified work schedules, breaks, and/or job rotation; moderate (group 2), characterized by job frustrations or stresses causing employee anger that were manageable by physician or therapist intervention with the employer; and major (group 3), including long-standing frustrations or anger associated with job and/or family stresses that could not be resolved. The review of patient data indicated that the psychosocial classification of the patient and current employment status are the most important factors in prolonging worker disability.

▶ It should come as no surprise that patients whose complaints are vague and nonanatomical are less likely to return to work, especially when job modification is difficult or job frustrations and/or chronic pain behaviors are present. What is reassuring is the number of patients whose clinical complaints are consistent with a specific anatomical diagnosis who can be maintained in the workforce despite significant ergonomic or psychosocial issues. I believe that this paper reflects the particular influence of 1 of the authors, the late Lewis Millender. If Boston were in Japan, Lewis would have been a *sensei*; if it were in India, he would have been a *guru*. Because he lived in the United States where we have no specific word to describe a special, thoughtful, compassionate, and considerate lover of truth and of his fellowman (and woman), *teacher and friend* will have to suffice. Thank you, Lewis, for 1 more gift.

P.C. Amadio, M.D.

Neurologic Manifestations of Cumulative Trauma Disorder
Uhl RL, Dubin A, Manseau C, et al (Albany Med College, NY)
Am J Orthop 25:478–480, 1996 10–2

Introduction.—Upper extremity pain and dysfunction without a single, specific injury may occur in individuals performing repetitive tasks. This situation has been described as cumulative trauma disorder, and symptoms are related to inflammation of muscles, joints, and tendon sheaths, and to neuropathy (or numbness, burning pain, tingling). Patients with neurologic manifestations of cumulative trauma disorders were reviewed to establish diagnostic criteria and treatment guidelines.

Patients.—Medical histories of 470 worker's compensation patients with upper-extremity pain were reviewed. Of these, 66 had no specific explanations for their pain, had neurologic symptoms related to repetitive activities, and some evidence of a discrete site of nerve compression. Electrodiagnostic studies were performed, and the patients were assigned into 1 of 2 groups: 24 had a clinical picture that fit the results of the electrodiagnostic study, such as numbness in the thumb and index finger, positive Tinel's sign at wrist, and/or compression of the median nerve at the wrist; 42 did not fit the electrodiagnostic study. The latter patients had numbness in the fingers, but had normal study results or results that showed median neuropathy when the patient complained of pain at the dorsal forearm.

Results.—All patients had a history of repetitive work for 2–13 years. After a change in job demands, 48 of 66 noticed their symptoms. All patients had conservative treatment first with rest, splinting, anti-inflammatory medication, steroid injections, and hand therapy. In 20 patients whose clinical picture fit the electrodiagnosis, surgical results were much

TABLE 1.—Response to Surgery

Category	Symptom Relief Reported by Patient
Complete relief	Preoperative symptoms gone, return to all activities
Substantial improvement	Some residual symptoms, some limitation of activities
Some improvement	Improvement in some preoperative symptoms, others not improved
No improvement	Preoperative symptoms remain or have completely recurred

(Reprinted by permission of the publisher from Uhl RL, Dubin A, Manseau C, et al: Neurologic manifestations of cumulative trauma disorder. *Am J Orthop* 25:478–480. Copyright 1996 by Quadrant Healthcom Inc.)

more predictable, with 80% getting good relief of symptoms (Table 1). The 42 patients with the more diffuse type of electrodiagnostic clinical picture had less relief of symptoms from surgery.

Conclusion.—Patients who do not have a clear electrodiagnostic clinical picture have less relief of symptoms from surgery; however, the role of electrodiagnostic studies in patients with neurologic complaints is still not well defined.

▶ The authors acknowledge that the term "repetitive" is arbitrary. They should also state that it is imprecise. Because there is no true definition in the medical literature of repetitive, the authors, in listing these groups of patients, should give the numbers of repetitions and force for the individual job. Electrodiagnostic studies are frequently mentioned in the literature, and there is now a standard—a criterion set up by the American Academy of Neurology. Not all electrodiagnostic tests are of equal quality, just as all radiographs are not of equal quality.

It should be emphasized that work and underlying medical conditions cannot be considered a cause of a specific diagnosis such as carpal tunnel syndrome. They would be considered risk factors.

The authors do not include job satisfaction in their criteria. In my opinion, this is the essential factor in getting patients back to work and free of symptoms.

The authors note that physical examination revealed multiple neuropathies, yet none of these patients was completely improved by surgery. What were the physical findings? Were atrophy or trophic changes noted?

The authors also failed to address how the patient's symptoms related to nonwork activities. If you carefully question these patients, you will find that their symptoms are aggravated equally by many household chores in addition to their work activities. I continue to believe that the term "cumulative trauma" is inappropriate and that the specific diagnoses should be listed.

This article fails to address individual personal health attributes and body characteristics that so greatly influence an individual's response to the job.

M.L. Kasdan, M.D.

Hand Problems in 100 Vibration-exposed Symptomatic Male Workers

Strömberg T, Dahlin LB, Lundborg G (Malmö Univ, Sweden; Kristianstad Central Hosp, Sweden)

J Hand Surg (Br) 21B:315–319, 1996 10–3

Introduction.—A substantial industrial problem exists with vibration-induced hand problems, expressed as a hand-arm vibration syndrome; the average prevalence of hand-arm vibration syndrome among workers exposed to vibration is 50%, according to the National Institute for Occupational Safety and Health. Neurosensory problems include vibration-induced white fingers, paresthesia, numbness, impaired manual dexterity, and carpal tunnel syndrome. In orthopedic and hand surgical practice, vibration-induced hand problems are not always sufficiently well recognized. The symptoms and clinical findings of 100 vibration-exposed male symptomatic workers were analyzed.

Methods.—Included were 100 vibration-exposed men ranging in age from 23 to 61 years who were exposed to vibration by hand-held tools up to more than 30 years before they were referred to a hand surgical department for neurosensory and vasospastic problems in the hand. The group included platers, grinders and welders, mechanics, concrete and stone workers, carpenters, electricians, and truck drivers. Their symptoms were numbness with or without tingling, intermittent or persistent numbness and reduced sensory perception, and intermittent or persistent numbness with reduced tactile discrimination and/or manipulative dexterity.

Results.—Forty-eight percent had isolated neurosensory symptoms, 20% had isolated vasospastic problems, and 32% had combined neurosensory and vasospastic problems. In 27% of the patients, there was abnormal cold intolerance, with pain and coldness without blanching of the fingers on exposure to cold. There was a greater predominance of neurosensory problems than vasospastic problems, particularly in the first 20 years of vibration exposure. Twenty-two of 80 patients with neurosensory symptoms had carpal tunnel syndrome.

Conclusion.—Neurosensory symptoms are not often related to carpal tunnel syndrome, and vibration-induced neurosensory and vasospastic symptoms can occur separately or together. In patients with vibration-induced neuropathy, the true level and nature of the nerve lesion must be defined before surgery is considered. A future study should be conducted on the neurophysiologic character of neuropathy in vibration-exposed patients.

▶ Although interesting, this article does not contain adequate information about the characteristics of the vibration exposure. Vibration can be measured. Force and time of exposure can also be measured. These should be assessed in this type of paper and should be a critical part of any type of evaluation related to peripheral vascular symptoms.

The diagnosis of carpal tunnel syndrome cannot be made on the basis of Tinel's sign or Phalen's test. These are strictly subjective and are often unreliable in a working population.

M.L. Kasdan, M.D.

Prevalence of Abnormal Median Nerve Conduction in Applicants for Industrial Jobs

Bingham RC, Rosecrance JC, Cook TM (Physical Medicine and Rehabilitation, Jackson, Tenn; Univ of Iowa, Iowa City)

Am J Ind Med 30:355–361, 1996 10–4

Introduction.—When carpal tunnel syndrome (CTS) is linked to an employee's job, workers' compensation usually pays the cost, which can reach $8,000–$10,000. Use of widely accepted objective testing for assessing abnormal median nerve conduction could be used to analyze the integrity of the median nerve segment within the carpal tunnel. New employees with evidence of abnormal median nerve conduction could be placed in jobs without CTS risk factors or have job tasks modified to decrease risk factor exposure. Nerve conduction tests were used to determine the prevalence of abnormal median nerve conduction across the carpal tunnel in applicants for industrial jobs.

Methods.—After a conditional offer of employment, 1,021 applicants underwent nerve conduction studies (NCS) in both hands in a private medical clinic. Applicants completed a self-administered symptom survey specific to the upper extremity. Mean age and average work years of applicants were 30.1 and 4.4 years, respectively. An 8-cm segment was used to determine sensory palmar latencies. The primary electrophysiologic measurement used to detect median neuropathy was the difference between the median and ulnar sensory latencies.

Results.—The prevalence of median neuropathy in job applicants was 17.5% in at least 1 hand. Only 10% of applicants with positive NCS admitted to symptoms associated with CTS. The incidence of median neuropathy in both hands was significantly higher in males than females: in males it was 13.5% and 10.3% in the right and left hands, compared to 12.3% and 7.23% in females. Applicants with work experience in the construction and production sectors had higher percentages of median neuropathy, compared to those not working and those in clerical/office or service jobs.

Conclusion.—Median neuropathy was detected in at least 1 hand in applicants for industrial jobs. These findings in applicants who have been given a conditional offer of employment raise public policy questions regarding whether or not employers should withhold employment on the basis of NCS positivity.

► This study demonstrates a useful technique for developing a baseline of NCS information on a group of industrial workers. The high prevalence of silent neuropathy (17.5%) indicates that there is much to be learned about the normal function of the median nerve, nerve slowing, and their relation to CTS. Bingham et al.'s article is useful because it highlights this present gap in knowledge. However, the authors also note that asymptomatic workers with more severe silent median neuropathy are more likely to have CTS than asymptomatic workers without severe silent median neuropathy. Their conclusion that "a large percentage of industrial workers have objective evidence of abnormal median nerve conduction within the carpal tunnel when hired" also contributes to the ongoing debate on the etiology of CTS. Most important, the authors' thoughtful discussion on the potential impact of prehire NCS measurements should be carefully scrutinized and digested by medical ethicists, and by clinicians and employers considering establishment of workplace nerve screening programs.

P.A. Nathan, M.D.

Diagnostics of Hand-Arm System Disorders in Workers Who Use Vibrating Tools

Gemne G (Stockholm)

Occup Environ Med 54:90–95, 1997 10–5

Introduction.—Symptoms that may be related to the use of hand-held vibrating tools are collectively referred to as the hand-arm vibration syndrome. The possible causes and effects of vibration, methods of assessment, and evaluation of exposures were discussed.

Disorders Possibly Caused by Vibration.—The circulation of the skin in the fingers may be disturbed, with reduced blood flow to the most exposed parts of the hand and development of "vibration white finger." Diffusely distributed finger neuropathy may be caused by damage to nerve fibers and receptors. Pain in the arm and hands may appear during work with low-frequency tools. There is less agreement on a causal relationship between exposure to hand-arm vibration and carpal tunnel syndrome. Although ergonomic factors are more important in this syndrome, some work with vibrating tools may contribute to its development. Vibration has also been linked to decreased muscle power and hearing deficits.

Assessment Methods.—Using clinical and laboratory findings and epidemiological data, the clinician must first determine that a hand-arm vibration syndrome is present. It must then be decided, on the basis of epidemiologic studies, whether the symptoms could be caused by vibration. If these inquiries are positive, it is necessary to decide whether the factual exposure is sufficiently harmful to have caused the patient's symptoms. White fingers can be assessed by recording the finger systolic pressure during cold provocation. Epidemiologic data are incomplete, however, regarding the quantitative association between vibration and both white finger and diffusely distributed neuropathy. In contrast, electrodiagnostic tests for carpal tunnel syndrome have sufficient validity.

Causality.—Determination of causality involves quantitative assessment of the dose of exposure. Time studies are important and should yield data on the duration, intermittency, and character of the vibration. If intermittency is not taken into account, duration and intensity are likely to be noncommensurable variables. To accurately assign causality, separate models for risk evaluation of vascular and neurologic disorders related to different types of work will have to be established. At present, thresholds for harmful exposure to vibration are unknown.

▶ This article is a useful resource for physicians involved in industrial medicine. The author, an international expert on the topic, sets forth practical, objective criteria for the investigation of upper extremity conditions suspected of coming from vibratory influences in the workplace. Equally important, he points out deficiencies in current methods available for assigning causation.

The author observes that the methods used to diagnose hand-arm vibration syndrome (HAVS) are neither particularly sensitive nor specific, and alternative diagnoses and etiologies are always possible. This latter is consistent with our clinical experience. The majority of the employed patients with Raynaud's phenomenon or carpal tunnel syndrome whom we have studied had no material exposure to vibration. Similarly, the overwhelming majority of workers exposed to vibration whom we have studied have not had Raynaud's phenomenon or carpal tunnel syndrome. We have found that analysis of personal and lifestyle factors—including body type, avocational exercise level, cold exposure, and cigarette smoking—is of far greater use in identifying patients with Raynaud's phenomenon or carpal tunnel syndrome than is the quantity, quality, or duration of vibratory exposure.

We would second the author's caution that thresholds for harmful exposure to vibration are unknown. Studies that show a clear, consistent univariate relationship between vibration exposure and Raynaud's phenomenon are rare. We are unaware of the existence of any multivariate studies that adjust for confounding personal and lifestyle factors and still show a clear and consistent relationship between vibratory exposure and upper extremity diagnoses clustered under the HAVS umbrella. The author has provided valuable observations that should prompt the clinician to carefully consider alternatives before embracing the diagnostic concept of HAVS and its implied etiology.

P.A. Nathan, M.D.

Injection Versus Surgery in the Treatment of Trigger Finger

Benson LS, Ptaszek AJ (Northwestern Univ, Chicago; Evanston and Glenbrook Hosps, Glenview, Ill)

J Hand Surg (Am) 22A:138–144, 1997 10–6

Background.—Conservative treatment for trigger finger (stenosing tenosynovitis of the digits) involves steroid injection into the tendon sheath, which can provide relief for a time. Surgical release of the A1 pulley uniformly produces permanent resolution. Injection and surgical treatment of trigger finger were compared with regard to symptom resolution, cost, and patient satisfaction.

Study Design.—A retrospective review was performed of the treatment of 109 trigger fingers in 102 patients. Surgical release was performed in 34 fingers and 75 were managed conservatively. The 2 treatment modalities were compared by retrospectively reviewing the clinical course, having patients complete a satisfaction questionnaire, and performing a cost analysis.

Study Group.—The study group consisted of 102 patients, with an average age of 61 years. The most commonly involved digit was the thumb. The mean follow-up time was 18 months.

Findings.—Of the 75 patients treated solely by injection, 22 underwent 2 injections and 6 underwent a third injection. Treatment with a single injection was successful in 60% of patients, although symptoms recurred in a minority of patients. Subsequent injections resulted in a diminishing level of success. Surgical treatment was completely successful, without recurrence and without complications. Surgical release cost Medicare patients $250.00 more than a second injection but resulted in permanent relief in all cases. All patients valued the permanent relief provided by surgical management.

Conclusion.—A single steroid injection is often successful in treating trigger finger and should be considered as initial therapy for the majority of patients, but further injections are less successful. Surgical management is uniformly successful in treating trigger finger. This suggests that if the first injection is insufficient to provide symptomatic relief, surgery should be considered. The additional cost of surgical treatment if offset by the permanence and completeness of symptomatic relief for this patient group.

▶ The simple fact, demonstrated by multiple studies, is that approximately 35% of patients will not gain relief from a single trigger finger injection and that further injections are even less effective. These patients require surgery, the cost of which is justified. The 65% success rate justifies this being the first line of treatment.

The authors' 60% success rate for a single injection is consistent with the known rate. A second injection was only successful in one third of their patients. After 2 failed injections, I proceed with surgery because few patients, in my experience, get relief from a third shot, few are willing to try a treatment that has already failed twice, and most just finally want the relief that surgery provides.

The cost issue not discussed is the use of percutaneous trigger finger release for fingers which repeatedly lock in flexion. Percutaneous release can provide immediate relief, and at the same cost as an injection. This saves the costs of an open surgical procedure altogether. Surgery is justified for the patient whose finger is locked and for the patient who has previously failed injection in another finger and, for this reason, is against having another.

J.M. Failla, M.D.

The Results of Surgical Treatment of Trigger Finger
Turowski GA, Zdankiewicz PD, Thomson JG (St Mary's Hosp, Waterbury, Conn; Yale Univ, New Haven, Conn)
J Hand Surg (Am) 22A:145–149, 1997 10–7

Background.—Trigger finger or stenosing tenosynovitis of the digital flexor tendon sheath is a common problem that is usually treated conservatively. There has been little research on the results of surgical treatment of the trigger finger. The results in a series of patients treated with surgery for trigger finger were reviewed.

Study Design.—A retrospective review of hospital charts and operative records was performed at St. Mary's Hospital, Waterbury, Connecticut. This review identified 75 patients treated surgically for trigger finger between 1987 and 1993. Of these 75 patients, 59 were available for a follow-up telephone interview and 46 were reexamined.

Study Group.—The study group consisted of 33 female and 26 male patients with an average age of 55 years. The average duration before surgery was 4 months. Seventeen patients had attempted conservative therapy. The operative procedures were performed by 3 orthopedists, 3 plastic surgeons, and 4 general surgeons. The average follow-up was 48 months.

Findings.—Surgical treatment was successful in all trigger finger patients in this series. Complete symptom resolution occurred in 97% and significant improvement occurred in the remaining patients. The recurrence rate was 3% and only 1 patient required reoperation. There were few complications resulting in minimal morbidity. There were no nerve injuries, tendon bowstringing, wound infections, or ulnar deviation of the digits in this patient group.

Conclusion.—Surgical treatment of advanced trigger finger has a high success rate, with minimal morbidity or recurrence. Although conservative therapy should remain the initial treatment for most patients with trigger finger, surgery continues to be a valid option after failure of conservative therapy or in patients with long-standing, advanced disease.

► The authors have filled a void in the literature by documenting what was only assumed to be true, that trigger finger release is successful in almost all patients. They also provide a rebuttal to the one report in the literature[1] that showed an abnormally high complication rate with trigger release, perhaps because of poor technique.

However, it is my clinical impression that it does take quite a long time (on the order of 6 months) for a small subset of patients to achieve this good result. I, therefore, warn these potentially slowly recovering patients preoperatively that this could be the case. In my experience, these patients are most often male, older than 50 years, very active in gripping sports such as tennis or golf, and tend to have thick palmar scars that are sensitive. At surgery, these patients appear to have a severe form of trigger finger, with bits of visibly frayed shreds of tendon and tenosynovium on the palmar surface of the flexor superficialis that are beneath the A1 pulley with the finger in flexion and move beneath the A2 pulley when the finger is passively extended. Perhaps this is caused by chronic shear forces between the tendon fascicles and a corresponding reparative process. When I see this pathology, I tangentially trim the frayed tendon shreds and tenosynovium with a tenotomy scissor and excise a central strip of A1 pulley to prevent adherence to the frayed area.

One of the 3 recurrences in this report may have involved this severe type of case. This patient was treated at reexploration with A1 pulley excision rather than simple division, and this may be why the second surgery was successful.

J.M. Failla, M.D.

Reference

1. Thorpe AP: Results of surgery for trigger finger. *J Hand Surg (Br)* 13B:199–201, 1988.

Suggested Reading

Labelle H, Guibert R: Efficacy of diclofenac in lateral epicondylitis of the elbow also treated with immobilization. *Arch Fam Med* 6:257–262, 1997.

▶ It is refreshing to see a well-designed, prospective, double-blinded, controlled study such as this one. Although the conclusions refute the effectiveness of diclofenac sodium for anything other than pain relief, they seem to support the effectiveness of immobilization alone. The high incidence of abdominal complaints with the use of diclofenac is concerning. Diclofenac and other NSAIDs are almost routinely prescribed in patients with lateral epicondylitis. The specter of a serious gastrointestinal complication, especially with elderly or medically complicated patients, should deter the use of such medications. Perhaps acetaminophen should be the drug of choice of pain relief in lateral epicondylitis.

K.A. Bengtson, M.D.

Pierre-Jerome C, Bekkelund SI, Mellgren SI, et al: Quantitative magnetic resonance imaging and the electrophysiology of the carpal tunnel region in floor cleaners. *Scand J Work Environ Health* 22:119–123, 1996.

▶ The purpose of this study was to look for subclinical evidence of median nerve pathology by comparing two groups of asymptomatic female workers (floor cleaners and referents) reportedly at differing risk for carpal tunnel syndrome (CTS) based on work exposure. The method involved comparing MRI and electrophysiologic findings between the two groups.

Although statistically significant differences were noted for a few variables, the mean values and ranges reported for both groups were well within the normal range for all variables. Thus, this study failed to demonstrate pathology in either group. In addition, no attempt was made to objectively evaluate work exposure. This being the case, any conclusions by the authors regarding the relationship between work exposure and subclinical median nerve pathology are questionable.

P.A. Nathan, M.D.

11 Arthritis

A New Metacarpal Osteotomy: Metacarpal Cervicocapital Shortening Osteotomy in the Rheumatoid Hand [French]

Leemrijse Th, Cadot B, Valtin B, et al (Hôpital Bichat, Paris)
Ann Chir Main Memb Super 15:132–137, 1996 11–1

Introduction.—Severe rheumatoid palmar and ulnar subluxations of the 4 long fingers are difficult to treat because of associated soft tissue retraction, which usually requires large releases. Weil's osteotomy, which was initially used to shorten the metatarsal head in painful rheumatoid feet, was adapted for use in patients with rheumatoid hand deformities.

> *Surgical Technique.*—Longitudinal skin incisions are made over the second and fourth intermetacarpal spaces. The dorsal veins at the level of the interdigital spaces are repaired. The metacarpal heads are exposed, and synovectomy is performed. The cervicocapital osteotomy is started 1–2 mm from the superior border of the cartilage head, and the oblique cut is continued in a proximal and palmar direction over a distance of 20–25 mm. The 2 parts are properly aligned, and Kirschner wires are used for temporary fixation. Two bone screws are inserted for permanent fixation. The overhanging bone edge is resected after permanent fixation (Fig 4).

Patients.—A 55-year-old woman with a lupus-like disorder and an 82-year-old woman with a 40-year history of rheumatoid arthritis underwent Weil's cervicocapital osteotomies. Both had excellent results.

Conclusion.—Weil's oblique cervicocapital osteotomy, when used to shorten the metacarpal bone, improves hand function in patients with severe rheumatoid hand deformities and avoids the need for extensive soft-tissue releases.

► This osteotomy allows bony release of intrinsic tightness without extensive proximal intrinsic soft-tissue release in severe rheumatoid palmar and ulnar subluxation of the metacarpophalangeal (MP) joint. The patients both had preservation of the MP joint articular surfaces and, thus, underwent soft-tissue realignment only. In the setting of the destroyed MP joint treated by replacement arthroplasty with a silicone prosthesis, the bone shortening entailed would obviously make this osteotomy unnecessary. However, in the

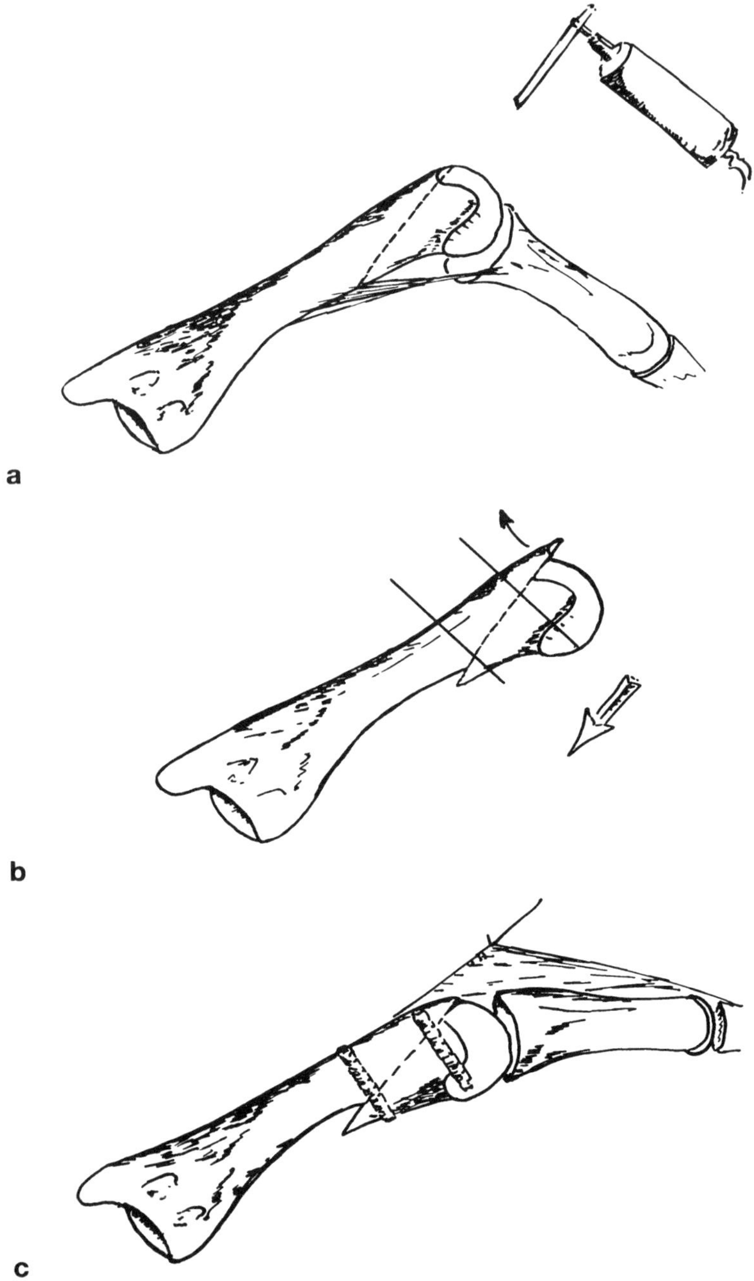

FIGURE 4.—**A,** lateral view: cervicocapital osteotomy. Intra-articular osteotomy, 1 or 2 mm from the superior border of the cartilage head; the direction is proximal and volar, 20–25 mm long. **B,** automatic positioning of the head. Temporary fixation is done with 2 Kirschner wires. Resection of the bone edge is accomplished after final fixation. **C,** final fixation with 2 screws. Fixation is without tension of the proximal phalanx and extensor tendon. (Courtesy of Leemrijse Th, Cadot B, Valtin B, et al: A new metacarpal osteotomy: Metacarpal cervicocapital shortening osteotomy in the rheumatoid hand. *Ann Chir Main Memb Super* 15:132–137, 1996.)

face of the current public outcry against silicone products, it is conceivable that silicone MP joint replacement will not be a popular option. In the event that no substitute prosthesis is available, the classic soft-tissue interposition athroplasties for the MP joint, which use extensor tendon or palmar plate, could be resurrected and could be supplemented with this metacarpal osteotomy.

J.M. Failla, M.D.

Non-cemented Replacement of the Trapeziometacarpal Joint

Wachtl SW, Sennwald GR (Chirurgie St Leonhard, St Gallen, Switzerland)

J Bone Joint Surg (Br) 78B:787–792, 1996 11–2

Background.—Several operations have been proposed to correct disabling osteoarthritis of the first trapeziometacarpal joint. Various cemented prostheses for trapeziometacarpal joint replacement have been described. The results with an uncemented trapeziometacarpal joint prosthesis were described.

Methods.—Forty-three patients with osteoarthritis of the basal joint of the thumb were included. There were 38 women and 5 men (mean age, 63 years). The Ledoux prosthesis was used in performing noncemented arthroplasty of the first carpometacarpal joint. This was a ball-and-socket design prosthesis with a titanium trapezial component and a polyethylene inlay. Osteotomy of the first metacarpal was performed perpendicular to the long axis of the medullary canal, about 7 mm distal to the joint. Passive motion was started after 2 weeks, and normal activity after 3 months.

Results.—There were 4 joint dislocations and 14 loosened implants. Reoperation was required in 17 patients at a mean of 9 months postoperatively. The likelihood of avoiding revision was 62% at 12 months and 59% at 16 months. Twenty-six of the 28 surviving prostheses were evaluated at a mean follow-up time of 25 months. On a 100-point scale, the patients' mean subjective evaluation was 79 points. Most of the patients reported problems with activities of daily living and tended to avoid using the hand. Three fourths of patients had pain on loading or movement or at rest. Trapeziometacarpal joint motion and wrist strength were significantly below normal. Stem subsidence within the first metacarpal and cup migration were apparent in follow-up radiographs (Fig 4). The stem was loose in 15% of patients and the cup in 46%.

Conclusion.—Based on these disappointing results, the authors no longer recommend the Ledoux prosthesis for noncemented replacement of the trapeziometacarpal joint. The prosthesis will eventually loosen because of design problems and insufficient anchorage. Prostheses for trapeziometacarpal joint replacement should be unconstrained and should retain the ligaments.

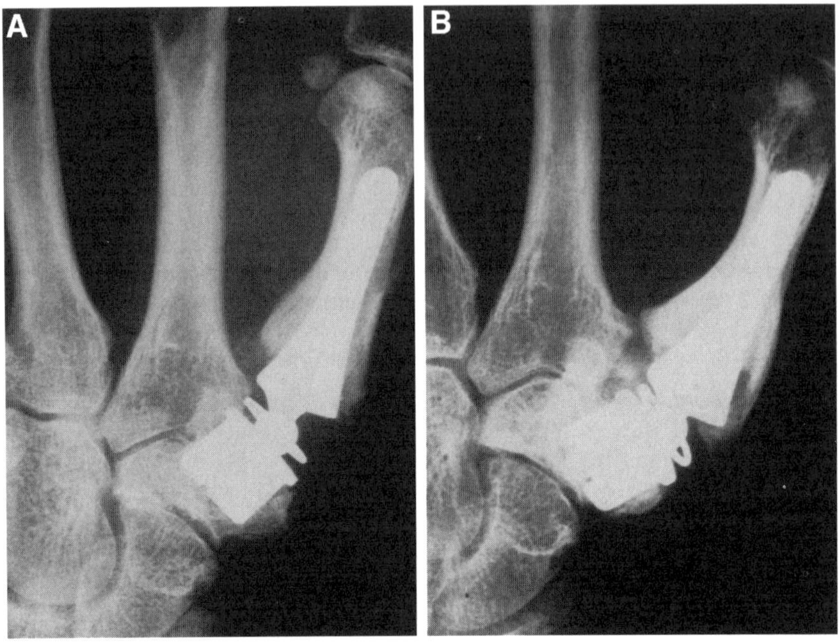

FIGURE 4.—Anteroposterior radiographs of a Ledoux prosthesis immediately after surgery (**A**) and 3 years after implantation (**B**). (Courtesy of Wachtl SW, Sennwald GR: Non-cemented replacement of the trapeziometacarpal joint. *J Bone Joint Surg [Br]*78B:787–792, 1996.)

► In the United States, aside from a brief period during which some surgeons were implanting the de la Caffinière prosthesis, there has been little enthusiasm for thumb carpometacarpal total joint arthroplasty. Our European colleagues have been stronger advocates of this approach. This article points out the shortcomings of a noncemented design. At the third European Congress of Hand Surgery, the congress of the Federation of European Societies for Surgery of the Hand, Wachtl and Sennwald together with Ledoux, the designer of the prosthesis, debated these issues. Ledoux's reported experience was far more favorable in outlook. The issue remains unresolved, and most of us will no doubt continue using some form of soft-tissue interposition for the present.

V.R. Hentz, M.D.

Anatomical and Biomechanical Studies of the Pathogenesis of Trapeziometacarpal Degenerative Arthritis

Najima H, Oberlin C, Alnot JY, et al (Univ of Paris V)
J Hand Surg (Br) 22B:183–188, 1997 11–3

Background.—The trapeziometacarpal joint is the biconcave and incongruous saddle joint which makes the wide circumduction motion of the thumb possible. Primary osteoarthritis of this joint can be disabling. There

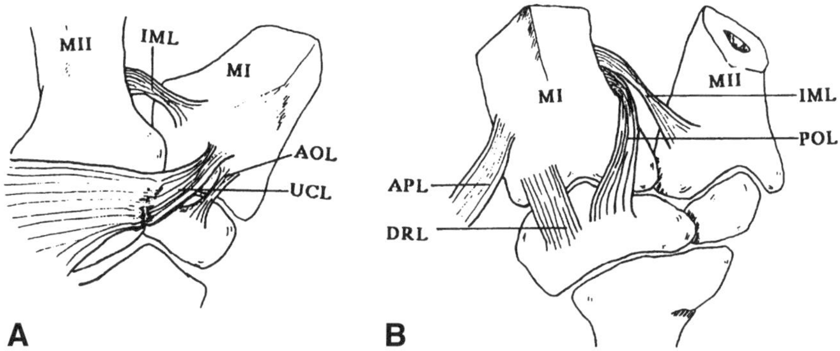

FIGURE 1.—Ligamentous anatomy of the trapeziometacarpal joint according to Pieron (1973). Palmar (**A**) and dorsal (**B**) views of the right first trapeziometacarpal joint. *Abbreviations: AOL,* anterior oblique ligament; *MI,* first metacarpal; *MII,* second metacarpal; *IML,* first intermetacarpal ligament; *APL,* abductor pollicis longus; *POL,* posterior oblique ligament; *DRL,* dorsoradial ligament; *UCL,* ulnar collateral ligament. (Courtesy of Najima H, Oberlin C, Alnot JY, et al: Anatomical and biochemical studies of the pathogenesis of trapeziometacarpal degenerative arthritis. *J Hand Surg [Br]* 22B:183–188, 1997.)

are 6 main hypotheses to explain the etiology of arthritis in this joint: ligamentous laxity caused by hormonal changes, hypoplasia of the joint surface, chronic joint stress, abductor pollicis longus abnormality, imbalance of synovial inflammatory mediators, and imbalance between the adductor pollicis and abductor pollicis longus acting on the first metacarpal. Ligamentous instability may result in large shear forces in the joint contact areas or mechanical stimulation of surrounding soft tissue; over time, this may lead to osteoarthritis in this area. To prevent progression, the joint is usually stabilized by ligamentous reconstruction. The joint contains 5 main ligamentous structures: the first intermetacarpal ligament (IML), the anterior oblique ligament (AOL), the ulnar collateral ligament, the posterior oblique ligament (POL), and the dorsoradial ligament (DRL) (Fig 1). This study was conducted to confirm the trapeziometacarpal ligamentous anatomy and to understand the mechanical properties of each component ligament.

Methods.—The study was performed on ligaments from 14 male and 18 female cadavers, with ages from 71 to 95 years. All samples were tested within 5 hours of excision. Ligaments were bound at the ends with silk thread and ultra-strength instant glue. The tensile properties of these ligaments were assessed by a strain-rate failure test in a material testing system. The articular surface of the joint was classified into 5 grades: grade 0, smooth; grade 1, superficial fibrillation; grade 2, deep fibrillation; grades 3 and 4, deep fibrillation with bone exposure. The maximum tensile strength of each ligament was correlated with the condition of the corresponding articular cartilage.

Results.—The maximum tensile strength of the AOL was decreased 51% when the condition of the joint cartilage decreased from grade 0 to grade 1. The maximum tensile strength of the first IML decreased 53%. The decrease in strength of the POL was closely correlated with the condition of the articular surface of the joint. These 3 ligaments also significantly decreased in strength with age.

Conclusion.—Anatomical and biomechanical studies of the ligaments of the trapeziometacarpal joint revealed that the POL and the DRL are the strongest and the first IML is the weakest of the 5 joint ligaments. The DRL is also the most elastic. The AOL, IML, and POL decrease significantly in strength with age. The AOL, IML, and POL play an important role in trapeziometacarpal joint stabilization. The decrease in strength of these 3 ligaments appears to be associated with the pathogenesis of osteoarthritis of this joint.

▶ The authors have looked at the pathogenesis of trapeziometacarpal degenerative arthritis in a rational manner. The attempt to correlate the diminishing strength of the AOL, IML, and POL with increasing stages of cartilage degeneration determined by gross examination is interesting. Presumably, the authors assigned the worst area of cartilage loss as the value used, but it is not clear whether this was on the trapezium metacarpal base or both. The method of using a silk suture in the strength to failure tests—even with the addition of cyanoacrylate—would seem, because of the possibility of slippage, a less reliable method than the bone-ligament-bone model currently most often advocated. The relatively low strain rate (0.08 mm/sec) may have contributed to the low ultimate loads recorded.

The description of the properties of the DRL is difficult to follow. The authors delineate the DRL as the strongest ligament but also the most elastic, at the same time describing it as being the primary restraint to dorsoradial subluxation of the first metacarpal. Without the stiffness calculations, these statements are difficult to accept. The AOL and "beak ligament" are deemed to be synonymous, but Pelligrini,[1] who coined the latter term, has not indicated his agreement. The other 4 ligaments are said to be nearly equal in lesser strength., but as the AOL, IML, and POL were attenuated in many of the samples, this also needs clarification. The study leaves unanswered the question of whether the ligament fatigue or dorsoradial displacement of the base of the metacarpal is primary in the pathogenesis. If the DRL is the strongest ligament and has a primary role in providing stability, why does not this ligament lose strength as well with progressive degenerative change?

The authors have omitted another causal factor from the 6 hypotheses stated in their introduction. That is trapezial tilt that may occur under axial compression from the fulcrum of its cantilevered purchase at the second metacarpotrapezoidal joint. An increasing tilt of the articular surface of the trapezium would increase the tangential force responsible for displacement of the first metacarpal base.

R.L. Linscheid, M.D.

Reference

1. Pelligrini VD Jr: Osteoarthritis of the trapeziometacarpal joint: The pathophysiology of articular cartilage degeneration. I. Anatomy and pathology of the aging joint. *J Hand Surg (Am)* 16A:967–974, 1991.

Hypermobility Associated With Osteoarthritis of the Thumb Base: A Clinical and Radiological Subset of Hand Osteoarthritis

Jónsson H, Valtýsdóttir STh, Kjartansson O; et al (Univ Hosp, Reykjavík, Iceland)

Ann Rheum Dis 55:540–543, 1996 11–4

Background.—Osteoarthritis (OA) of the hand, a common condition seen primarily in postmenopausal women, causes much morbidity. A major determinant of disability is the severity of involvement of the first carpometacarpal joint (CMC 1). Evidence suggests that laxity of the volar ligaments with secondary joint instability may play an important role in the development of CMC 1 OA. However, no one has found a connection with generalized articular hypermobility.

Methods and Findings.—Hypermobility was assessed in 50 consecutive women with clinical hand OA and thumb base symptoms using the Beighton criteria. Thirty-one patients showed the features of hypermobility, with Beighton scores of 2 or greater. Seventeen patients fulfilled 4 or more criteria. In a control group of 94 women, the corresponding figures were 30 and 9, respectively. Patients with hypermobility features had fewer and less severely involved interphalangeal joints on clinical and radiologic assessment. Two subsets were evident radiologically, the first characterized by severe interphalangeal OA, and the second by predominant involvement of the CMC 1. In the first subset, the prevalence of hypermobility was similar to that in the control group. Most of the patients in the second subset had hypermobility.

Conclusions.—Articular hypermobility is causally associated with the development of thumb base OA. Further, hypermobility-associated hand OA constitutes a definite clinical and radiologic subset of hand OA. Clinically, most patients with hand OA and hypermobility can be identified by applying the hypermobility criterion of a 90-degree or greater passive dorsiflexion of the fifth finger.

▶ The authors assert the existence of 2 phenotypically different types of hand OA: with predominant involvement of the distal interphalangeal joints without associated hypermobility, and another with prevalent thumb basal joint OA associated with evidence of diffuse systemic hypermobility of the joints. Although the authors do not prove cause and effect but only an association between hypermobility and the prevalence of the thumb basal joint OA, their hypothesis is provocative and deserving of further consideration. Further, experimental evidence from our laboratory suggests that hyperextension of the thumb metacarpophalangeal joint can overload the volar compartment of the trapeziometacarpal joint in a manner identical to that observed in patients with osteoarthritic disease in the presence of an incompetent palmer beak ligament. Similarly, these data suggest that stabilization of the thumb metacarpophalangeal joint to prevent hyperextension can favorably alter the loading patterns in the trapeziometacarpal joint and perhaps alleviate the early symptoms of basal joint arthritis.

V.D. Pellegrini, Jr., M.D.

Extensor Carpi Radialis Longus Tendon Arthoplasty in the Treatment of Primary Trapeziometacarpal Arthrosis

Atroshi I, Axelsson G (Hassleholm-Kristianstad Hosps, Hassleholm, Sweden)

J Hand Surg (Am) 22A:419–427, 1997 11–5

Background.—A large number of procedures have been described for treatment of arthrosis of the trapeziometacarpal (TMC) joint. However, there have been few prospective studies measuring patient outcomes such as pain, satisfaction, and activities of daily living (ADL) or comparing objective measurements with a control population. A study attempted to address these shortcomings.

Methods and Findings.—Seventeen patients undergoing trapezial excision and extensor carpi radialis longus tendon arthroplasty for primary TMC arthrosis were assessed preoperatively and at 12 and a mean 39 months postoperatively. At the final follow-up, complete or significant pain relief and patient satisfication with outcomes were documented. Postoperative residual pain was more likely to occur in patients with a longer history of thumb pain and more advanced preoperative radiographic changes. Mean ADL scores improved significantly compared with preoperative values. Mean pulp and key pinch strength were 93% and 100%, respectively, of the preoperative values, although they were significantly lower than mean pinch strengths in an age-matched control group. Four patients, who still had some thumb pain with light work, had substantial proximal migration of the first metacarpal during maximal pinch. Scaphotrapezoid arthrosis was unassociated with residual pain after surgery.

Conclusion.—Extensor carpi radialis longus tendon arthroplasty is a technically easy, safe procedure for the treatment of TMC arthrosis requiring surgery. This procedure can provide good pain relief and a high degree of patient satisfaction.

► This article adds to the body of literature and, for the most part, coincides with what we have seen at the Mayo Clinic in Rochester, Minnesota regarding tendon arthroplasty and TMC arthrosis. Confirmation of a high degree of satisfaction goes along with the objective findings of alleviation of pain and preservation of strength at approximately 80% of expected values. We have found that the loss of strength caused by biomechanical alteration has been offset by the reduction in pain, essentially allowing patients to maintain their preoperative condition, albeit in a more comfortable manner. What remain to be seen with respect to TMC arthritis are the outcomes of patients who are operated on at an earlier age and what role reoperation plays with respect to long-term function.

C.H. Johnson, M.D.

Determinants of Hand Function in Patients With Rheumatoid Arthritis

Vliet Vlieland TPM, van der Wijk TP, Jolie IMM, et al (Univ Hosp Leiden, The Netherlands)
J Rheumatol 23:835–840, 1996 11–6

Background.—Rheumatoid arthritis often affects the function of the hands in activities of daily living (ADL). Which clinical variables contribute to the function of the hand in ADL, and to what extent, was investigated.

Methods.—Hand function in ADL in 50 patients with rheumatoid arthritis was assessed by 3 methods: (1) the dexterity items of the Arthritis Impact Measurement Scales, (2) direct observation of these items by an occupational therapist, and (3) the Jebsen hand function test. Muscle strength, deformity and destruction, range of motion, and local arthritis activity were also assessed.

Results.—Pinch and grip strength, the patient's assessment of hand pain and stiffness, thumb and finger flexion, wrist range of motion, metacarpophalangeal joint alignment, swan neck and Z deformities, and Larsen erosion score were significantly correlated with most of the measures of hand function. Pinch strength, hand stiffness, and Z deformity and ulnar deviation accounted for 78% of the variance of the combined hand function factor.

Conclusions.—In setting goals for conservative or surgical treatment of the rheumatoid hand, pinch and grip strength should be carefully considered. Other consistent indicators of impaired hand function were reported hand stiffness, metacarpophalangeal joint malalignment, and thumb flexion and deformity. Measurements of the level of hand function in ADL should be included in the evaluation of the effectiveness of treatment for rheumatoid arthritis of the hands.

Flexor Tenosynovectomy and Tenolysis in Longstanding Rheumatoid Arthritis

Tolat AR, Stanley JK, Evans RA (Wrightington Hosp, Lancashire, England)
J Hand Surg (Br) 21B:538–543, 1996 11–7

Background.—Forty-two percent to 55% of patients with rheumatoid arthritis (RA) have flexor tendon involvement. Improvement in flexor tendon pull-through is very beneficial in such patients. The long-term outcomes of flexor tenosynovectomy and tenolysis in patients with long-standing RA were reported.

Methods.—Forty-three patients with 49 affected hands and 424 affected flexor tendons were included. The duration of RA at the time of surgery was more than 15 years. Patients were clinically assessed at a mean of 5.7 years. The main indications for surgery were pain and inability to flex actively despite good passive range of motion.

Findings.—Excellent sustained pain relief was achieved. Patient satisfaction with the outcome of the procedure was high. Pulp-to-pulp (opposition) and key pinch ability were adequate in 81%. In 45%, the range of finger motion was excellent to good, and in 22%, it was fair. Thirty-three percent of results were judged to be poor. Poor results were associated with significant joint disease, preoperative tendon ruptures, extensive digital surgery, readhesions, and combinations of operative procedures that adversely affected the rehabilitation program.

Conclusions.—Flexor tenosynovectomy appears to be a useful procedure in patients with long-standing RA. Recurrences are rare. However, patients with tendon ruptures preoperatively, except for the flexor pollicis longus, have poor prognoses.

▶ This important study looks at the results of flexor tenosynovectomy in patients having long-standing RA. The difficulty of examining the flexor aspect of the hand is properly pointed out in this paper. However, hand surgeons need to keep in mind the high incidence of flexor tenosynovitis, as well as compression of the median nerve in the carpal tunnel, when evaluating patients with RA. This study also points out the increased difficulty in achieving good results when patients already have peritendinous scarring and joint damage. The evaluation of the patients, the technical aspects of surgery and therapy, and a logical approach to follow-up evaluation of the patients are all well-described in this paper.

E. Fleegler, M.D.

Primary Metacarpophalangeal and Proximal Interphalangeal Arthrosis of the Hand: Indications and Results of 27 DJOA Arthroplasty [French]

Condamine JL, Fourquet M, Marcucci L, et al (CHU côte de Nacre, Caen, France)

Ann Chir Main 16:66–76, 1997 11–8

Background.—Arthritis of the proximal interphalangeal (PIP) joint is the third most common type of arthritis of the hand. Although more rare, arthritis of the metacarpophalangeal (MP) joint also prompts many patients to seek treatment. Experience in using digital joint arthroplasty to treat PIP and MP joint osteoarthritis was reported.

Methods.—The PIP joint ($N = 19$) or the MP joint ($N = 8$) was replaced in 20 patients (mean age, 58 years; range, 49 to 84 years) between 1985 and 1994. Digital joint arthroplasty implants are shown in Fig 5. The

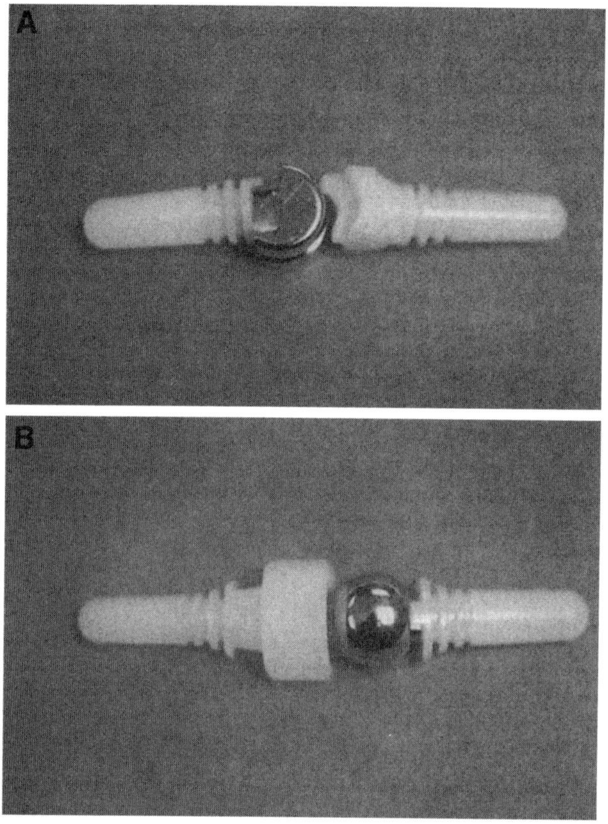

FIGURE 5.—A, second-generation digital joint arthroplasty 3, proximal interphalangeal model. B, second-generation digital joint arthroplasty 3, metacarpophalangeal model. (Courtesy of Condamine JL, Fourquet M, Marcucci L, et al: Primary metacarpophalangeal and proximal interphalangeal arthritis of the hand. Indications and results of 27 digital joint arthroplasties. *Ann Chir Main* 16:66–76, 1997.)

average elapsed time from the onset of symptoms to the time of surgery was 34 months (range, 12 to 72 months). The dorsal operative approach was used in all but 6 procedures.

Findings.—Three complications were observed, all involving the PIP implant. In 1 patient, acute septic ulceration that required ablation developed. In another patient, acute subluxation requiring surgical reduction of the implant developed. Axial deviation over the course of 3 months developed in the third case. Pain and grip strength improved in almost all cases. Mobility, however, improved only slightly, with range of motion of 35 degrees to 50 degrees for the MP joints and 50 degrees for the PIP joints. Radiologic evaluation over 2 years of follow-up revealed the development of periarticular ossifications; ossification of the proximal shank of the implant, in particular, was associated with less mobility.

Conclusion.—Proximal interphalangeal and MP implants did improve pain and grip strength, but the effects on mobility were disappointing. One case of axial deviation occurred, which is consistent with reports in the literature. Their experience has led these authors to adopt an anterolateral surgical approach to the PIP joint, which avoids the extensor apparatus and enables reduction of the flexor muscles postoperatively.

▶ Silicone implant arthroplasty of the finger joints was first proposed as a solution to finger joint arthritis some 30 years ago. It remains the standard today. This is truly a remarkable record of endurance, but the troublesome incidence of lateral deformity, the limited arc of motion usually provided, and the high rate of implant fracture over time have all prompted a search for a new type of arthroplasty. A variety of pretenders to the throne have appeared over the years only to slink back into the shadows as complications of implant wear, loosening, and breakage have accumulated.

This report describes a new contender—digital joint arthroplasty. The results, as far as pain relief and range of motion are concerned, have little to offer over silicone arthroplasty, although lateral stability seems perhaps better. The 50% incidence of implant subsidence at an average follow-up of just over 2 years is certainly worrisome, however. I believe we still have far to go before we can identify finger joint arthroplasty with the favorable characteristics associated with hip and knee joint arthroplasty.

P.C. Amadio, M.D.

Long-term Follow-up of 50 Duke Silicone Prosthetic Fingers

O'Farrell DA, Montella BJ, Bahor JL, et al (Duke Univ, Durham, NC)

J Hand Surg (Br) 21B:696–700, 1996 11–9

Introduction.—Emotional and physical trauma may result from the loss of a digit. Because of the high visibility of the hand, patients who undergo amputation of a finger may view themselves as deformed or different. Patient satisfaction and functionality of custom-made digital protheses were assessed.

Methods.—Digital protheses were made for 33 patients who underwent a total of 50 digital amputations. Amputation was necessitated by digital trauma in most patients; tumor or congenital defects was the cause in 3. The prostheses were made from casts of each patient's hand using a hard dental stone and dental base-plate wax. After removal from the mold, the prosthesis was ground smooth and painted to match the patient's skin tone. Suction held the prosthesis to the affected finger.

Results.—Twenty-two of 33 patients wore the prosthesis. Twenty-five patients returned to work; 19 of these returned to their previous work and 12 of them wore the prosthesis while working. The occupations of these 12 patients included typist or account keeper, machine operator, medical technician, teacher, social worker, factory worker, and housekeeper. The 8 patients who did not return to work had multiple digit amputations. Most patients were satisfied with the appearance, fit, and color of the prosthesis. Twenty-six patients stated that the prosthesis was helpful psychologically, and 31 patients believed that the prosthesis improved their appearance. Activities such as writing, typing, and holding a cup were thought to be aided by the prosthesis.

Conclusion.—Overall, most patients were satisfied with the prosthesis, although one third of the patients did not wear the device. The prosthesis was helpful psychologically and functionally for most patients, improving activities such as writing, typing, or holding light objects.

► Prosthetic fingers are a good option for many people after the loss of fingers. Most of the 33 people fitted with these prostheses accepted and used them. However, one third did not and ended up as nonwearers. At an average cost of $1,200 per digit and a significant amount of time invested in the fabrication and fitting, care must be taken in the assessment of each individual before recommendation.

Cosmesis is the primary benefit, and function is secondary. It is important that these patients receive proper counseling regarding their loss and training in the use of the prostheses. If prosthetic fingers are indicated, the surgeon should leave as much length as possible in the digit to enhance fitting and should bury nerve endings to minimize the formation of neuromas. The article cites a significant reference for additional reading.[1]

M. LeBlanc, M.S.M.E., C.P.

Reference

1. Alison A, MacKinnon SE: Evaluation of digital prostheses. *J Hand Surg (Am)* 17A:923–926, 1992.

Posterior Interosseous Neuropathy in Rheumatoid Arthritis

Kishner S, Biundo JJ Jr (Louisiana State Univ, New Orleans)

J Clin Rheumatol 2:29–32, 1996 11–10

Introduction.—Entrapment or compressive neuropathies are complications of rheumatoid arthritis. Carpal tunnel syndrome and ulnar neuropathy at the elbow and wrist are the most common. Entrapment neuropathy of the posterior interosseous nerve is characterized by the inability to extend the fingers. It is uncommon, but occurs in patients with rheumatoid arthritis of the elbow.

Differential Diagnosis.—Other conditions that can result in the inability to extend the fingers are extensor tendon rupture, dislocation of the extensor tendons into the intermetacarpal space, and subluxation of the metacarpophalangeal joints.

Treatments and Case Reports.—Sixteen cases of posterior interosseous neuropathy in rheumatoid arthritis have been reported. Steroid injection of the elbow joint and nerve decompression with or without synovectomy are the 2 primary forms of therapy. In 43% of these 16 patients, steroid injection was effective. Nerve decompression produced good results in the patients for whom steroid injection was unsuccessful. Nerve decompression was performed in 10 patients. In 1 patient, it was done 1 year after symptom onset and was unsuccessful.

Discussion.—Surgical decompression should be considered if conservative treatment is unsuccessful. Prevention through control of synovitis of the elbow, anti-inflammatory medication, and supplemental steroid injection of the elbow is recommended. Diagnostic testing was also discussed.

▶ Posterior interosseous neuropathy and rheumatoid arthritis must be differentiated from digital extensor tendon rupture or subluxation into the intermetacarpal space and from C-6 radiculopathy. The authors comprehensively and clearly review how this is accomplished by physical and electrodiagnostic examinations.

Surgical decompression of the nerve at the arcade of Frohse that proximally borders the superficial layer of the supinator muscle is the most reliable treatment. This can be done initially and should be considered quickly after an unsuccessful response to steroid injection to minimize the risk of permanent nerve damage. Either an anterior or posterior approach can be used. The latter is preferred when simultaneous radial head excision is contemplated. Tendon transfers are reserved for unsuccessful decompression, usually in late (more than 2 years) cases, in which there is severe permanent nerve damage.

A.A. Freeland, M.D.

High Implant Fracture Incidence With Sutter Silicone Metacarpophalangeal Joint Arthroplasty

Bass RL, Stern PJ, Nairus JG (Univ of Cincinnati, Ohio)

J Hand Surg (Am) 21A:813–818, 1996 11–11

Background.—The Sutter silicone metacarpophalangeal joint implant was introduced in 1987. In 1992, it was reported that 50 degrees of motion or more was obtained reliably with this implant. Outcomes of the Sutter metacarpophalangeal joint implant were reported, with particular emphasis on the incidence of implant failure and recurrence of clinical deformity.

Methods.—Thirty-four patients with rheumatoid arthritis were included. One hundred sixty-eight implants were used in 42 hands. The mean follow-up time was 27 months.

Findings.—At the final follow-up assessment, 20% of the implants were definitely fractured. Forty-five percent of those followed up for more than 3 years were definitely fractured (Fig 2, C). The mean ulnar drift in intact implants was 11 degrees at final follow-up; in the fractured implants, it was 23 degrees. However, implant fracture and patient satisfaction were uncorrelated. Eighty percent of the patients stated that they would undergo the procedure again.

Conclusions.—Although patient satisfaction in this series was unrelated to radiographic findings, the incidence of implant fracture was high. Be-

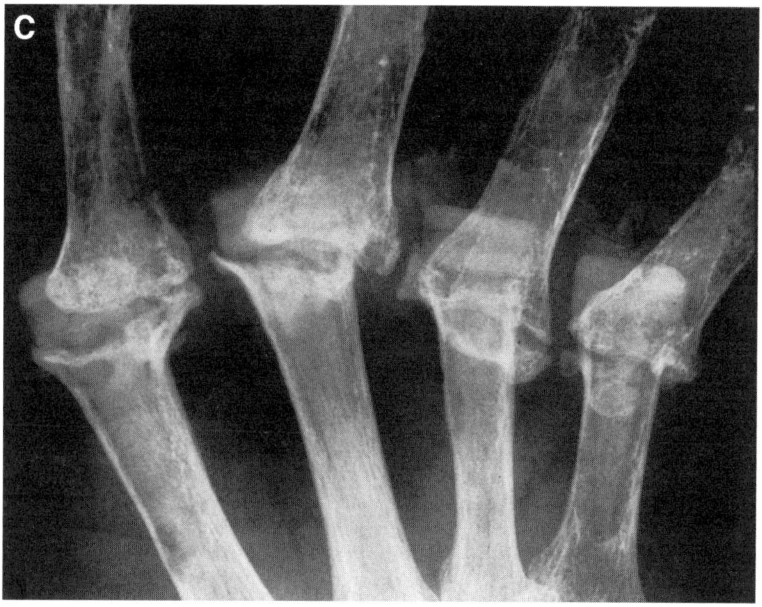

FIGURE 2, C.—Implant deformation and failure over 4 years. At 4 years, implants in middle, ring, and small metacarpophalangeal joints are definitely fractured, with proximal translation of the base of the proximal phalanx of more than one half the width of the midportion of the implant. The index finger is severely deformed. (Courtesy of Bass RL, Stern PJ, Nairus JG: High implant fracture incidence with Sutter silicone metacarpophalangeal joint arthroplasty. *J Hand Surg [Am]* 21A:813–818, 1996.)

cause of this high incidence and the recurrence of deformity, the use of this implant design should be reconsidered.

► The authors report an alarmingly high fracture rate at relatively short follow-up (mean, 27 months) with the Sutter silicone implant used in the metacarpophalangeal joints of patients with rheumatoid arthritis. Although the overall fracture rate was 20% of 168 implants, even more worrisome was an implant failure rate of 50% of 30 implants observed for a minimum of 3 years after operation. This latter rate is more than twice the fracture rate reported in several series of Swanson silicone metacarpophalangeal joint implants observed for a longer period of time. As might have been predicted, recurrence of ulnar drift was associated with radiographic evidence of implant fracture.

Unfortunately, the authors do not tell us the relative fracture rates between the radial and ulnar digits so that we might discern whether radial to ulnar loading in the index ray had any bearing on the observed increased fracture rate with this device. Similarly, fluoroscopic studies during active motion of the digit would provide information relative to the fixation of the implant stems as it might also relate to the observed increased fracture rate. Without any of this information, the authors' recommendation to abandon this implant design awaits confirmation of their data by another series.

V.D. Pellegrini, Jr., M.D.

Suggested Reading

Damen A, van der Lei B, Robinson PH: Carpometacarpal arthritis of the thumb. *J Hand Surg (Am)* 21A:807–812, 1996.

▶ In this series of CMC arthoplasties with trapezium excision and FCR tendon interposition, the authors have a lengthy average follow-up (8 years, 7 months). The overall complication rate was 18%. It appears that the results of this procedure do not deteriorate over time and that thumb metacarpal-scaphoid impingement does not occur. The results of this study are comparable with those reported with a number of other techniques, but other studies do not use the same methods to document their results. If results are indeed similar regardless of technique, one should favor the simplest technique.

E.R. North, M.D.

Hollevoet N, Kinnen L, Moermans JP, et al: Excision of the trapezium for osteoarthritis of the trapeziometacarpal joint of the thumb. *J Hand Surg (Br)* 21B:458–462, 1996.

Lins RE, Gelberman RH, McKeown L, et al: Basal joint arthritis: Trapeziectomy with ligament reconstruction and tendon interposition arthroplasty. *J Hand Surg (Am)* 21A:202–209, 1996.

▶ The authors demonstrate good to excellent functional results in approximately 90% of patients following LRTI reconstruction for basal joint osteoarthritis. Likewise, they noted a 50% increase in grip strength over preoperative measurements and a 43% increase in lateral pinch. Despite these excellent functional results, the authors express concern over the restoration of only one half of the trapezial space compared to normal thumbs without evidence of osteoarthritis; similarly, there is a 33% decrease in the trapezial space ratio when compared to preoperative values in the operated thumb.

While these observations speak to the incomplete restoration of the trapezial space by the LRTI procedure, they have little bearing on the anticipated longevity of this operation. An assessment of the "change" in trapezial space ratio is as a reflection of the durability of the LRTI reconstruction would more accurately compare the trapezial space at follow-up with that noted on the first x-ray taken following removal of the temporary K-wire fixation. By all available accounts, the LRTI reconstruction would appear to be durable and associated with a significant increase in grip and pinch strength. The relationship between ligament reconstruction, restoration of the trapezial space, and increase in grip and key pinch as observed with LRTI compared with simple trapeziectomy remains to be proven by a rigorous prospective clinical trial.

V.D. Pellegrini, Jr., M.D.

Menon J: Arthroscopic management of trapeziometacarpal joint arthritis of the thumb. *Arthroscopy* 12:581–587, 1996.

Rothwell AG, Cragg KJ, O'Neill LB: Hand function following silastic arthroplasty of the metacarpophalangeal joints in the rheumatoid hand. *J Hand Surg (Br)* 22B:90–93, 1997.

▶ Functional testing showed lasting improvement in a variety of prehension tasks following arthroplasty. Range of motion was not improved, but the arc of motion was altered: less ulnar deviation and more extension.

P.C. Amadio, M.D.

Schemitsch EH, Ewald FC, Thornhill TS: Results of total elbow arthroplasty after excision of the radial head and synovectomy in patients who had rheumatoid arthritis. *J Bone Joint Surg (Am)* 78A:1541–1547, 1996.

▶ This report on the unconstrained capitellocondylar design shows worse results when arthroplasty is performed in patients who had previously had a radial head excision and synovectomy. This is likely due to the unconstrained design and the fact that this particular implant does not have a radial head component. Thus, balancing soft tissues is more difficult in the absence of the radial head. Such problems would be less of a concern with semiconstrained designs, such as the Coonrad elbow.

P.C. Amadio, M.D.

12 Tumors and Tumor-like Conditions

Giant Cell Tumors of the Bones of the Hand

Athanasian EA, Wold LE, Amadio PC (Mayo Clinic and Found, Rochester, Minn)

J Hand Surg (Am) 22A:91–98, 1997 12–1

Introduction.—Giant cell tumor of the bone is seen in about 5% of bone tumors; of those, only 2% to 5% are tumors of the hand. Compared to other giant cell tumors of the bone, giant cell tumors of the hand occur at an early age, have a shorter duration of symptoms, recur more rapidly, and are multicentric. Curettage is less effective in these tumors. Treatment methods of giant cell tumors of the hand associated with oncologic success or failure and observations of earlier reports were reviewed.

Methods.—Data from medical records and radiologic, pathologic, and surgical reports were analyzed in a review of 14 patients with giant cell tumor of the bones of the hand. These patients were seen in a single institution from 1944 to 1994. Mean patient age was 32.7 years and mean follow-up was 5.8 years. Patients were most commonly seen initially for swelling of the hand (85%) or pain (62%). A mass was detected on physical examination in 7 patients. Radiographs were available in 10 patients: 4 patients had grade 2 lesions and 6 had grade 3 lesions. Histologically, 2 tumors were grade 2 and remaining tumors were grade 1.

Results.—Eight of 10 patients initially treated with curettage with or without bone grafting had recurrent disease. Mean duration to recurrence was 5.9 months. Of 3 patients treated with either wide excision or ray resection, 1 was complicated by gross intralesional contamination (Fig 4). Local and systemic recurrences occurred at 17 months. Regardless of procedure, local recurrence was observed in 6 of 8 patients treated for primary recurrent disease. Five patients underwent either local excision, wide excision, amputation, or ray resection after initial recurrence. Lung metastases were detected in 2 patients after or concurrent with local recurrence. Multicentricity was not observed in this patient series.

Discussion and Conclusion.—Earlier reports indicate high risk of local recurrence of giant cell tumors of the hand. Local recurrences of the hand range from 50% to 86% and are higher than local recurrence in long

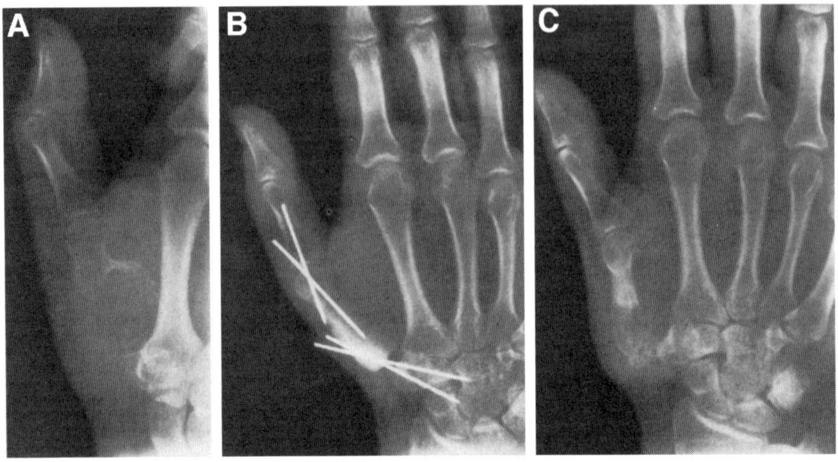

FIGURE 4.—A, lytic expansile lesion involves thumb metacarpal base; B, wide excision followed by reconstruction with iliac dowel graft; C, proximal lysis and destruction suggest recurrence. (Courtesy of Athanasian EA, Wold LE, Amadio PC: Giant cell tumors of the bones of the hand. *J Hand Surg [Am]* 22A:91–98, 1997.)

bones; some authors condemn use of curettage in these patients. Adequate treatment requires understanding of this tumor's behavior, local aggressiveness, and potential for disease-related death.

▶ This 50-year record review makes some useful and important points, but is also a disappointing study in that it communicates far less useful data and more confusing detail than one would expect from this institution.

The major point is that giant cell tumors of bone in the hand are likely to recur if treated by intralesional excision (80% of those treated primarily, and 75% of those treated for recurrent disease). However, this did not stop some of the "10 surgeons" who operated on these patients from additional curettage, local burring, phenolization, and radiation—all of which, when added to curettage in primary lesions, did not seem to affect outcome in a positive way.

The real value of this report is that it further confirms that en-bloc excision of the affected bone is needed to minimize the risk of recurrence of giant cell tumor of bone in the hand; and anything less will *not* do!

It would have been both useful and interesting to learn whether surgeons at this institution have learned their own published lesson; and if the most recently treated of the patients received proper care—sadly, those data were not discernible to this reviewer. One must accept that excision and bone replacement—or limited amputation—is the realistic and proper treatment for this relatively uncommon but well-known aggressive local bone tumor.

C.A. Peimer, M.D.

En Bloc Resection of Tumors of the Distal End of the Ulna
Cooney WP, Damron TA, Sim FH, et al (Mayo Clinic and Found, Rochester, Minn)
J Bone Joint Surg (Am) 79-A:406–412, 1997 12–2

Background.—Patients with tumors of the distal end of the ulna sometimes require *en bloc* resection. It has been suggested that this operation should be followed by reconstruction of the osseous defect. The results of *en bloc* resection of the distal end of the ulna, without subsequent reconstruction, are reviewed.

Patients.—The experience included 8 patients undergoing *en bloc* resection for malignant tumors or aggressive benign tumors of the distal end of the ulna. None of these patients had reconstruction of the osseous defect. The oncologic and functional results were reviewed a mean of 79 months after surgery. The tumor was a giant-cell tumor in 4 patients, a low-grade osteogenic sarcoma in 2, a hemangioendothelioma in 1, and a soft-tissue epithelioid sarcoma with osseous involvement in 1. The resection removed between 3 and 9 cm of bone from the distal end of the ulna. The amount of bone removed in the 4 patients with malignancy was at least 7.5 cm, to ensure an adequate proximal margin. For the patients with benign tumors, no more than 6.6 cm of bone was removed. Four patients, including 3 of those with malignant tumors, had extraperiosteal resection; the rest had subperiosteal resection (Fig 1).

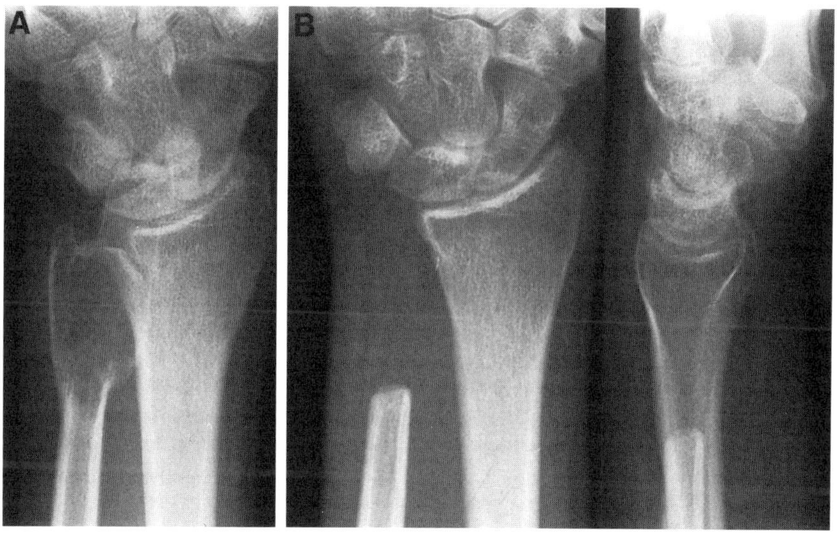

FIGURE 1.—Case 7. A, initial oblique posteroanterior radiograph of a 19-year-old man who had a destructive, expansile, lytic lesion of the distal end of the ulna. A biopsy demonstrated a giant-cell tumor. B, postoperative posteroanterior and lateral radiographs, made after subperiosteal removal of the distal 4.6 centimeters of the ulna. The functional result was excellent. (Courtesy of Cooney WP, Damron TA, Sim FH: *En bloc* resection of tumors of the distal end of the ulna. *J Bone Joint Surg [Am]* 79A:406–412, 1997.)

Outcomes.—During follow-up, no patient had local or systemic evidence of tumor recurrence. Six patients were rated as having an excellent functional result, while the other 2 had a good result. There were no problems with radiocarpal instability, as signaled by "clunking" or laxity, or with limited range of motion. The operation caused a 15% reduction in grip strength, compared with the unoperated side. This change was not directly related to the amount of bone resected, however.

Conclusions.—These patients had good oncologic control and functional results after *en bloc* resection for tumors of the distal end of the ulna, without osseous reconstruction. Such reconstruction does not appear to be necessary on a routine basis; it may add additional risk and morbidity without functional gain. The good results were achieved in patients with no history of wrist fracture, ligamentous laxity, or rheumatoid arthritis.

▶ The authors have clearly shown that in a tumorous condition without a history of trauma and disruption of the interosseous membrane or of the relationship of the radial carpal ligaments to the carpal bones, that resection of the distal ulna for tumorous conditions can be accomplished without the need for reconstruction and stabilization of the distal ulna. Orthopedists are aware of the fact that resection of excessive length of the ulna in posttraumatic situations can be associated with significant instability between the radius and the ulna. It is important to note that in the tumorous situation, this is not a problem and the ulna can be resected without significant morbidity.

R.D. Beckenbaugh, M.D.

The Treatment of Enchondromas in the Hand by Endoscopic Curettage Without Bone Grafting

Sekiya I, Matsui N, Otsuka T, et al (Nagoya City Univ, Japan)

J Hand Surg (Br) 22B:230–234, 1997 12–3

Introduction.—The usual treatment of enchondroma of the hand involves curettage and filling the resultant bone cavity with cancellous bone. The technique of endoscopic curettage without bone grafting was performed in 9 patients with enchondromas in the hand.

> *Surgical Technique.*—After making a 2- to 3-mm incision at the level of the lesion, the cortex of the bone over the tumor is fenestrated utilizing a Kirschner wire. The bulk of the tumor is removed (and sent for histologic examination) without endoscopic assistance using a small curette. A second incision is made at the opposite side of the lesion and the cortex of the bone and the dorsal cortex of the bone over the tumor are fenestrated. An 18-gauge needle is inserted for irrigation and flushed for several minutes with normal saline solution. A 1.5-mm diameter endoscope is inserted into the bone cavity and curettage of the tumor is performed.

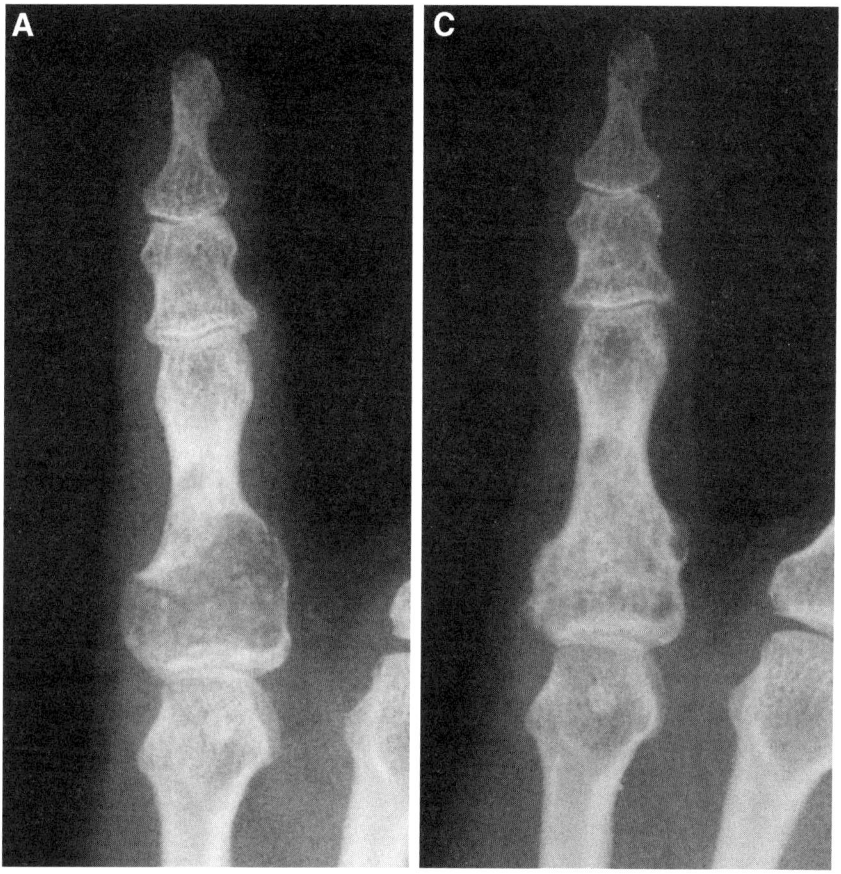

FIGURE 5.—Case 2. A 47-year-old woman with enchondroma of the proximal phalanx of the left little finger. **A**, preoperative view; **C**, x-ray film 1 year after surgery showing good remodeling of the lesion. (Courtesy of Sekiya I, MatSui N, Otsuka T: The treatment of enchondromas in the hand by endoscopic curettage without bone grafting. *J Hand Surg [Br]* 22B:230–234, 1997.)

Portals are exchanged to ensure complete observation of the interior of the cavity. After complete visualization of the area and total removal of the lesion, the medullary cavity is irrigated and one stitch is used to close the incision. A compression dressing is applied for about 3 days and the patient is cautioned about the risk of pathologic fracture.

Results.—The diagnosis of enchondroma was confirmed by histologic evaluation. No postoperative fractures, infections, or complications were observed. On the average, full recovery was achieved within 5.6 weeks after surgery. New bone formation was detected on an average of 2.4 months after surgery and remodeling of the lesion was seen 4.1 months after surgery (Fig 5).

Conclusion.—The use of bone grafting in the treatment of enchondromas of the hand is controversial. Endoscopic curettage of enchondroma in the hand with no bone grafting offers a magnified image and decreased blind area with the endoscope, complete curettage through the portals, and early functional recovery.

▶ This series represents another interesting application of endoscope-assisted surgery; but, as the authors note in the full text, the enchondromas are actually *not* removed endoscopically. The *title is misleading,* therefore. Nonetheless, the use of 2 small portals for enchondroma curettage does offer the advantage of a less invasive surgical insult, and especially where their methodology has already imposed one full disability interval related to the pathologic fracture (which is how 95% of enchondromas present).

My own preference continues to be to treat the enchondroma and the fracture simultaneously, thereby reducing the disability to a single interval; internal fixation with K-wires (which can be done percutaneously with fluoroscopic assistance) is added as necessary, and used in most such cases. The endoscope could also be used to assist curettage in acute cases, where irrigation and suction allow adequate visualization.

The other issue in this paper is whether or not one grafts the curetted defect. This and other articles confirm that bone grafting is not necessary in the small bones of the hand. However, unlike the authors' allegation that final radiographs show "good remodeling," I find that their illustration—and my own experience—confirms that the major advantage of grafting to the clinician and patient is that a grafted zone becomes homogeneous, making appreciation of residual, slow-growing, and/or recurrent enchondromas much less speculative by imaging criteria. (Of additional note in their illustrated case is the diffuse primary osteoarthritis and congenital brachymesophalangia, the latter raising issues of possible systemic enchondral ossific problems.)

One awaits the day when we need only inject bone morphogenic protein into such a curetted cavity and merely wait a few minutes for the gel to set before discharging the patient.

C.A. Peimer, M.D.

Subungual Exostosis: Case Report and Review of the Literature
Davis DA, Cohen PR (Univ of Texas, Houston)
Pediatr Dermatol 13:212–218, 1996 12–4

Background.—Subungual exostosis is an uncommon bony tumor that is usually acquired, benign, and located under the distal medial nail of the hallux. A patient with this tumor was described, and the literature on it was reviewed.

Case Report.—Boy, 16 years, was brought for medical care of a nodule on the distal medial aspect of his left first toenail. The nodule had been growing for 5 months. One year earlier, the boy had dropped a barbell on that part of his foot. The lesion was tender to palpation on physical assessment. Radiography showed a bony lesion with a broad-based contiguous cortex and a thin cartilaginous cap, which confirmed the clinically suspected diagnosis of subungual exostosis. The exostosis was removed surgically under local anesthesia. Lesion reduction was performed with a rongeur. The underlying bone was curetted to create a shallow, saucer-shaped defect in the hallux. Adequate lesion removal was verified on intraoperative radiographs. During 10 months of follow-up, there was no evidence of recurrence.

Conclusions.—Including the current patient, 321 patients with subungual exostosis have been reported in the English language literature between 1857 and 1994. Subungual exostosis occurs in a female–male ratio of 2:1. Although these lesions are most often seen in adults in their early 20s, they may also occur in children and adolescents. Most lesions affect the first hallux and are associated with trauma. The diagnosis can be suspected clinically and confirmed radiographically. Surgery is indicated.

▶ This is a useful review to be reread when confronted by the differential diagnosis of bony masses involving phalanges.

E. Fleegler, M.D.

The Surgical Treatment of the Forearm in Multiple Hereditary Osteochondromas [Italian]

Manzotti A, Memeo A (Università degli Studi—Milano, Italia)

Minerva Ortop Traumatol 47:663–667, 1996 12–5

Background.—Multiple hereditary osteochondromatas is the most frequent benign bone tumor. In these patients, deformities of the forearm are the most common cause of functional impairment. The authors' experience with surgical treatment of the forearm in patients with multiple hereditary osteochondromatas was described. The cases of 14 patients were reviewed.

Methods.—In these 14 patients, 3 types of forearm were identified by Masada's classification: 9 were type I, 2 were type II, and 3 were type III. Four surgical techniques were used in 70 procedures: simple excision of osteochondromatas; corrective osteotomy of the radius; corrective osteotomy of radius and ulna with open reduction of the radial head; and lengthening of the ulna with an external circular fixator. The follow-up was 2 to 10 years.

Discussion.—The primary goal of surgical treatment of multiple hereditary osteochondromatas is to restore full range of motion in the forearm, despite the esthetic deformity.

► A rather large series of patients was reviewed by these authors. Points of interest include the classification of the deformities, done according to the works of Masada et al. and Bock and Reed,[1] and the different surgical options applied, which were related to the proposed classification. In the majority of the cases, a simple excision of the osteochondromata was able to improve function by restoring pronosupination. In 2 cases, symptoms related to compression of neurovascular structures were resolved. In 1 case, open reduction of the radial head could not improve elbow range of motion. In 1 case, ulna lenghtening was obtained using the Ilizarov distraction technique.

M. Ceruso, M.D.

Reference

1. Bock G, Reed MH: Forearm deformities in multiple cartilaginous exostoses. *Skeletal Radiol* 20:483–486, 1991.

Infantile Haemangiopericytoma of the Hand

Templeton PA, Gordon DJ, O'Hara MD (Royal Belfast Hosp for Sick Children, Northern Ireland; Queen's Univ, Belfast, Northern Ireland; Royal Victoria Hosp, Belfast, Northern Ireland)

J Hand Surg (Br) 21B:121–123, 1996 12–6

Background.—Infantile hemangiopericytomas (IHPs) are rare subcutaneous tumors that arise from pericytes and appear to be locally invasive, although their prognosis is better than that of adult hemangiopericytomas. Diagnosing these tumors is difficult. A 7-week-old boy with IHP of the hand was described.

Case Report.—On examination, the boy was found to have an ulcerated tumor affecting the index finger of the right hand. The tumor, first noticed at birth, had grown quickly to envelope the entire index finger and had displaced the other fingers. He had no other significant medical or family history. Radiography confirmed a soft-tissue tumor. Three days after this referral, the tumor ulcerated and began to hemorrhage. The bleeding increased after hospitalization, and despite blood transfusion, the hemoglobin level dropped to less than 9 g/dL. The affected digit was amputated as an urgent, life-saving measure. The distal part of the second metacarpal was included in the excision. The resulting wound was partly sutured, and the remainder was covered with a full-thickness graft taken from the right groin. The infant's recovery was rapid and uneventful. After 36 months of follow-up, there was no evidence of local recurrence or distant disease. Hand function was good.

Conclusions.—Radical surgery is the treatment recommended for hemangiopericytoma, which has serious implications when the tumor occurs in the hand. The patient described had good hand function despite major resection, partly because second digit and ray amputation is less debilitating than many other digital amputations and partly because of the adaptability of infants.

▶ This valuable case report widens our understanding of the behavior of hemangiopericytomas. One must keep in mind that the patient had emergency surgery because of hemorrhaging. When considering the approach to this patient, one must keep in mind the standard approach to patients with tumors. This includes appropriate biopsy after the evaluation of the patient by other means in association with staging. Normally, this sequence is part of the orderly care of the patient with a tumor. Although maintaining as much hand function as possible after tumor treatment is desirable, the primary goal is adequate treatment to save the patient's life.

E. Fleegler, M.D.

Congenital Neuroepithelioma in an Infant Hand

Erdmann D, Brown RE, Rumbolo PM (Southern Illinois Univ, Springfield, Ill)
J Hand Surg (Br) 21B:117–121, 1996 12–7

Background.—Although neuroepithelioma arising from the CNS is relatively common in children, a peripheral nerve origin is very rare. An infant with a congenital peripheral neuroepithelioma of the hand was described.

Case report.—The boy was born with a soft-tissue mass of the left palm. At physical examination at 6 weeks, the tumor was noted to be a well-circumscribed purple mass, measuring 2 × 1.5 × 0.5 cm, at the base of the index and middle fingers with no fixation to surrounding tissues (Fig 1). Clinically, the tumor was diagnosed as a hemangioma. When the infant was seen again 6 weeks later, significant enlargement of the mass was observed (Fig 2). Radiologic assessment showed separation of the second and third metacarpal heads but no bony erosion or invasion. Normal vascularity was seen on intraoperative angiography. The mass measured 4 × 2.5 ×1.5 cm on exploration. Histologically, the tumor was found to consist of small round cells with clear margins. The diagnosis of peripheral neuroepithelioma was confirmed by electron microscopy and immunohistochemistry. No metastases were found on a CT scan of the chest, on a bone scan, or in a bone marrow aspirate. Chemotherapy was initiated. Three months after tumor resection,

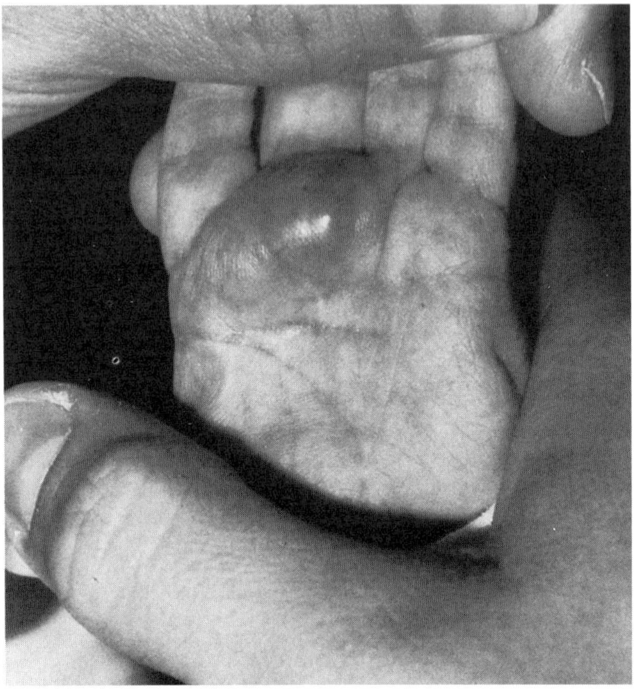

FIGURE 1.—Appearance at 6 weeks of age. (Courtesy of Erdmann D, Brown RE, Rumbolo PM: Congenital neuroepithelioma in an infant hand. *J Hand Surg [Br]* 21B:117–121, 1996.)

a second-look procedure showed no sign of recurrence. Follow-up to 4 years of age revealed no evidence of recurrent disease. Hand function was normal.

Conclusions.—This patient had a primitive malignant tumor of neuroepithelial origin found very rarely in newborns. There have been no previous reports of peripheral neuroepithelioma of the hand.

▶ Reviews of rare hand tumors are important. Such articles help us when we encounter these unusual cases and also contribute to the information available for analysis when significant numbers of the same type of cases collect in the literature. In this case, the ease with which a very serious malignant tumor could be confused clinically with a hemangioma is emphasized. It seems that the principle of the follow-up re-evaluation "saved the day" in this patient's case. However, more follow-up re-evaluation will be necessary for us to learn the outcome for the patient presented. The actual resection of the tumor is only briefly alluded to in this article in Figure 5 (see original article).

E. Fleegler, M.D.

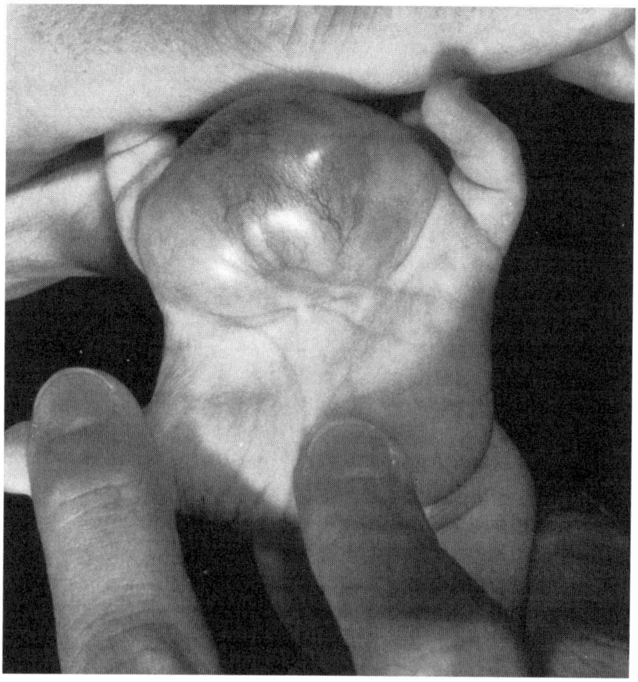

FIGURE 2.—Appearance at 12 weeks of age just before surgery. (Courtesy of Erdmann D, Brown RE, Rumbolo PM: Congenital neuroepithelioma in an infant hand. *J Hand Surg [Br]* 21B:117–121, 1996.)

Subungual Glomus Tumours: A Different Approach to Diagnosis and Treatment

Ekin A, Özkan M, Kabaklioglu T (Dokuz Eylül Univ, Izmir, Turkey)

J Hand Surg (Br) 22B:228–229, 1997 12–8

Introduction.—Subungual glomus tumors tend to recur, even after complete removal. One of the major problems after surgery is postoperative nail deformity. A transillumination test for diagnosis and a surgical technique designed to prevent postoperative nail deformity were developed.

Methods.—Nine patients with subungual glomus tumors had a mean duration of 28 months of symptoms (mostly pain and subungual discoloration). The tumor was in the proximal part of the nail under the lunula in 6 patients and at the distal end of the nail in 3 patients. All patients had positive reactions to cold provocation tests. Seven patients were given a transillumination test; they were taken to a dark room and light was projected under the pulp. The tumor was able to be localized and its size estimated because it gave a different color than normal tissue.

Surgical Technique.—For tumors in the proximal end of the nail, 2 incisions were made in the lateral paronychial folds at 90 degrees to the eponychium. The eponychial flap was elevated and a window was opened on the nail that was a little bit bigger in diameter than the tumor. The matrix was opened with an H incision and a small curette was used to remove the tumor. An absorbable 6/0 suture was used to close the matrix, the eponychial flap was closed on the nail, and the paronychial incision was closed. The window was made larger than the tumor and the same procedure was performed for distal tumors.

Results.—All patients had pain relief postoperatively. One patient had repeat surgery for a recurrent tumor. There were no deformities or cosmetic problems in the nail. One patient experienced softening of the lunula.

Conclusion.—Transillumination is a new diagnostic method helpful in determining the location and estimating the diameter of subungual glomus tumors. The surgical technique described makes it easy to reach the glomus tumor under the proximal ungual bed and minimizes any defect. With nail growth, the defect disappears in 4–6 weeks.

▶ This is a report of an interesting method to elucidate clinical diagnosis of glomus tumors developed by these authors. The *Journal* took the added expense of publishing a color photograph to make their method of transillumination (simply done in a dark room using a "laser pointer") visible for the article.

I had the good fortune to have heard this paper at the International Federation of Societies for Surgery of the Hand in Helsinki, Finland in 1995, and then had the chance to see the authors' color slides and discuss the presented material. This is a small but thoughtful and innovative "clinical trick" that can be helpfully applied in this pesky and painful, frequently occult subungual neoplasm.

C.A. Peimer, M.D.

The Management of Pigmented Lesions of the Nail Bed

Glat PM, Spector JA, Roses DF, et al (New York Univ)
Ann Plast Surg 37:125–134, 1996 12–9

Introduction.—Correct diagnosis of pigmented lesions of the nail bed is essential because the differential diagnosis ranges from hematoma to melanoma. These lesions are often categorized as melanonychia striata, which refers to any linear tan-brown-black pigmentation of the nail bed. The management of these lesions was discussed and a retrospective review of 30 cases provided.

Treatment.—The nail bed biopsy is important for proper diagnosis. Melanonychia striata can range from a dark streak to a completely pigmented nail bed, and the cause can either be neoplastic or nonneoplastic. In whites with single digit involvement, nail bed biopsy is essential. If the lesion can be removed at biopsy and is benign, no further treatment is required. Recurrences are monitored for changes in size. In the absence of a clear margin, recurrence after nail growth, or in the case of melanoma in situ, total nail bed excision is carried out followed by reconstruction. Management of these lesions in nonwhites is controversial because of their high incidence. Lesions should be monitored for changes. Those lesions that are seen during adulthood, are broader than 6 mm, are either variegated or very dark, and are accompanied by periungual pigmentation are more likely to develop into melanoma and should be carefully monitored. When seen in multiple digits, the condition is usually not a neoplasm.

Study Population.—A retrospective review was performed on 30 patients with malignant melanoma treated at New York University between 1982 and 1995. There were 8 patients with cutaneous melanoma and 22 patients with subungual melanoma. There were 9 men and 21 women with an age range of 13 to 82 years. Although lesions occurred on each digit, the thumb was the most common. Seven patients had long-standing lesions on the melanoma site, whereas 23 had no previous lesions. The average delay between the patient noticing the lesion and diagnosis was 31 months. Misdiagnosis was involved in 41% of these cases of delay. The average invasion depth was 1.36 mm in cutaneous lesions and 3.68 mm in subungual lesions. Ulceration was more common in the subungual group.

Treatment.—Patients with intermediate-thickness lesions had elective lymph node dissection. All the invasive cutaneous lesions were treated with wide excision until negative margins were obtained, followed by grafting. All invasive ungual lesions were treated with amputation 1 joint proximal to the lesion. There was 1 recurrence at the site of the excision. All patients with cutaneous melanoma survived without evidence of disease at 14 months' to 12 years' follow-up. There was 1 death in the subungual melanoma group, which had a follow-up of 6 months to 9 years.

Conclusion.—Pigmented lesions of the nail bed are difficult to diagnose, but correct diagnosis is essential because the conditions potentially responsible for this type of lesion differ considerably in their treatment. Excisional biopsy is the diagnostic tool of choice for melanonychia striata lesions.

▶ This article provides useful information regarding a management algorithm for pigmented lesions of the nail bed. Especially useful information is provided regarding the discussion of melanonychia striata. The article, in general, confirms what appears to be a gradual shift toward a more conservative management approach to subungual melanoma. Several articles now exist in the literature which confirm the fact that level of amputation does not affect survival or outcome. In fact, the level of amputation in the past has been practiced by tradition only, with minimal scientific substantiation.

Our recent review of the Mayo Clinic experience (accepted for publication in *Plastic and Reconstructive Surgery*) confirms the adequacy of conservative amputation. In fact, survival was not significantly affected by the depth of the primary lesion, and data supported the use of local excision for lesions of 3 mm or less, with conservative amputation for those greater than 3 mm.

Because the vast majority of all subungual lesions in all series are found in the thumb, the condition takes on critical functional impact. We currently strive for a conservative resection, which is adequate treatment for the primary disease while preserving as much function as possible of the thumb. For those lesions greater than 3 mm which cannot be treated with local excision and histologic clear margins, my current practice regarding the thumb is complete excision of the nail bed, with distal resection at the level of the mid portion of the distal phalanx. A volar pad of thumb is preserved and rolled up to the dorsum of the thumb for an adequate soft-tissue closure, maintaining as much length as possible.

In my mind, it has become quite clear that the treatment of subungual melanoma is moving in similar fashion to more conservative resection margins, much in the same way the treatment of melanoma has been changed with respect to other cutaneous locations throughout the body. The recommended size of excision margins has decreased over the years from that which was obtained by pure anecdotal evidence to more conservative measurements that are more data based.

C.H. Johnson, M.D.

Micrographic Surgery for Subungual Squamous Cell Carcinoma

de Berker DAR, Dahl MGC, Malcolm AJ, et al (Royal Victoria Infirmary, Newcastle Upon Tyne, England)

Br J Plast Surg 49:414–419, 1996 12–10

Background.—Subungual squamous cell carcinoma (SCC) is a relatively rare tumor involving the nail bed distally and the matrix proximally. Although the diagnosis often is delayed, the tumor rarely spreads to other parts of the body. It can be difficult to distinguish between invasive and in situ subungual SCC. An experience with Mohs micrographic surgery for the treatment of subungual SCC was reviewed.

Methods.—The experience included 8 patients with subungual SCC: 4 men and 4 women; mean age, 61 years. The disease had been present for a mean of 5 years. All patients were treated as outpatients using Mohs micrographic surgery. In this procedure, an excision specimen is divided and examined, and the results are used to map the location of any residual tumor in the wound margin. It ensures complete removal of tumor while preserving uninvolved tissue. After the final procedure, the wounds were allowed to heal by secondary intention. The patients were followed up yearly thereafter.

Results.—The patients required 2 to 6 Mohs procedures, with a median of 3. The mean period required to achieve tumor clearance was 7 days. A mean of 14 specimens were examined per patient. The distal phalanx was preserved in all cases. The patients were followed up for a mean of 3 years, during which time there have been no recurrences. All of the operated digits have remained functional. There were no healing complications, and the cosmetic results were good except for loss of the nail plate.

Conclusions.—In patients with subungual SCC, Mohs micrographic surgery offers a safe and useful alternative to amputation, as long as bone is not involved. The Mohs procedure preserves the function and cosmetic appearance of the digit. Healing can occur by secondary intention, even in patients with exposed bone.

▶ Mohs micrographic surgery is not what the hand surgeon, regardless of the surgeon's base specialty, considers when a patient has a finger with a lesion suspicious for SCC, especially a subungual lesion. The plastic surgery–trained hand surgeon is familiar with this technique in the management of lesions that affect valuable facial structures such as the eyelid or nose, where limiting the amount of normal tissue to be excised is paramount. However, the authors show the applicability of this technique in the digit. The outcome in terms of local disease control is excellent, amputation is avoided, and the wounds remaining from the Mohs surgery are allowed to heal by secondary intention, which they apparently do well.

V.R. Hentz, M.D.

Intraneural Biphasic Synovial Sarcoma: An Alternative "Glandular" Tumor of Peripheral Nerve

Connell JX, Browne WL, Gropper PT, et al (Univ of British Columbia, Vancouver; Richmond Hosp, BC)

Mod Pathol 9:738–741, 1996 12–11

Background.—Tumors consisting of heterologous tissue arising in peripheral nerves are relatively rare. A patient with a biphasic synovial sarcoma arising in a digital nerve in the hand was described.

> *Case Report.*—Girl, 16 years, was evaluated for a slow-growing, painful lump on the palm of her hand. The lump had been present for 1 year. On physical examination, a small, tender, 2-cm mass was noted on the radial aspect of the palm at the level of the third metacarpal. Surgical exploration revealed a firm, 2.5-cm tumor arising from the common digital nerve. The tumor and some adherent nerve bundles were resected. The tumor was diagnosed as a synovial sarcoma based on its typical light microscopic appearance and immunohistochemical staining profile. The middle finger, including the distal two thirds of the metacarpal, was resected.

Conclusions.—This patient had a primary intraneural biphasic synovial sarcoma arising in the common digital nerve of the hand. This tumor can resemble glandular peripheral nerve sheath tumors because both consist of a mixture of spindled mesenchymal cells with admixed glandular epithelial elements.

▶ This report emphasizes the dangers posed by a lump in the finger. The size of the tumor in this 16-year-old patient with a 1-year history of an enlarging and painful lump should arouse clinicians' suspicions. In addition to the history, physical examination, and routine x-ray evaluation studies, an MRI before surgically altering the area is valuable. This study may give us additional information about the characteristics of the tumor as well as supply details of the anatomical extent of the lesion.

Considering all of the features that have accumulated through the evaluation of such a patient, the surgeon will then approach the biopsy in a manner that will limit the soiling of surrounding tissue with tumor cells. In addition to the value of reporting cases such as this, the long-term follow-up results will also be extremely important to other clinicians.

E. Fleegler, M.D.

Dupuytren's Disease and the Relationship Between the Transverse and Longitudinal Fibers of the Palmar Fascia: A Dissection Study

Holland AJA, McGrouther DA (Univ of London)

Clin Anat 10:97–103, 1997 12–12

Background.—The surgeon operating on patients with Dupuytren's disease must understand the anatomy of the palmar fascia. The fibers of the palmar fascia may be classified as longitudinal, transverse, and vertical in their orientation to the plane of the palm; the longitudinal fibers are the ones of greatest interest in Dupuytren's disease. In the distal palm, the longitudinal fibers are found in 3 separate layers: the superficial, intermediate, and deep layers. The relationship between the longitudinal and transverse fibers of the palmar fascia was assessed in a cadaver study.

Methods and Findings.—An operating microscope was used in the dissection of 10 fixed cadaver hands. In each hand, the deepest longitudinal fibers passed toward the dorsum of the hand, proximal to the transverse fibers of the palmar fascia, and into the vertical septa separating the flexor tendons. To the naked eye, the deep fibers seemed to pass toward the metacarpals. The authors discerned 1 deep layer of longitudinal fibers passing dorsally distal to the transverse fibers and another passing dorsally proximal to the transverse fibers (Fig 6).

Conclusions.—The deep longitudinal fibers of the palmar fascia can be further divided into 2 sublayers, the deepest of which passes dorsally and proximal to the transverse fibers of the fascia. Any surgery that preserves the transverse fibers will also conserve the deepest layer of the longitudinal fibers. Even the most radical surgery for Dupuytren's disease, which would run the risk of damaging the digital neurovascular bundles, is likely to preserve at least part of this layer.

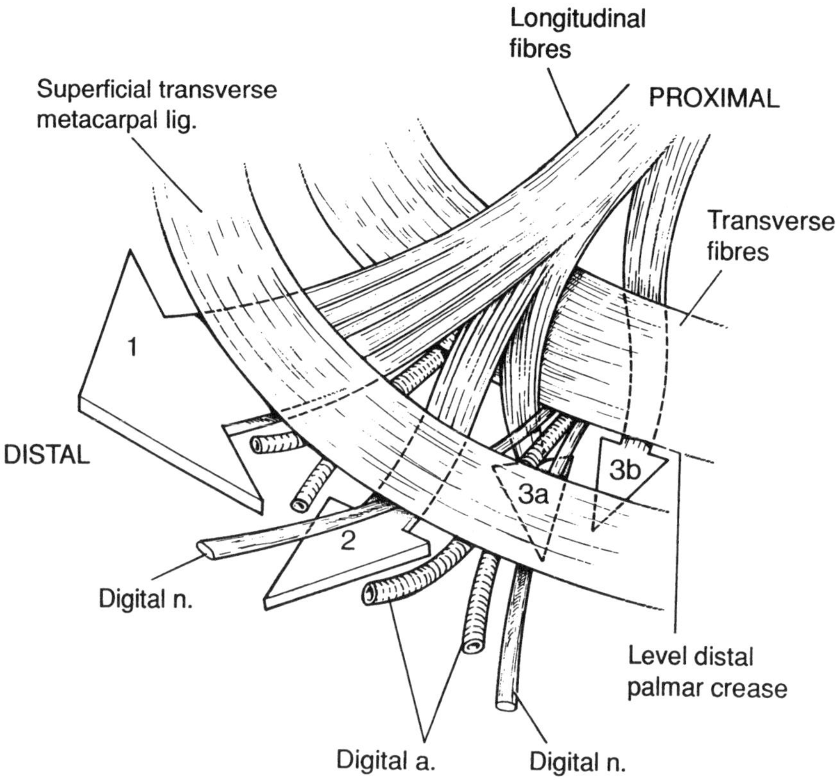

FIGURE 6.—Diagrammatic representation of the relationship of the longitudinal and transverse fibers of the palmar fascia. Superficial fibers (*layer 1*) insert into the skin, the intermediate fibers (*layer 2*) spiral around the neurovascular bundles, and the deep fibers pass dorsally distal (*layer 3a*) and proximal (*layer 3b*) to the transverse fibers. *Abbreviations: lig.*, ligament; *digital n.*, digital nerve; *digital a.*, digital artery. (Courtesy of Holland AJA, McGrouther DA: Dupuytren's disease and the relationship between the transverse and longitudinal fibers of the palmar fascia: A dissection study. *Clin Anat* 10:97–103. Copyright 1997, Wiley-Liss, Inc. Reprinted by permission of Wiley-Liss, Inc., a subsidiary of John Wiley & Sons.)

▶ This elegant anatomical study helps explain the difficulty of excising all the diseased tissue in Dupuytren's disease. The recent popularization (and success, in selected cases) of percutaneous cordotomy, without excision of either diseased nodule or cord, should encourage us to rethink our approach to this condition.

P.C. Amadio, M.D.

Long-term Results After Segmental Aponeurectomy for Dupuytren's Disease

Moermans JP (Clinique du Parc Léopold, Brussels, Belgium)
J Hand Surg (Br) 21B:797–800, 1996 12–13

Background.—Some authors have proposed the use of segmental aponeurectomy for Dupuytren's disease to reduce the incidence of wound complications and stiffness associated with wide dissections. How segmental aponeurectomy compares with other techniques, the stability of the contracture correction associated with this procedure, and the incidence of recurrences were determined.

Methods.—One hundred seventy-three segmental aponeurectomies performed in 141 patients were reviewed. This represented 59% of the total number done at the author's institution. Surgery had been performed a mean of 2.9 years before the review.

Findings.—Segmental aponeurectomy resulted in a lasting correction of the contracture. The follow-up values were even slightly better than the immediate postoperative measures in hands that did not show any sign of disease progression. The proportions of recurrences, extensions, and hands free of disease were comparable to those associated with other procedures. The recurrence rate was 38%. Type of surgery is apparently unassociated with the progression of Dupuytren's disease.

Conclusions.—The outcomes of segmental aponeurectomy for the treatment of Dupuytren's disease compare favorably with the outcomes of other procedures. An analysis of the late results in this series showed a lasting correction of the contracture.

▶ The authors propose that a less extensive surgical exposure for Dupuytren's contracture would limit wound complications and stiffness associated with wider dissections. Unfortunately, they did not define the extent of their "segmental aponeurectomy" in terms of number or location of the incisions. Their results do show that the incidence of recurrence and extension were similar to those after more extensive operations. The follow-up period averaged only 2.9 years. No data were given to support their hypothesis that wound complications or postoperative stiffness were lessened by their technique.

W. Engber, M.D.

Pharmacologic Regulation of Dupuytren's Fibroblast Contraction In Vitro

Rayan GM, Parizi M, Tomasek JJ (Univ of Oklahoma, Oklahoma City)
J Hand Surg (Am) 21A:1065–1070, 1996 12–14

Introduction.—Dupuytren's diseased tissue has been found to contain fibroblasts, which are thought to be responsible for contraction of palmar fascia. The effect of different pharmacologic agents on the contraction of Dupuytren's fibroblasts was evaluated.

Methods.—Two groups of pharmacologic agents were evaluated: agonists that promote Dupuytren's fibroblast contraction and antagonists that inhibit contraction. Agonists included angiotensin II, serotonin, prostaglandin $F_{2\alpha}$, and lysophosphatidic acid (LPA). The antagonists were nifedipine, verapamil, and prostaglandin E_1 and E_2. Dupuytren's fibroblasts were cultured in a stabilized type I collagen lattice and were contraction assayed. Agonists and antagonists were added to the culture during 2 separate experiments. Fibroblast contraction was assayed by measuring the change in the diameter of the lattice.

Results.—Angiotensin II, serotonin, LPA, and prostaglandin $F_{2\alpha}$ were found to significantly induce fibroblast contraction compared with no agonist. Of the 4 agonists, LPA was found to promote the most fibroblast contraction compared with the other agonists and was at least 1,000 times as active as the other agonists. Nifedipine, verapamil, and prostaglandin E_1 and E_2 all inhibited LPA-induced fibroblast contraction to some degree. Prostaglandin E_2 was found to inhibit LPA-induced fibroblast contraction to a greater extent than did prostaglandin E_1.

Conclusion.—All agonists evaluated produced some degree of contraction of Dupuytren's fibroblasts; LPA was the most potent inducer of fibroblast contraction. Both calcium channel blockers and prostaglandin E_1 and E_2 inhibited the contraction induced by LPA.

▶ Dr. Rayan and co-workers have performed an elegant study on the pharmacologic regulation of myofibroblasts in Dupuytren's disease. Using in vitro methods, they have expanded on the earlier work of Hurst et al.[1] The latter study showed that prostaglandins $F_{2\alpha}$ and E_2 promote contraction and relaxation of Dupuytren's myofibroblasts in vitro. Dr. Rayan and co-workers have found that LPA, an agonist of smooth-muscle contraction, significantly promoted myofibroblast contraction compared with other smooth-muscle agonists tested. In addition, prostaglandins E_1 and E_2 and nifedipine and verapamil inhibited LPA-promoted myofibroblast contraction.

In their discussion, the authors speculated that increased LPA and decreased prostaglandin E may contribute to contraction of Dupuytren's palmar fascia. Although this is an intriguing possibility, the micro-environment of the palmar fascia may be subject to multiple, endogenous pharmacologic signals, such that a cascade of cellular signals may play a role as myofibroblasts proliferate and form a Dupuytren's nodule and cord. It will be a formidable task for any investigator to unravel the cellular biology leading to development of therapeutic agents. For example, should therapies be cell directed to interfere with myofibroblast proliferation or contraction or with their transmembrane anchoring strands, or should therapies be directed toward collagen proliferation? Finally, the difficulties of drug delivery, mode of administration, frequency, safety, and efficacy are attendant with development of any new therapeutic agent. Dr. Rayan and co-workers have provided a good basis for future studies in these areas.

M.A. Badalamente, Ph.D.

Reference

1. Hurst LC, Badalamente MA, Makowski J: The pathobiology of Dupuytren's contracture: Effects of prostaglandins on myofibroblasts. *J Hand Surg (Am)* 11A: 18–23, 1986.

Suggested Reading

Burge P, Hoy G, Regan P, et al: Smoking, alcohol and the risk of Dupuytren's contracture. *J Bone Joint Surg (Br)* 79-B:206–210, 1997.

▶ People with Dupuytren's contracture who have surgery are more likely to smoke or drink than people without Dupuytren's who have surgery. What does this mean?

P.C. Amadio, M.D.

Keilholz L, Seegenschmiedt MH, Sauer R: Radiotherapy for prevention of disease progression in early-stage Dupuytren's contracture: Initial and long-term results. *Int J Radiation Oncology Biol Phys* 36:891–897, 1996.

▶ This study from Nuremberg, Germany, describes the rate of progression in 130 patients with Dupuytren's disease treated at an early stage by radiation (total dose of 30 Gy). Fifty-four patients were followed for more than 5 years. Forty-four showed no progression to a more advanced stage of the disease. According to these results, radiotherapy is effective in preventing progression of disease. Safety is another issue. Radiation oncologists in the United States do not advise radiation for this benign disease.

V.R. Hentz, M.D.

Lanzetta M, Morrison WA: Dupuytren's disease occurring after a surgical injury to the hand. *J Hand Surg (Br)* 21B:481–483, 1996.

▶ Three case reports of finger flexion contracture and palmar fibrosis occurring after surgery do not make an epidemic, but they do serve to question the dogma that Dupuytren's disease is not brought on by or aggravated by trauma. Either intraoperative difficulty or postoperative dystrophy was involved in each case. In one patient, a subsequent elective procedure did not result in any aggravation, though no special precautions were taken.

P.C. Amadio, M.D.

Sanjay BKS, Raj GA, Younge DA: Giant cell tumours of the hand. *J Hand Surg (Br)* 21B:683–687, 1996.

▶ The results from this study of 7 patients treated by aggressive surgery, usually en bloc resection and appropriate skeletal reconstruction, should be compared to the results reported from the Mayo Clinic series (Abstracts 12–1 and 12–2). In this aggressively treated group, only 1 patient developed a local recurrence. This patient also developed pulmonary and skeletal metastases.

V.R. Hentz, M.D.

13 Congenital Problems

Surgical Treatment and Postoperative Splinting of Recessive Dystrophic Epidermolysis Bullosa
Ladd AL, Kibele A, Gibbons S (Stanford Univ, Calif)
J Hand Surg (Am) 21A:888–897, 1996 13–1

Background.—Three types of epidermolysis bullosa (EB) have been identified: EB simplex, characterized by mild intraepidermal blisters; junctional EB, which causes generalized blistering; and dystrophic EB. Scarring does not occur in the first 2 types but is the hallmark of dystrophic EB. Dystrophic EB is commonly inherited as a recessive trait, known as recessive dystrophic EB (RDEB). Scarring of the hands and fingers in children with RDEB leads to pseudosyndactyly, an adducted thumb, and digital contractures. The role of surgical intervention, hand therapy, and postoperative splinting was assessed is 7 children with RDEB.

Methods.—The mean age of the patients was 5 years 8 months; 6 were boys and 1 was a girl. Nine hands were affected, and 3 of the children had severe contractures. The goal of surgery was to achieve simple grasp and pinch, primarily by release of the adducted thumb. Using a technique of epidermal degloving, the hand and fingers are "de-cocooned." This procedure is followed by further release of web and flexion contractures. Full-thickness skin grafts are taken from areas free of blistering, usually the abdomen. Perioperative antibiotics are administered as 3 doses of IV cefazolin. Patients are discharged the day after surgery and readmitted 10 to 14 days later for cast removal and wound debridement. Postoperative splinting and wound care requires 1 to 5 days in the hospital. A splint is worn at night for an indefinite period and an elastic compressive custom-made glove is used during the day.

Results.—All skin grafts healed successfully and no wound infections occurred. Surgery released the pseudosyndactylies and contractures in all patients, but mild contractures persisted or developed. Two children had moderate recurrence of contractures because of poor compliance with the postoperative regimen. Five children (7 hands) obtained a functional grasp and release.

Discussion.—The treatment protocol for the hand deformities of RDEB requires an interdisciplinary team of physicians, surgeons, therapists, and nurses. Compliance by the child and supportive parents are also essential for a successful outcome. Early and aggressive surgical release of the contractures allows the child to achieve relatively normal psychomotor development.

▶ The authors provide a detailed description of their approach to treating children with RDEB. Although this condition is rare, many of their conclusions are useful to most surgeons who operate on children. The authors stress the importance of a multidisciplinary team that includes the hand surgeon, appropriate consulting physicians, a pain service, therapists, and a supportive family. There is a detailed description of surgical treatment and postoperative care, which is important information in obtaining the authors' goals of improved simple grasp and pinch. Overall, this is an excellent and extensive review of the treatment for children with RDEB.

J.A. Katarincic, M.D.

Classification of Ulnar Deficiency According to the Thumb and First Web

Cole RJ, Manske PR (Orthopaedic Clinic, Memphis, Tenn; Washington Univ, St Louis)

J Hand Surg (Am) 22A:479–488, 1997 13–2

Introduction.—There are 6 different classification systems used to define abnormalities on the ulnar side of the forearm in ulnar-deficient upper extremities, but they do not adequately address the hand, where the most significant problems occur. Medical records and radiographs of 55 involved extremities of 45 patients treated for ulnar deficiency were reviewed retrospectively to evaluate hand abnormalities and develop a classification system of ulnar deficiencies according to the thumb and first web.

Methods.—Records were reviewed for information regarding demographics; characteristics of elbow, ulna, and hand morphology; and recommended surgical treatment. Four classification types were proposed as follows, based on progressive involvement of the thumb and first web: type A, thumb and first web are normal; type B, the first web has mild deficiency, the thumb has mild hypoplasia, extrinsic tendon function is intact, and opposition is present; type C, moderate to severe first web and thumb deficiency, potential loss of opposition, malrotation of the thumb into the plane of other digits, thumb-index syndactyly, absent extrinsic tendon (Fig 4); and type D, absent thumb. Forty of 55 hands (73%) had thumb and first-web abnormalities. There were 15, 10, 20, and 10 type A, B, C, and D hands, respectively. The Ogden, Bayne, and Swanson classification systems incorporate elbow and ulna characteristics, but still do not adequately address hand abnormalities. As an example, an extremity with an atypical pattern of ectrodactyly, no active motion of the thumb, and partial aplasia of the ulna would be classified as a thumb/first web type C, an Ogden II-C, a Bayne II-C, or a Swanson I-C (Fig 7).

Conclusion.—The proposed classification system describes the anatomy of the forearm and/or elbow, supplemented by the hand classification type.

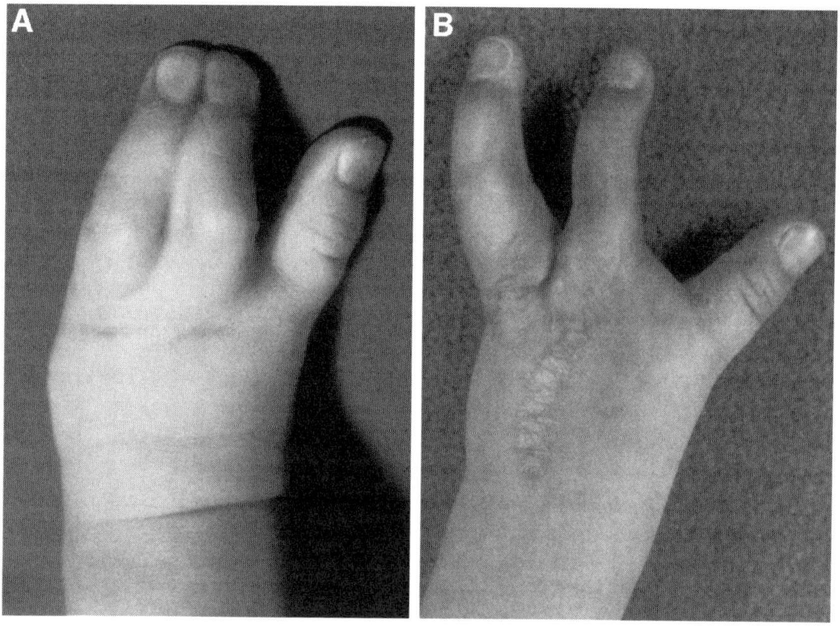

FIGURE 4.—Type C hand. **A,** preoperative clinical appearance of a type C hand revealing severe narrowing of the first web space and associated malrotation of the thumb ray toward the plane of the other digits. Remaining index and long fingers are involved by a complex syndactyly. Opposition is not present. **B,** postoperative clinical appearance after 2-stage operation reconstruction, including syndactyly release followed by first web deepening using a dorsal pedicle flap and rotational osteotomy of the thumb metacarpal. (Courtesy of Cole RJ, Manske PR: Classification of ulnar deficiency according to the thumb and first web. *J Hand Surg [Am]* 22A:479–488, 1997.)

This system is based on progressive deficiency of the thumb and first web and correlates well with progressive incidence of ulnar ectrodactyly and increasing incidence of other hand abnormalities.

▶ Congratulations to the authors for codifying a generally accepted surgical practice, that of using thumb-first web status as a most important guide in selecting surgery for any congenital hand problem, but particularly in the so-called "ulnar deficiency" group. The many classifications of this group seem to ignore this problem, although it is the most common surgical need in the group. The authors' types B and C may yet be subcategorized, particularly when results (not a part of this presentation) are being given. For initial acceptance, however, the considerable disparity within types B and C (see figures for the wide variety in type C) is best downplayed for ease of acceptance.

Almost as useful in this article is demonstration that the many classifications of ulnar deficiency are insufficient and that there is considerable doubt that "ulnar deficiency" is a suitable name for this condition, which includes not only ulnar but *central and radial* deficiency, not only distal but also proximal limb deficiency (some conditions designated *phocomelia* and most of those designated *pterygium cubitale* could be included), and not only

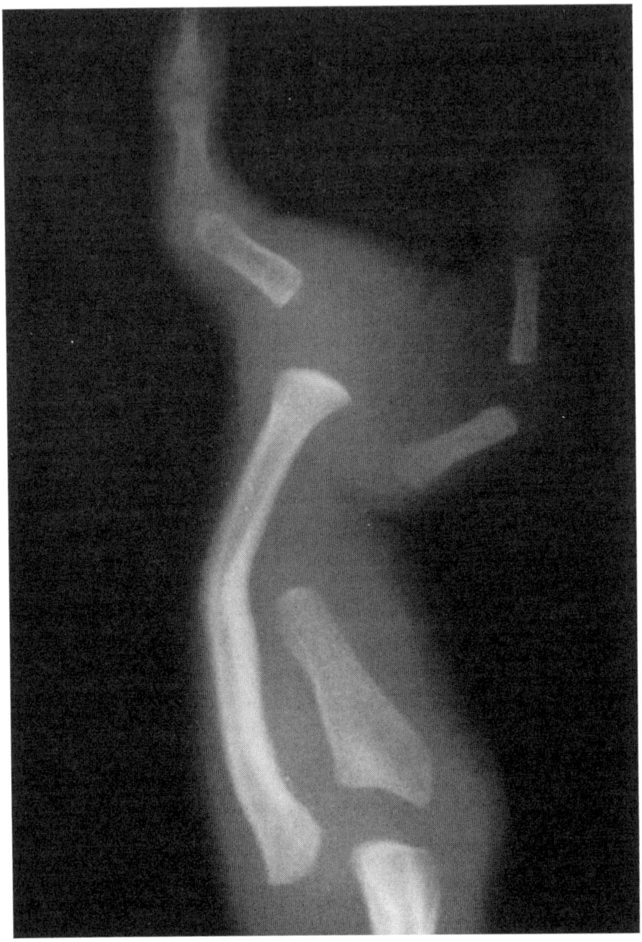

FIGURE 7.—X-ray film of an extremity with partial absence of the ulna and an atypical pattern of ectrodactyly consisting of a single ulnar digit and proximal take-off of the thumb. Clinically, this thumb has no active tendon function, resulting in classification as a thumb/first web type C or as an Ogden II-C, a Bayne II-C, or a Swanson I-C. (Courtesy of Cole RJ, Manske PR: Classification of ulnar deficiency according to the thumb and first web. *J Hand Surg [Am]* 22A:479–488, 1997.)

barely detectible anomalies (hypoplasia of a single ulnar digit) but also such severe hypoplasia as distal amputation. Obviously, a total reclassification is needed, but for now we will happily accept a clarification aimed at focusing attention on a major functional problem, which has many satisfactory solutions.

J.H. Dobyns, M.D.

Toe to Hand Transfer in Children, Part 2: Functional and Psychological Aspects

Kay SP, Wiberg M, Bellew M, et al (St James's Univ, Leeds, England)
J Hand Surg (Br) 21B:735–745, 1996 13–3

Introduction.—Part 1 of this 2-part series on toe-to-hand transfer in 40 children focused on technical aspects of the procedure. The functional and psychological aspects were addressed in the same series of children.

Methods.—At a mean follow-up of 45 months, 37 of the 40 children and their parents returned for evaluation by a hand therapist, an independent surgeon, and a clinical psychologist. Fourteen and 26 children, respectively, underwent single or double microvascular transfer of toes to the hand. Secondary procedures were common (Fig 4). Functional evaluation included motor recovery, sensory recovery, and assessment of donor site problems. Psychological assessments were conducted via interviews of patients and parents.

Results.—All except 3 children had an active range of movement in their transfer(s). There was a significant difference between total active and total passive range of movement that diminished slightly with time. Grip function, particularly resisted grip function, was poor in children with the lowest total active range of movement. It seemed that range of motion was better in children who were older at the time of transfer. Protective sensibility was recovered in all transfers and most (73%) recovered good levels of 2-point discrimination and light touch perception. Five of 40 children had minor problems at the donor site. Toe transfers were judged to improve appearance of the hand by 84% of parents and 88% of children and hand function by 92% of parents and all the children. Most parents thought other childrens' reactions to their child did not change because of surgery, but most children reported their peers were more positive. Most parents were very satisfied with surgical results.

Conclusion.—Survival of toe-to-hand transfer in children is good. The psychosocial results are encouraging. Psychosocial well-being did not worsen because of toe transfers, but actually improved. The authors encourage integrating children as normally as possible into their peer groups and harboring normal and reasonable expectations for the future.

▶ This is the follow-up counterpart to the earlier paper on technique. It monitors the results of the second toe transfers at a mean of 3 1/2 years. As expected with any nerve surgery in young children, excellent functional sensation was obtained almost independent of the number of nerves repaired. Active range of motion in the transfer was an average of 60 degrees, with the older children gaining slightly more motion. The authors attribute this fact to possibly better therapy cooperation of the older child. In fact, it most likely relates to the way in which these transfer digits are used, i.e., for basic opposition grasp as opposed to complete flexion.

It also may relate to the fact that the transferred digits were like a standard pollicization, treated with longitudinal Kirshner wire fixation and emphasis on

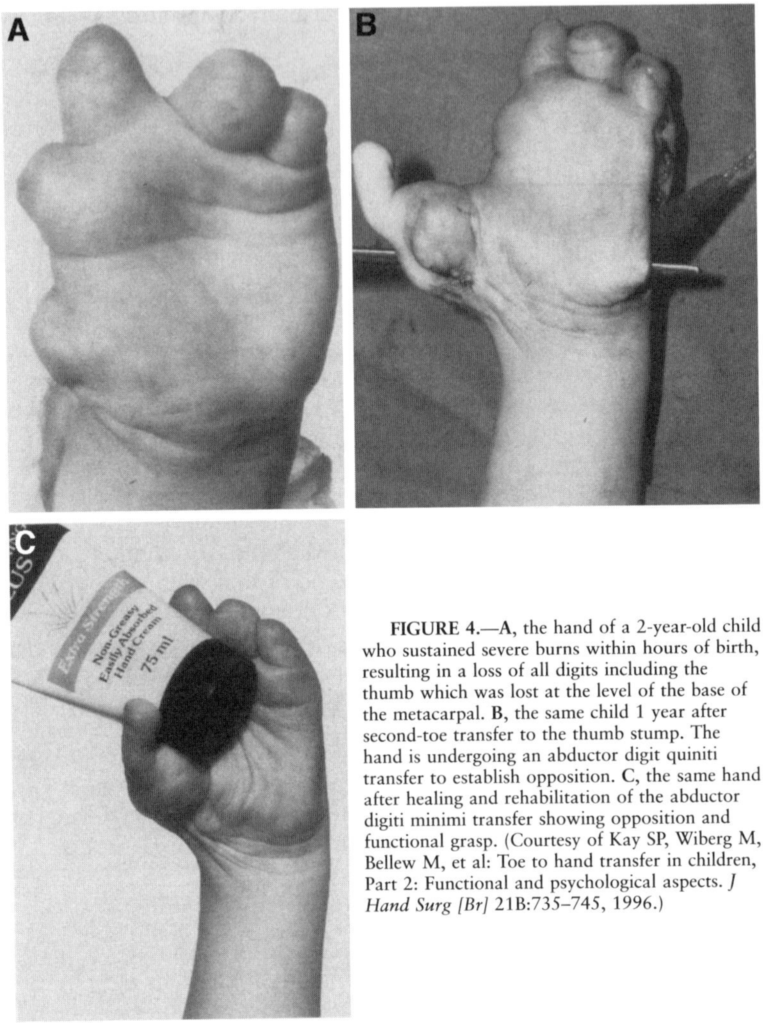

FIGURE 4.—**A**, the hand of a 2-year-old child who sustained severe burns within hours of birth, resulting in a loss of all digits including the thumb which was lost at the level of the base of the metacarpal. **B**, the same child 1 year after second-toe transfer to the thumb stump. The hand is undergoing an abductor digit quiniti transfer to establish opposition. **C**, the same hand after healing and rehabilitation of the abductor digiti minimi transfer showing opposition and functional grasp. (Courtesy of Kay SP, Wiberg M, Bellew M, et al: Toe to hand transfer in children, Part 2: Functional and psychological aspects. *J Hand Surg [Br]* 21B:735–745, 1996.)

tight extensor repairs. This may have lessened the motion but helped to avoid the so-called hook distal interphalangeal joint which can be seen in second-toe transfer. The paper emphasizes the fact that secondary procedures to further balance the hand and transfer tendons are to be expected. Tenolysis, however, did not offer expected gains and was not, in general, worthwhile.

Overall, 71% of the children regularly used their transferred toes. Both the child and the family were satisfied with the transfer. Foot donor problems were minor but were present in 12% of patients, and in 2 patients, caused difficulty in shoe wear. Like its lead article, this follow-up provided further data to support the use of microvascular toe transfer when the option of local digital rearrangement is not present.

A.L. Osterman, M.D.

Toe to Hand Transfer in Children, Part 1: Technical Aspects

Kay SP, Wiberg M (St James's Univ, Leeds, England)

J Hand Surg (Br) 21B:723–734, 1996 13–4

Introduction.—As microvascular surgery has improved technically, its uses have widened. A consecutive series of 40 children who underwent microvascular toe transfer to the hand is reported.

Methods.—The mean patient age was 5 years, 2 months. Fourteen children underwent single toe transfer and 26 had 2 second toes transferred during 1 surgical procedure.

> *Surgical Technique.*—All procedures began with dissection and exploration of the hand. Transfer was taken at the level of the base or proximal phalanx in the foot and either arthrodesed or chondrodesed to the recipient ray of the hand in most patients. Toe harvest began distally at the confluence of the dorsal and plantar systems. Transplants were harvested with only 1 vein and 1 artery. The plantar digital nerves were split from the common digital nerve of an adjacent toe, and flexor tendons were harvested through the dorsal extension of the wound. After harvest of the toes and repair of the donor site, the transfers of the first ray were usually joined to the radial artery or its remnant, transfers to the fifth ray were usually joined to the ulnar artery, and transfers of the central rays were usually joined to the radial artery, palmer arch, or ulnar artery.

Results.—There were no transfer failures, but 75% of children underwent additional staged procedures to improve appearance and function (Fig 9).

Discussion/Conclusion.—The focus of surgical planning in children undergoing toe-to-hand transfer is establishing a prehension pattern that is not already present. Function is the first priority, but creation of a more functional hand may create a more bizarre appearance than already existed. The hand, like the face, is constantly in view and is used for communication. Thus, a balance must be reached between function and

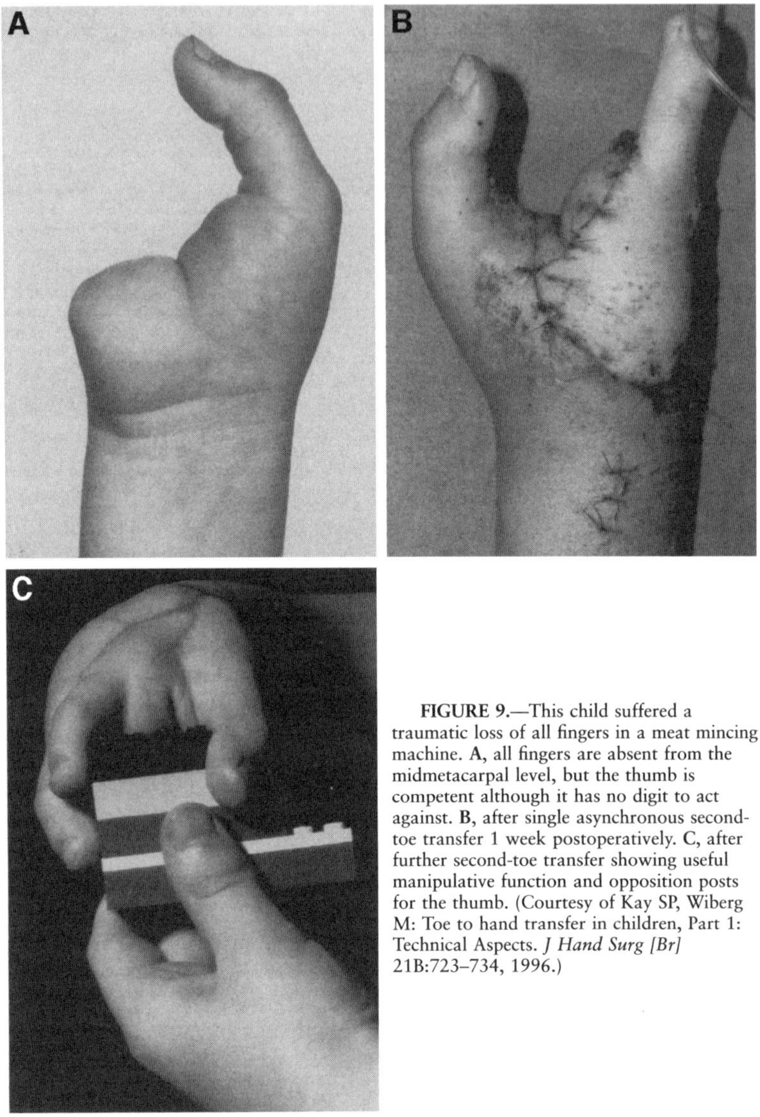

FIGURE 9.—This child suffered a traumatic loss of all fingers in a meat mincing machine. **A**, all fingers are absent from the midmetacarpal level, but the thumb is competent although it has no digit to act against. **B**, after single asynchronous second-toe transfer 1 week postoperatively. **C**, after further second-toe transfer showing useful manipulative function and opposition posts for the thumb. (Courtesy of Kay SP, Wiberg M: Toe to hand transfer in children, Part 1: Technical Aspects. *J Hand Surg [Br]* 21B:723–734, 1996.)

appearance. The key to transfer success is careful execution of each operative stage.

► This article proves that microvascular toe transfer in children is not only technically feasible but highly successful (100% survival after 5 emergency re-explorations). Forty successive transfers of a single or dual second-toe transfer are richly detailed. These transfers were done at an early age (less than 6 years) and in short order (average operating room time, 5½ hours for single transfer, 7½ hours for double transfer).

Does such technical virtuosity mean that pollicization is passe? Emphatically, the answer is "no." I agree with the authors that the reconstructive goal is to increase the versatility of the hand, giving both fine and grasp function whenever possible. Pollicization does this for a 3- or 4-fingered hand without much inherent risk and without the technical demands of this procedure.

The indications for microvascular toe transfer, therefore, exist when there are insufficient digits to allow for local digital rearrangement to accomplish these basic prehensile goals (see figure). In reviewing the authors' cases, I found myself agreeing with their plan in 60% of cases, uncertain in 25%, and likely to use standard techniques in 15%. The paper emphasizes some important technical points, with which I agree, as follows: (1) preoperative angiographic studies were not necessary, (2) transverse defects usually have some reconstructable recipient parts, and (3) the use of the second toe, either singly or in pairs, is better as compared with a monoblock of second and third toes.

Growth in the transplanted part averaged 91% of the normal toe with a 10% premature closure rate. This compares favorably with that of pollicization and should be taken into account in length designs of these transfers.

A.L. Osterman, M.D.

Postaxial Type-B Polydactyly: Prevalence and Treatment

Watson BT, Hennrikus WL (Naval Hosp, San Diego)

J Bone Joint Surg (Am) 79-A:65–68, 1997 13–5

Introduction.—Duplication of the small finger (postaxial polydactyly) is classified as type A when the extra digit is fully developed and as type B when the extra digit is rudimentary. The true prevalence of postaxial type B polydactyly is uncertain because many rudimentary digits are tied off by the physician and not recorded. A prospective screening study investigated the prevalence of this anomaly and the results of treatment with suture ligation.

Methods.—The study included 11,161 consecutive infants who were being screened for instability of the hip and were also given a general orthopedic screening. The racial mix of the group was 6,694 white, 2,008 black, 1,618 Asian, and 589 Hispanic; 252 newborns were classified as other or mixed race. Treatment of postaxial type B polydactyly consisted of ligation at the base of the digit, performed without anesthesia. Fifteen of the 21 newborns with a rudimentary extra digit (28 fingers) were reexamined at an average age of 20 months.

Results.—The prevalence of postaxial type B polydactyly was 1 in 531 live births. Twelve infants (57%) were boys and 9 (43%) were girls. The anomaly was more common in blacks (67%) than in whites (24%); 2 infants (10%) had 1 black parent and 1 white parent. No Asian or

Hispanic children were affected. Eighteen infants (86%) had a family history of the anomaly and 16 (76%) had the extra digit on both hands. No syndromes were identified in any of the infants. The average time for an extra digit to fall off after ligation was 10 days. One infant, whose extra digit had a large base, needed an operation when a blackened digit had not fallen off after 1 month. There were no deformities or limitations in range of motion at follow-up. Some infants had residual bumps; the average diameter was 2 millimeters and the largest bump was 6 millimeters.

Discussion.—Postaxial polydactyly was confirmed to be more common in black than in white infants. A dominant mode of inheritance was evident, with 18 of 21 infants having a parent with the anomaly. Suture ligation at the base of the pedicle appears to be a simple, safe, and effective treatment.

► In a prospective study, the authors define the actual prevalence of postaxial type B (rudimentary and pedunculated) to be one in 531 live births. The previously reported black-to-white ratio of 10 to 1 is repeated here. Concerns about exsanguination are alluded to, but it is stated that there is no case report in the literature. With none of these children having associated syndromes, the concerns I have with bleeding are lessened, but in the white children with no family history of the anomaly caution is warranted. The authors do a nice job of quantifying the residual cosmetic deformity which averaged 2 mm in diameter. Acceptance of the deformity by the patients, is quite high. This may be the result of the lack of functional deficit and of social acceptance, with 86% of the patients having a family history of the anomaly. On a technical note: I prefer to use a ligaclip for removal because it is easier to apply and may leave less of a bump.

J.A. Katarincic, M.D.

Surgical Treatment of Camptodactyly [French]

Glicenstein J, Haddad R, Guero S (Hôpital Robert Debré, Paris)
Ann Chir Main Memb Super 14:264–271, 1995 13–6

Background.—Camptodactyly is a flexion disorder of the flexor-extensor equilibrium in the proximal interphalangeal joint. The deformity may involve 1 or more fingers. It is caused by neither trauma nor paralysis, but it cannot be defined as a congenital anomaly because it often first occurs in adolescence. Camptodactylies can be isolated, primitive, or associated with other hand malformations. A clinical experience with camptodactyly was reported.

Patients.—Between 1975 and 1989, 59 patients received a diagnosis of camptodactyly of 1 or more fingers. Fifty-six of the anomalies were isolated, and 3 were associated with other hand malformations. Eleven children were not treated but were followed up, and their involved fingers were manipulated. Seventeen children (27 fingers) were treated with static or dynamic splints, and 31 children (43 fingers) were operated on. In all surgically treated patients, the procedure consisted of a total anterior tenoarthrolysis with lengthening of the skin by a rotation flap. Patients wore a static splint for 4–6 weeks, then a dynamic splint for at least 3 months.

Results.—After a follow-up of at least 1 year, 5 patients (20 fingers) treated by manipulation only were available for evaluation. Eleven fingers were improved, 7 remained the same, and 2 had deteriorated. In 9 patients who had a total of 24 fingers treated with splints, 14 fingers were improved, 5 remained the same, and 5 had deteriorated. Of 39 surgically treated fingers in 29 patients, 30 were improved, 7 remained stable, and 2 had deteriorated.

Conclusions.—This procedure is not suitable for all patients with camptodactyly, but it is particularly effective for reducing or correcting this hand deformity in young children. Adolescents and adults with articular blockage will only benefit from corrective osteotomy.

▶ The authors review their experience with 59 patients with camptodactyly, typically as an isolated deformity. Their work calls into question some ideas that are ingrained in our thinking, particularly the notion that an abnormal lumbrical insertion is a frequent cause. The authors view the problem as an imbalance between the extensor and flexor systems as they affect the proximal interphalangeal joint. They use a rotation flap plus a full-thickness graft to overcome volar skin shortage. They caution against applying techniques that succeed in children to adolescents with the same problems. For significant contractures in the latter age groups, correctional osteotomy seems best.

V.R. Hentz, M.D.

Radial Opening Wedge Osteotomy in Madelung's Deformity

Murphy MS, Linscheid RL, Dobyns JH, et al (Mayo Clinic and Found, Rochester, Minn)

J Hand Surg (Am) 21A:1035–1044, 1996 13–7

Background.—Managing symptomatic Madelung's deformity of the wrist can be very challenging. Biplanar radial opening wedge osteotomy is a nonablative procedure aimed at restoring a more normal anatomy to relieve pain and improve function and appearance. One experience with this procedure was described.

Methods and Outcomes.—Twelve wrists in 11 female patients, aged 9–31 years, with Madelung's deformity underwent radiopalmar opening wedge osteotomy. In 5 patients, radiographic findings met the criteria for generalized dyschondrosteosis. The patients were unhappy with the appearance of their affected wrists. The primary motion deficits were in radiocarpal extension and forearm pronosupination, which were associated with varying degrees of discomfort with sustained activity. Decreased radioulnar angle, lunate subluxation shown radiographically, and varying

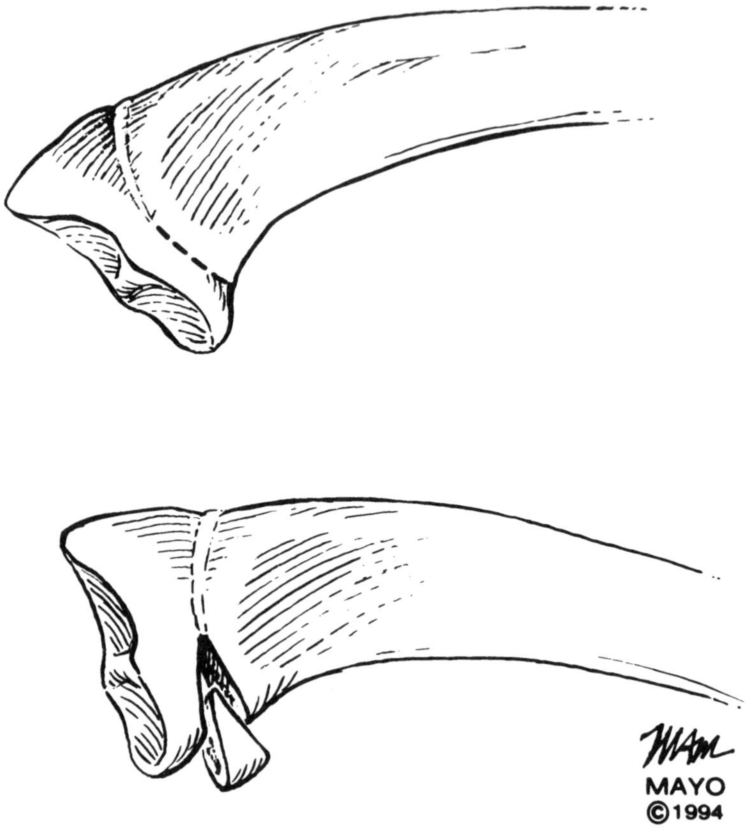

FIGURE 3.—Technique for physeal osteotomy. In the immature radius, the physis is identified as a thin white line. The osteotomy is directed from the ulnopalmar cul-de-sac to the ulnar aspect of the physis before wedging open with interpositional material. (Reprinted by permission of Mayo Foundation, from Murphy MS, Linscheid RL, Dobyns JH, et al: Radial opening wedge osteotomy in Madelung's deformity. *J Hand Surg [Am]* 21A:1035–1044, 1996.)

degrees of dorsal subluxation of the ulnar head were noted in all patients. Surgery was indicated for pain, limited motion, appearance, and, in 2 girls, progressive deformity. Iliac crest graft was used in the biplanar corrective opening wedge osteotomy of the radius. Fixation was achieved with a plate or Kirschner wire. Six patients had supplementary distracting external fixation. Mean follow-up time was 48 months. All patients had satisfactory pain relief. There were no changes in range of motion or grip strength. The radioulnar angle was improved by 11 degrees. However, lunate subluxation showed minimal change. Forearm length and the bowed appearance of the forearm were improved. Radioulnar joint reduction was improved but remained incongruous (Fig 3).

Conclusions.—Biplanar opening wedge osteotomy can be effective in selected patients with Madelung's deformity and disabling pain at the radiocarpal and radioulnar joints. The goal of this procedure is to correct abnormal anatomy based on biomechanical principles.

► Classic Madelung's deformity results from premature closing of the ulnar palmar aspect of the distal radial physis. The radial and dorsal aspect of the physis continue to grow, creating the retinographic and clinical defomity. Most patients have ulnar-sided wrist pain secondary to the normal growth of the ulna, which becomes disproportionate to the radial length. The ulnar head displaces dorsally as the carpus displaces ulnarly and palmarly. Seldom do patients have pain at the radiocarpal joint but rather have pain secondary to ulnocarpal abutment. Pain is often relieved by ulnar shortening with ablation of the ulnar physis; however, to correct aesthetic deformity, a distal radial osteotomy is necessary.

P. Dell, M.D.

Extremity Gangrene In Utero

Carr MM, Al-Qattan M, Clarke HM (Hosp for Sick Children, Toronto)
J Hand Surg (Br) 21B:652–655, 1996 13–8

Background.—Neonatal extremity gangrene is rare. An infant born with evidence of intrauterine vascular occlusion was described.

Case Report.—Boy, born at 35-weeks' gestation, weighed 2.22 kg at birth. The pregnancy had been normal until week 34, when the mother noticed reduced fetal movements; shortly thereafter she went into labor. Placental abnormalities included multiple infarcts and several sclerotic chorionic villi. The neonate was found to have a large necrotic area on the ulnar border of the right forearm and hand. The tips of his right thumb, ring finger, and little finger were ischemic. The thenar eminence was edematous. No ulnar pulse at the wrist was noted on Doppler assessment, although the radial pulse was palpable. The initial diagnosis was hyperviscosity syndrome, resulting in ulnar artery thrombosis.

Partial exchange transfusion was performed, decreasing the infant's hematocrit level from 0.7 to 0.52. Débridement of the necrotic areas was done at 3 weeks of age. The ring and little fingers were amputated, and pathologic assessment showed coagulative necrosis. Physiotherapy and right hand splinting were begun. At 7 months, the physiotherapist noted increased tone and neglect on the left side. A CT scan showed multiple large cystic lesions in the right cerebral hemisphere, suggesting massive intrauterine infarction in the right anterior and middle cerebral artery distribution. At 1 year of age, the infant underwent a 4-flap Z-plasty of the first web space and release of the ulnar aspect of the wrist with a full-thickness skin graft. Although splints were used after surgery, progressive ulnar deviation of the forearm and wrist developed. At 3 years of age, his dominant right hand was functioning well. The left hand was used for 2-handed tasks. The ulnar wrist flexion deformity was more pronounced at this time. Repeat radiographs showed little increase in the length of the right radius.

Conclusions.—Extremity gangrene resulting from intrauterine embolization of infarcted placental substances is a rare entity believed to be most commonly a manifestation of embolic phenomenon during maturation of the neonatal circulatory system. Neonatal gangrene is managed conservatively, and amputation is delayed as long as possible, because the line of demarcation tends to migrate distally. Before definitive treatment, evidence of multiple emboli should be sought carefully.

► The authors have thoroughly reviewed this rare condition. They provide good circumstantial evidence that the cause of gangrene in their patient was emboli from placental infarcts. They address their future treatment plans very briefly and do not specifically refer to their plans for treating the growth arrest. I have treated older children who sustained a similar perinatal injury, and who have growth arrest, forearm contractures similar to Volkmann's diffuse lipomatous infiltration, or a combination of these. In my experience, growth arrest is the most intractable problem, because the injury occurred at such an early age, and because the forearm contractures limit distraction lengthening.

M.A. James, M.D.

Suggested Reading

Glicenstein J, Guero S, Haddad R: Median clefts of the hand: Classification and therapeutic indications based on a series of 29 cases [French]. *Ann Chir Main* 14:253–263, 1995.

► This review of 20 patients (9 bilateral) supports Barsky's technique of reconstruction for simple cases. Often, however, complex deformities are present (superdigits, transverse bones in the cleft, complex syndactylies) which will require a custom approach.

P.C. Amadio, M.D.

Holten IWR, Smith AW, Bourne AJ, et al: The Apert syndrome hand: Pathologic anatomy and clinical manifestations. *Plast Reconstr Surg* 99:1681–1687, 1997.

► This paper is not of general interest and furthermore is of less value if it is abstracted, since its principal value is in its own abstracting of the current relevant literature about Apert and similar syndromes. However, for those with a special interest in these conditions, the paper is a treasure trove of information about the causes (from genetic to phenotypic to morphologic to dysfunctional amplification) of the basic mesenchymal to musculoskeletal abnormalities. For those with such interests, the paper in its entirety belongs in their files.

J.H. Dobyns, M.D.

Işik S, Selmanpakoğlu N, Açikel C: The use of tissue expanders in syndactyly repair. *Eur J Plast Surg* 19:225–228, 1996.

▶ This paper reports on the use of tissue expanders to avoid the need for skin grafting in adults with untreated syndactyly. The average age of the 11 patients treated was 20 years. I would agree that expanders are a good option in adults. Their use in children is more problematic because of both the small size and patient compliance.

P.C. Amadio, M.D.

14 Rehabilitation, Occupation, and Sports

Grip Strength and Finger Dexterity Across Five Styles of Commercial Wrist Orthoses

Stern EB (Univ of Minnesota, Minneapolis)
Am J Occup Ther 50:32–38, 1996 14–1

Background.—Commercial orthoses properly adjusted to patients' needs are thought to be effective in the treatment of temporary wrist pain, weakness, or mild inflammation while allowing functional use of the splinted hand. The power grip strength and finger dexterity of 5 types of commercial static wrist extensor orthoses were compared.

Methods.—Twenty-three women participated in the crossover study. The orthoses studied were the Kendall-Futuro #33, AliMed Freedom Long, AliMed Freedom Short, Smith & Nephew Rolyan D-Ring, and LMB Wrist Rest (Table 1).

Findings.—The finger dexterity associated with the Futuro, AliMed Short, Rolyan, and LMB did not differ significantly from that of the free hand. Finger speed was slower with the AliMed Long orthosis than with the LMB and the free hand. The power grip strength of the Rolyan orthosis was comparable to that of the free hand. The other 4 orthoses decreased grip strength compared with the Rolyan and with the free hand (Figs 2, 3).

Conclusions.—These different styles of orthoses affect power grip and finger dexterity differently. Clinicians should consider these data when choosing an orthosis, although the patient's medical needs and preference should be the overriding factors in the final decision.

Faster					Slower
17.9 (1.1)	17.9 (2.3)	17.3 (1.5)	17.3 (1.6)	16.9 (1.7)	16.7 (1.6)
Free Hand	LMB	Rolyan	Futuro	AliMed Short	AliMed Long

FIGURE 2.—Mean numbers of Purdue Pegboard pins placed (standard deviations) across conditions. Note that there is no significant difference in grip strength between or among the underlined conditions. Significance established a priori at $P<0.05$ for post hoc analyses. (Reprinted with permission from Stern EB: Grip strength and finger dexterity across five styles of commercial wrist orthoses. *Am J Occup Ther* 50:32–38. Copyright 1996 by the American Occupational Therapy Association, Inc.)

TABLE 1.—Comparison of Orthoses

Splint	Design	Wrist Support	Material	Distal End Fingers	Distal End Thumb	Length	Closures
Rolyan	Circumferential gauntlet; dorsal opening	Volar metal stay	Padded cotton with stockinette lining	At or proximal to distal palmar crease	Between thenar and MCP creases	½ forearm	D-ring; hook-and-loop self-fasteners
AliMed Short	Gauntlet; dorsal-radial opening	Volar metal stay	Elasticized	Proximal to distal palmar crease	Between thenar and MCP creases	½ forearm	Hook-and-loop self-fasteners
Futuro	Gauntlet; dorsal opening	Volar metal stay	Elasticized	Between distal palmar crease and MCP creases	Between thenar and MCP creases	½ forearm	Hook-and-loop self-fasteners
AliMed Long	Gauntlet; dorsal-radial opening	Volar metal stay	Elasticized	Proximal to distal palmar crease	Between thenar and MCP creases	⅔ forearm	Hook-and-loop self-fasteners
LMB	Wire foam and elasticized strap	Dorsal radial wire foam with palmar distal transverse arch support	Wire foam	Proximal to distal palmar crease	Clears thenar crease	≤ ½ forearm	Elasticized "z" strap; hook-and-loop self-fastener

Abbreviation: MCP, metacarpophalangeal.
(Reprinted with permission from Stern EB: Grip strength and finger dexterity across five styles of commercial wrist orthoses. *Am J Occup Ther* 50:32–38. Copyright 1996 by the American Occupational Therapy Association, Inc.)

Stronger					Weaker
30.6 (5.5)	29.8 (7.1)	25.6 (9.1)	25.1 (8.5)	24.4 (6.7)	24.0 (6.6)
Free Hand	Rolyan	Futuro	AliMed Short	LMB	AliMed Long

FIGURE 3.—Mean grip strength (standard deviation) in kilograms across conditions. Note that there is no significant difference in grip strength between or among the underlined conditions. Significance established a priori at $P<0.05$ for post hoc analyses. (Reprinted with permission from Stern EB: Grip strength and finger dexterity across five styles of commercial wrist orthoses. *Am J Occup Ther* 50:32–38. Copyright 1996 by the American Occupational Therapy Association, Inc.)

▶ This article gives us insight into the use of commercially available splints and their effectiveness when custom fit is not required. The author has chosen the most commonly available splints and shown us their use and drawbacks. This study also clearly demonstrates that when grip strength and function are the most important considerations, a choice of a shorter arm splint is preferable. Commercial splints, if chosen and fitted properly, can be cost- and time-efficient in the management of hand injuries.

P. Lalwani, O.T.R., C.H.T.

Training of Muscle Excursion After Tendon Transfer

Schreuders TAR, Stam HJ, Hovius SER (Univ Hosp Rotterdam Dijkzigt, The Netherlands)

J Hand Ther 9:243–245, 1996 14–2

Objective.—Discrepancies in excursion between the muscle to be replaced and the transferred muscle are common in tendon transfer (TT) surgery. In patients undergoing TT to replace the wrist extensors in radial palsy, the length of the pronator teres (PT) muscle must be doubled to permit full wrist movement. This raises questions about whether and how postoperative training programs can facilitate muscle fiber lengthening. Wrist flexion of 10 to 20 degrees is generally considered an excellent result of TT for radial palsy. The case of a patient who achieved particularly good wrist motion with postoperative training after TT for radial palsy was reviewed.

Case Report.—Man, 25, had wrist drop caused by radial palsy after humerus fracture 6 years previously. After TT and 4 weeks of immobilization, the patient was given a thermoplastic splint that held the wrist and proximal interphalangeal joints in extension and the metacarpophalangeal joints in slight flexion. The patient wore the splint day and night, except for 30 min/day of active, supervised contraction of the TT. The patient gradually gained control of the transferred muscles and was allowed to start exercising at home after 6 weeks. He was to remove the splint for 15 minutes 3 or 4 times per day to perform active contraction exercises.

By 2 months, the patient was wearing the splint only at night. Every 2 hours, he was to put the wrist in maximum palmar flexion and to contract the PT against moderate resistance; this exercise was designed to improve strength, excursion, and speed. One year after TT, his grip strength was 23 kg. His active range of motion was 0 to 65 degrees for wrist flexion and 0 to 60 degrees for wrist extension. He could extend all of the metacarpophalangeal joints with the wrist in extension, and he had full finger flexion.

Conclusions.—In this patient with TT for radial palsy, postoperative therapy provided especially good wrist motion. A program of serial splinting and static contraction against resistance in a lengthened position may increase excursion of the PT and other transferred muscles. These techniques should be evaluated further in patients with TT. Also, a universal classification of the results of TT is needed for standardized comparisons.

▶ This case study invites comments because of the remarkable postoperative outcome. There are many unanswered questions regarding how best to rehabilitate the patient after TT. Are there methods that might be useful in preconditioning a muscle before transfer? Can exercises, done in specific positions of the muscle or against specific resistances, result in added sarcomeres before transfer?

V.R. Hentz, M.D.

Botulinum Toxin in Writer's Cramp: Objective Response Evaluation in 31 Patients

Wissel J, Kabus C, Wenzel R, et al (Virchow Klinikum and Charité, Berlin)
J Neurol Neurosurg Psychiatry 61:172–175, 1996 14–3

Background.—Although previous studies have demonstrated that botulinum toxin is effective in the treatment of writer's cramp, most of these reports did not include objective or quantifiable response variables. The effects of local botulinum toxin injections have now been quantified using a newly developed rating scale of writing performance and a computer-assisted analysis of writing speed.

Methods and Findings.—Thirty-one patients who were undergoing botulinum toxin therapy were studied. A mean dose of 133.2 units Dysport, divided between 2 forearm muscles, was injected per session. A total of 124 injection sessions were performed during 1 year. Weakness was the most common adverse effect, reported during 72% of the follow-up visits. Scores on the Writer's Cramp Rating Scale were improved significantly after treatment. Pen movement speed also significantly increased.

Conclusion.—Quantifiable scales were used to determine the effects of botulinum toxin treatment in patients with writer's cramp. Botulinum toxin was found to induce significant improvements.

▶ This article will primarily interest physicians who treat patients with writer's cramp and other focal limb dystonias. It describes an instrument—the Writer's Cramp Rating Scale (WCRS)—for documenting the severity of abnormal posture and writing disability. The authors report the results of botulinum toxin injection in 31 patients with writer's cramp. In addition to the WCRS, they used subjective patient assessment of improvement and a computer-based measure of writing speed.

Injections were performed under electromyographic (EMG) guidance. It is not clear, however, whether muscle selection was based on IM EMG confirmation of the role of butulinum toxin in initiation of dystonic movement, as opposed to compensatory contraction. Regardless, the majority of patients reported subjective improvement. A significant correlation was found between WCRS and computer measurements. Interrater reliability, however, was low for a third of the WCRS subscales and moderate or substantial for the others. Revision of the WCRS to improve interrater reliability appears necessary before widespread acceptance.

Patients in this series who produced interconnected "l" letters at greater than 2 per second had the best subjective outcomes. Frequencies below 1 Hz predicted a poorer outcome. This observation deserves confirmation because it may assist in selection of patients for chemodenervation.

Note: The dosages reported in this article are for the European product Dysport. Botox, the preparation commonly used in the United States, is dispensed in units based on a different standard. Fewer units of Botox are required for equivalent potency.

C. Burgar, M.D.

Self-reported Carpal Tunnel Syndrome: Predictors of Work Disability From the National Health Interview Survey Occupational Health Supplement

Blanc PD, Faucett J, Kennedy JJ, et al (Univ of California, San Francisco)
Am J Ind Med 30:362–368, 1996 14–4

Introduction.—In recent years, carpal tunnel syndrome (CTS) has become a leading source of occupational illness. Most previous studies have focused on the diagnosis and prevention of CTS. However, little is known about how frequently CTS causes work disability and what the relevant risk factors are. Risk factors for work disability in patients with CTS were analyzed.

Methods.—The study used data from the 1988 Occupational Health Supplement to the National Health Interview Survey, a nationwide, population-based survey of public health. The respondents included 544 individuals with self-reported CTS and 32,688 without CTS. All participants in both groups were aged 18 to 64 years and had a history of participation in the labor force. Work disability was analyzed as a dependent variable, defined as cessation of work with no attributed cause or cessation of work or a job change attributed specifically to CTS. Ergonomic risk of work disability was analyzed as a dependent variable, defined according to the amount of repetitive hand and wrist bending at the participant's most recent job.

Results.—Eleven percent of the participants with CTS reported work disability attributed specifically to CTS. The corresponding national prevalence of CTS-related work disability was estimated at 240,578 individuals. Ergonomic risk at the participant's last job was a significant predictor of work disability, even after adjustment for sociodemographic factors and health status. The odds ratio for work disability was 1.7 per 120 minutes of daily exposure to repetitive hand or wrist bending.

Conclusions.—Work disability is common in individuals with CTS. Work disability may be predicted by ergonomic conditions on the job, specifically by repetitive hand and wrist bending. Although the findings can be generalized to the United States population, the limitations of the study must be acknowledged, particularly the reliance on case self-reporting.

▶ The title of this article, carefully read, speaks volumes. From this survey of a huge population (33,232), 544 individuals said that they had CTS. They answered yes to the question, "Do you have a condition called carpal tunnel syndrome?" Thus, they are self-reported: no physician diagnosis was required. Given this possibly overwhelming limitation (think about how many patients come to your office or clinic with any hand pain or numbness and ask, "Is this the carpal doctor?"), this study found that these 544 individuals also were more likely to view themselves as in fair/poor health than the non–self-reporting individuals with CTS and were 3 times more likely to state that they had other non-CTS musculoskeletal disorders.

Clearly, ergonomic demands may impair an individual's ability and motivation to work at the same job or to continue working at all, especially, as this study implies, when the job involves more than 3 hours per day of repetitive hand activity, here defined as occupational hand bending. Interestingly, nonwhite individuals who were self-reporters and said they had CTS had an increased likelihood of work stoppage by a factor of almost 3. Perhaps this is a unique cohort deserving of further study.

V.R. Hentz, M.D.

Reliability of the Manual Dynamic Mode of the Baltimore Therapeutic Equipment Work Simulator

Coleman EF, Renfro RR, Cetinok EM, et al (Spartan Motors Inc, Charlotte, Mich; TRW Space and Electronics Group, Redondo Beach, Calif; AK Enerji Electric Energy Auto Producer Group Inc, Istanbul, Turkey; et al)
J Hand Ther 9:223–237, 1996 14–5

Introduction.—The Baltimore Therapeutic Equipment Work Simulator (BTEWS) (Baltimore Therapeutic Equipment Co., Hanover, Md.) has been marketed for the assessment and treatment of upper extremity problems. It can operate in static mode, to provide maximum resistance for isotropic exercise, and in dynamic mode, to provide resisted isotonic exercise in either manual or automatic status. Although the BTEWS has proved reliable in the static mode, its reliability in the dynamic mode has been questioned. The reliability of the manual dynamic mode of the BTEWS was studied.

Methods.—Twelve different BTEWS units were each tested by repeated observations of exercise-head resistance in the manual dynamic mode using a previously described timed–weight-drop test. Fifty measurements were made at weight levels of 5–40 lb. Resistance was held consistent at 92% of the applied weight. Any change in weight-drop times between observations reflected a change in the resistance of the exercise head. Weight-drop time was evaluated as the sole dependent variable at each load level, within and between machines.

Results.—There was considerable variation in resistance between trials. Causes of variation in weight-drop times included failure of the weight to drop and times that were unrecognized by the electronic timing system. The measurable times varied from 0.75 to 16.97 sec. For 10 of the 12 units tested, weight-drop times exceeded ± 3 standard deviations (SD) from the mean. Eight units had times ± 4 SD from the mean, and 4 had times ± 5 SD from the mean. The printout provided by the units did not give an accurate indication of the resistance produced by the exercise head. The printout data suggested intermachine correlations of +1.0 to +0.9906. In contrast, correlations based on weight-drop times ranged from +0.9866 to −0.9956.

Conclusions.—The manual dynamic mode of the BTEWS does not provide constant weight-drop times for a constant externally supplied torque. The resistance readings are inconsistent, both within and between BTEWS units. The manual dynamic mode of this device should not be used for clinical assessments that require consistent resistance. Patients should be monitored closely when the manual dynamic mode is used for exercise sessions. Use of the BTEWS should be discontinued if increased inflammation, decreased sensation, or increased pain is noted.

► It is becoming more and more apparent. Our system of health care delivery is becoming increasingly scrutinized. The demands on us as health care practitioners have changed immensely in this past decade. No longer are we able to administer treatment or assessment as we once did—we are called to objectively substantiate that which we deem necessary for our injured or disabled patients, based on an accurate evaluation. Our tools used in assessment must be both reliable and valid. This scientific article by Coleman et al. examines 1 of the instruments more commonly used in a hand therapy clinic for assessment, the BTEWS. This is often used for upper quadrant strengthening, functional capacity evaluations, work simulation, and work-hardening evaluations.

The purpose of this study was to assess the manual dynamic mode calibration of 13 BTEWS units by using a timed–weight-drop test to determine the consistency of resistance produced by the exercise head. First, F-tolerance metal weights were suspended from a wire wrapped around a 12-inch diameter pulley that was attached to the simulator exercise shaft. Then the pulley was locked into position with a slide bolt to prevent pretest rotation. The elapsed time for the weight to rotate the cylinder through 1 complete revolution was timed using a Brower Speedtrap II timing system (Brower Timing Systems, Draper, Utah). This uses a infrared beam trigger and a receiver timer that is certified accurate to 1/100 of a second. Fifty weight-drop trials at 5, 10, 20, 30, and 40 lb were each individually timed. Before each weight-level change, resistance was reset at 92% of the suspended weight to be used in the series of 50 weight drops. The variations in weight-drop times were used as an indication of changes in the resistance produced by the exercise head. Of 13 BTEWSs, 1 unit was untestable at all weight levels because of strong static resistance and not used for this study.

Results showed a large variation in the manual dynamic mode in all 24 machines, with weight-drop times fluctuating from 0.75 to 16.97 sec at all given resistances. The resistance fluctuations with machines seemed to be random. When comparing intersimulator total performance, it was found that the console printout data generated by the simulators did not accurately reflect the actual resistance produced by the exercise head. Also, if the end test button was activated during the dynamic mode, all weights would come to an abrupt halt.

In summary, this study found that the resistance produced by the manual dynamic mode was inconsistent both within and between simulators. Serious doubts are raised regarding the reliability of the dynamic mode if used in clinical assessments. The authors state that the method described by the manufacturer as a dynamic test is actually a measurement of static torque applied in a dynamic mode.

This study is valuable because we must conclude that patients for whom the BTEWS is used for assessment or for treatment must be carefully selected to avoid adverse reactions. Is it possible that the resistance variations in the dynamic mode may detrimentally affect those whose injuries have not yet attained mature tensile strength, those with unstable joints, where sensation is compromised or where an inflammatory state exists? Each patient session must be screened and monitored.

K. Colbert, O.T.R., C.H.T.

The Hand Therapy Certification Examination: Results of the First Five Years

Roth LP, Kasch MC, Fullenwider L, et al (Professional Examination Service, New York; Hand Rehabilitation Ctr of Sacramento, Calif; Eastside Hand Rehabilitation, Kirkland, Wash; et al)

J Hand Ther 9:213–217, 1996 14–6

Background.—The Hand Therapy Certification Commission (HTCC), established in 1989, was founded to test and recognize the knowledge and skills of occupational and physical therapists specializing in upper-extremity rehabilitation through certification and recertification. The results of the first 5 years were reported.

Results.—The Hand Therapy Certification Examination (HTCE) has now been given 5 times, taken by 3,252 candidates. A total of 2,211 have

TABLE 1.—Percentages of Candidates Reporting Association Memberships

	1991 (%)	1992 (%)	1993 (%)	1994 (%)	1995 (%)	1991–95 (%)
AOTA	79.8	50.4	66.0	61.0	53.8	62.2
APTA	9.7	7.4	6.4	8.2	8.8	8.1
ASHT	23.4	13.4	29.2	35.9	44.1	29.2
AAHS	*	*	2.6	3.9	3.4	3.3
State OT/PT association or chapter	*	*	51.7	56.9	55.6	54.7

*These data not collected for the year cited.

Abbreviations: AOTA, American Occupational Therapy Association; *APTA*, American Physical Therapy Association; *ASHT*, American Society of Hand Therapists; *AAHS*, American Association of Hand Surgeons; *OT*, occupational therapy; *PT*, physical therapy.

(Courtesy of Roth LP, Kasch MC, Fullenwider L, et al: The Hand Therapy Certification Examination: Results of the first five years. *J Hand Ther* 9:213–217, 1996.)

TABLE 2.—Percentages of Candidates Working in Particular Facility Types

	1991 (%)	1992 (%)	1993 (%)	1994 (%)	1995 (%)	1991–95 (%)
Inpatient or outpatient hospital-based treatment	38.2	46.9	45.5	48.8	49.4	45.8
Therapist-owned practice	33.9	27.8	25.3	22.6	24.8	26.9
Physician-owned practice	17.4	12.9	14.1	11.7	7.4	12.7
Corporate-owned practice	*	*	10.0	13.6	15.0	12.9
Other	9.6	12.4	5.1	3.4	3.4	6.9

*These data not collected for the year cited.

(Courtesy of Roth LP, Kasch MC, Fullenwider L, et al: The Hand Therapy Certification Examination: Results of the first five years. *J Hand Ther* 9:213–217, 1996.)

TABLE 3.—Candidate Job Titles

	1993 (%)	1994 (%)	1995 (%)
Staff therapist	44.3	49.5	47.8
Senior therapist	21.4	19.6	20.3
Clinic supervisor	9.5	11.2	10.4
Department supervisor	12.1	11.4	10.6
Facility supervisor	4.4	3.9	5.8
Educator	1.0	0.2	0.4
Researcher	0.5	0.2	0.0
Student	0.0	0.0	0.0
Other	7.2	3.9	4.8

(Courtesy of Roth LP, Kasch MC, Fullenwider L, et al: The Hand Therapy Certification Examination: Results of the first five years. *J Hand Ther* 9:213–217, 1996.)

TABLE 4.—Candidate Years of Occupational or Physical Therapy Licensure/Certification

	1991 (%)	1992 (%)		1993 (%)	1994 (%)	1995 (%)
Licensed in 1975 or earlier	23.0	13.1	Licensed 21 years or more	3.1	5.5	7.2
Licensed in 1976–1980	33.6	23.7	Licensed 14–20 years	15.5	18.5	19.2
Licensed in 1981–1986	43.5	49.2	Licensed 8–13 years	34.3	31.5	28.8
Licensed in 1987 or later	0	14.0	Licensed 5–7 years	47.2	44.5	44.7

(Courtesy of Roth LP, Kasch MC, Fullenwider L, et al: The Hand Therapy Certification Examination: Results of the first five years. *J Hand Ther* 9:213–217, 1996.)

become certified hand therapists (CHTs). Demographic data indicate that the candidates belonged to a variety of associations (Table 1) and worked in numerous treatment settings (Table 2). About half were working as staff therapists (Table 3). During the 5 years of testing, candidates have reported decreasing amounts of experience (Table 4). The number of candidates with upper-extremity caseloads for 6 years or less also declined (Table 5). The examination has performed reliably. Mean scores have declined annually between 1991 and 1995.

Conclusions.—In general, the results of the first 5 years of the HTCE administration have been very good.

▶ The definition of hand therapy seems to have become quite complex over the last 5–10 years. Changes in the health care industry associated with managed care have further complicated the role of the therapist. The HTCC and Professional Examination Services have established objective testing criteria for the designation of a physical or occupational therapist who specializes in the field of upper-extremity rehabilitation as a CHT. These objective standards give referring physicians and their patients a more accurate accounting as to the knowledge and expertise of accredited therapists. The accreditation "CHT" is a valuable reference in indicating a particular level of specialized education and experience, much as the "CPA" is to the accounting industry or the "CLU" is to the insurance industry. Because the designation of CHT is valuable in the industry, the criteria for attaining and maintaining the designation are constantly evolving. This article provides

TABLE 5.—Percentages of Candidates Who Have Maintained Caseloads of 50% or More Upper-extremity Patients

	1991 (%)	1992 (%)		1993 (%)	1994 (%)	1995 (%)
			1–2 years	11.2	11.2	8.4
5 years or less	34.9	51.7	3–4 years	37.0	33.7	32.1
			5–6 years	32.9	26.6	34.7
6 to 10 years	44.7	39.4	7–10 years	18.6	18.9	16.1
11 years or more	19.2	16.4	11 years or more	0.0	9.6	8.8

(Courtesy of Roth LP, Kasch MC, Fullenwider L, et al: The Hand Therapy Certification Examination: Results of the first five years. *J Hand Ther* 9:213–217, 1996.)

valuable insight regarding the creation and evolution of the standards required to acquire the CHT designation. The article provides strictly objective information. It is insightful and I recommend it to those interested in gaining a deeper understanding of the testing and certification process required for becoming a CHT.

C. Gordon, O.T.R., C.H.T.

Upper Extremity Angular Kinematics of the One-handed Backhand Drive in Tennis Players With and Without Tennis Elbow

Knudson D, Blackwell J (Baylor Univ, Waco, Tex; Univ of San Francisco, Calif)

Int J Sports Med 18:79–82, 1997 14–7

Introduction.—The term tennis elbow (TE) is used to describe medial and lateral elbow pain caused by a variety of activities. A more limited definition of TE is lateral epicondylitis, an overuse injury of the extensor carpi radialis brevis that develops in up to 50% of tennis players. Affected players often have a 1-handed backhand. Three groups of tennis players participated in a study of wrist and elbow angular kinematics and impact acceleration of the racket during 1-handed backhand execution.

Methods.—Sixteen men with a mean age of 35 years took part in the study. All were right-handed and normally used a 1-handed backhand. Five were tennis professionals with no history of TE (PRO group), 6 were intermediates with no history of TE (−TE group), and 5 were intermediates with a history of medically confirmed TE (+TE group). Using an instrumented racket, and with additional measurement devices placed on their racket arm, the players were instructed to execute 1-handed backhands down the center of an indoor court. Tennis balls were projected from a machine at a frequency and speed similar to those of a baseline rally. The first 10 strokes with central impacts were analyzed for angular kinematics and racket acceleration at impact.

Results.—All players used correct technique, with the elbow almost completely extended during the stroke. The 3 groups did not differ significantly in the mean impulse after impact or in the mean elbow angular position or velocity after impact. There was a significant difference, however, between the PRO group and the +TE group in mean wrist angular velocity after impact (−4.04 rad/sec of extension vs. 0.42 rad/sec of flexion, respectively).

Conclusion.—In this group of professional and intermediate tennis players, all had correct 1-handed backhand technique at the elbow. But whereas the PRO and −TE players maintained concentric action of the wrist extensor muscles after impact, the +TE players tended to have eccentric muscle actions of the wrist extensors after impact.

▶ The authors provide data that support existing data in the literature suggesting that there may, indeed, be altered biomechanics in patients predisposed to TE. A small number of tennis players who have had TE, players who have not, and professional tennis players were compared. It was found that in the normal 1-handed backstroke, a professional tennis player is in the process of extending the wrist at the point of ball impact and continues to do so immediately thereafter. Patients who have a history of tennis elbow experienced wrist flexion immediately after ball impact, which caused eccentric loading of the common extensor group. Whether this is cause or effect is unknown. However, a group of amateur players who did not have a history of tennis elbow did not have the same biomechanics. There could be a causal role. However, it is also possible that this is an adaptive response in players who have had a problem in the past.

S.W. O'Driscoll, M.D.

Suggested Reading

Fleisig GS, Barrentine SW, Escamilla RF, et al: Biomechanics of overhand throwing with implications for injuries. *Sports Med* 21:421–437, 1996.

▶ This article summarizes the chain of kinematic events (position and motion) of the arm and the rest of the body associated with overhand throwing. Joint and muscle forces associated with throwing are also mentioned, though cursorily. Relationships between these events and pathophysiological consequences at the elbow (e.g., overstress in the ulnar collateral ligament, spur formation) and shoulder (rotator cuff tears, entrapment of the labral) with overuse are reviewed. Unfortunately, the scientific basis for these associations is weak, consistent with the conclusion of the article. Thus, no new insights into treatment and rehabilitation are really presented, though the authors do state, rightfully so, that knowledge of the biomechanics of throwing should help coaches to teach proper technique and clinicians to deliver optimal treatment.

F.M. Zajac, Ph.D.

Giacobetti FB, Sharkey PF, Bos-Giacobetti MA, et al: Biomechanical analysis of the effectiveness of in-line skating wrist guards for preventing wrist fractures. *Am J Sports Med* 25:223–225, 1997.

▶ Wrist guards may prevent scrapes but probably do not materially increase the force needed to break a wrist.

P.C. Amadio, M.D.

Necking LE, Lundström R, Dahlin LB, et al: Tissue displacement is a causative factor in vibration-induced muscle injury. *J Hand Surg (Br)* 21B:753–757, 1996.

▶ The study has little relevance to the worker using vibrating tools. The 2-day only exposure for the rats with constant vibration for 5 hours is an inappropriate model for study. The human factory worker would not be exposed to 5 hours of constant vibration. To translate the 5 hours over 2 days in a rat muscle to a human muscle is an ill-advised correlation.

M.L. Kasdan, M.D.

Rennie HJ: Evaluation of the effectiveness of a metacarpophalangeal ulnar deviation orthosis. *J Hand Ther* 9:371–377, 1996.

▶ It is a beautiful split. Unfortunately, this study shows it makes no impact on function or pain.

K.A. Bengtson, M.D.

Stiens SA, Haselkorn JK, Peters DJ, et al: Rehabilitation intervention for patients with upper extremity dysfunction: Challenges of outcome evaluation. *Am J Ind Med* 29:590–601, 1996.

▶ This article provides an excellent overview on rehabilitation intervention for patients with upper extremity dysfunction with the perspectives of impairments, disabilities, and handicaps for each patient. Understanding the dysfunctions and their impact on each individual is critical to develop an intervention program to help that person. Key points in outcome measures and research have also been nicely pointed out in this paper.

P. Wu, M.D.

Toth-Cohen S, Petralia PB, Miller KS: Therapists' experiences with computer-assisted instruction in hand therapy. *J Hand Ther* 10:41–45, 1997.

▶ Computer technology for self-study and continuing education will become increasingly more important as managed care and low reimbursement for hand therapy services cause a decrease in funding for continuing education. This year the American Society of Hand Therapists has canceled all continuing education courses because of poor attendance, the direct result of funding cuts for continuing education with hospitals and clinics across the country. The ASHT is developing an internet presence that will facilitate a new venue for education, but the problems of maintaining the continuing education units required by the Hand Therapy Certification Commission may not be solved by this mode of instruction. Alternate methods of instruction will need to address this issue.

R.B. Evans, O.T.R./L., C.H.T.

15 Microsurgery

Replantation of Ring Avulsion of Index, Long, and Ring Fingers

Tseng OF-Y, Tsai Y-C, Wei F-C, et al (Shin Kong Wu Ho-Su Mem Hosp, Taipei, Taiwan; Chang-Gung Mem Hosp, Lin Kou, Taiwan; Emory Univ, Atlanta, Ga)

Ann Plast Surg 36:625–628, 1996 15–1

Objective.—Ring avulsion injuries can range from simple circumferential tearing of the skin to denuding of a finger to complete amputation of the finger. Reports suggest that only about 50% of degloved finger amputations are successfully salvaged. Successful replantation was done in 1 case of a patient with complete degloving of the index, middle, and ring fingers.

Case Report.—Man, 23, had complete degloving amputation of the index, middle, and ring fingers of his left hand in a roller machine accident. The finger joints were preserved, including the bony framework, tendons, and pulleys, but the neurovascular bundles were avulsed. Replantation surgery was done 12 hours after the accident. Sensation was maintained by anastomosing the proximal stump of the neurovascular bundle on the ulnar side to the distal stump of the radial side. After anastomosis of 2 arteries and 2 dorsal veins, the skin was loosely closed, with a porcine skin graft covering the remaining skin defect. The patient received Dextran-40 infusion for 1 week in the hope of enhancing microcirculation.

Additional débridements and skin grafts were required on the severely crushed middle finger. Osteomyelitis of the distal phalanx of this digit ultimately necessitated amputation of the distal phalanx. The patient returned to work after 6 months of rehabilitation. Surgical release and coverage with a first web space flap was required for flexion contracture of the proximal interphalangeal joint of the left middle finger. At 18 months, the patient had nearly complete range of motion of the fingers and about 80% power grasp. He had intact light touch sensation of the index and ring fingers, although only protective sensation of the middle finger. The aesthetic results were good.

Discussion.—Good results were reported with a 3-finger replantation after a degloving amputation in a laborer. Good motion and strength were maintained, and sensation was preserved by transpositional digital nerve transfers. The aesthetic results of this technique are superior to those of other reconstruction methods.

▶ This report describes a functional result after treatment of a 3-finger degloving injury with replantation and a secondary flap for contracture. The result is an example of how aggressive replantation and sophisticated secondary surgery can be successfully applied to an injury usually defined as irreparable.

W.L. Lineaweaver, M.D.

Clinical Outcome of Digital Replantation Using the Fibrin Glue-assisted Microvascular Anastomosis Technique

Isogai N, Cooley BC, Kamiishi H (Kinki Univ, Osaka, Japan; Med College of Wisconsin, Milwaukee)

J Hand Surg (Br) 21B:573–575, 1996 15–2

Background.—Once the decision has been made to replant an amputated extremity, restoration of blood flow is the immediate objective. The time needed for replantation becomes a major factor in patients with multiple-digit amputations. A number of techniques have been suggested to shorten the time needed for replantation, specifically for faster microvascular anastomoses. Putting fibrin glue around the anastomosis may reduce the number of microsutures required, thus shortening repair time. An experience with fibrin glue around microvascular anastomoses during digital replantation surgery was reviewed.

Methods.—The experience included 36 finger replantations in 21 patients during a 4-year period. There were 14 single-digit and 7 multiple-digit replantations. All replantations were done by a standardized technique. Vascular anastomoses were usually done with 4 sutures in the arteries and veins distal to the distal interphalangeal joint and 6 sutures in vessels proximal to this site. After completion of each anastomosis, fibrin glue was applied. Ten seconds later, the microvascular clamps were released to permit blood flow. All patients received continuous IV infusion of urokinase and PGE for 10 days after surgery.

Results.—Thirty-two of the 36 digits survived with satisfactory functional outcomes. This was comparable to the results reported with conventional microvascular anastomosis. All 4 failed replantations involved crushed or avulsed digits. It took an average of 3.2 hours to replant each digit, compared with 4.5 hours with conventional anastomosis.

Conclusions.—Topical application of fibrin glue can assist microvascular anastomosis in replanted digits. The use of fibrin glue shortens operative time by reducing the number of microsutures required. There are no adverse effects on replant outcome.

▶ The authors show that the use of fibrin glue does not alter survival rates in digital replantation, and it shortens operative times. Unfortunately, in the United States, at least at this time, there are no commercially available products for this purpose. The blood bank can take a measure of an individual patient's blood and manufacture a fibrin-fibrinogen extract that can be mixed with thrombin at the correct time, but this is probably not practical in replant circumstances.

V.R. Hentz, M.D.

Two-stage Toe-to-thumb Reconstruction in Pollicized Second Metacarpal and Useless Fingers

Sastre N, Caravantes MI, Mayoral-Garcia C (Universidad Nacional Autonoma de Mexico)

J Reconstr Microsurg 12:431–437, 1996 15–3

Background.—A toe may be transplanted to the hand when the thumb is amputated near the metacarpophalangeal joint or with partial loss of the metacarpal, when second or third fingers are damaged at the proximal phalanx level, or when there are complicated defects of the second to fifth fingers or combinations of severe injury to the thumb, fingers, and hand. A patient was described in whom a toe was transplanted because 2 fingers had been lost, including the entire first ray.

> *Case Report.*—Farm worker, 25, sustained injuries to both hands from a cartridge powder explosion. Initial treatment at a rural hospital consisted of amputation of the complete first ray of the right hand at the metacarpal–trapezium joint. Every phalanx from the index finger and distal phalanges of the third and fourth fingers were resected. Seven months later, on referral, a 2-stage surgical reconstruction was planned. The initial stage consisted of transfer of the second metacarpal to the trapezium, creating the first web space, which was covered with skin from a reverse radial forearm flap. In the second stage, the right big toe was transferred to the hand with anastomoses of the first dorsal metatarsal artery to the radial artery (end-to-end) and the veins to the radial vena comitans and cephalic vein in the flap (reverse flow). Excellent functional and cosmetic outcomes resulted.

Conclusions.—This case report demonstrates that partial pollicization of a ray can be combined with a big toe transfer when no structure remains distal to the trapezium. The transfer provides stability, strength, and mobility to the new thumb. In addition, the radial forearm flap has great potential for covering large defects of the hand, is capable of being a useful vessel carrier, and is capable of receiving a second transferred structure through microsurgical anastomoses.

▶ The authors show that a reversed, pedicled radial forearm flap can be used as a source of recipient vessels for a microsurgical flap. The recipient vessels sustain flow that is reversed from their physiologic direction, but the vessels clearly sustained the flap. If this observation proves to be a general one, the radial forearm flap after transposition can serve as a donor site in complex hand reconstruction, which means that, in some cases, multiple free flaps and vein grafts would be unnecessary.

W.L. Lineaweaver, M.D.

Metacarpal Hand: Classification and Guidelines for Microsurgical Reconstruction With Toe Transfers

Wei F-C, El-Gammal TA, Lin C-H, et al (Chang Gung Mem Med College, Taipei, Taiwan; Chang Gung Mem Hosp, Taipei, Taiwan)

Plast Reconstr Surg 99:122–128, 1997 15–4

Background.—A hand that has lost its prehensile ability through amputation of all fingers, with or without the thumb, is called a *metacarpal hand.* A variety of microvascular toe transfer techniques can be performed to restore function. When deciding which procedure to use, the surgeon must consider the level of amputation of the fingers as well as the functional status of the remaining thumb. A classification scheme for the various patterns of the metacarpal hand and guidelines for selecting the proper toe transfer procedure were presented.

TABLE 1.—Type I Metacarpal Hand

Subtype	Level of Finger Amputation	Recommendations
IA	Distal to the metacarpophalangeal joint	1. Bilateral second toes for amputations distal to the web space. 2. Combined second and third toes for amputations proximal to the web space (transproximal phalanx transfer)
IB	Through the metacarpophalangeal joint with intact metacarpal articular surface	Combined second and third toes (composite joint transfer)
IC	Through the metacarpophalangeal joint with damaged metacarpal articular surface or transmetacarpal amputation	Combined second and third toes (transmetatarsal transfer)

(Courtesy of Wei F-C, El-Gammal TA, Lin C-H, et al: Metacarpal hand: Classification and guidelines for microsurgical reconstruction with toe transfers. *Plast Reconstr Surg* 99:122–128, 1997.)

TABLE 2.—Type II Metacarpal Hand

Subtype	Level of Thumb Amputation	Recommendations
IIA	Distal to the metacarpal neck	Whole or trimmed great toe transfer (transproximal phalanx transfer)
IIB	Proximal to the metacarpal neck with adequate thenar muscle function	1. Preliminary distraction lengthening or interpositional bone graft followed by whole or trimmed great toe transfer, or 2. Transmetatarsal second toe transfer
IIC	Any level with inadequate thenar musculature	1. Thumb reconstruction in a second stage following finger reconstruction, and 2. Tendon transfer to restore opposition
IID	Any level with damaged carpometacarpal joint	Same as in IIA and IIB, but aiming at reconstructing immobile thumb post

(Courtesy of Wei F-C, El-Gammal TA, Lin C-H, et al: Metacarpal hand: Classification and guidelines for microsurgical reconstruction with toe transfers. *Plast Reconstr Surg* 99:122–128, 1997.)

Classification and Guidelines.—Type I hands are characterized by the amputation of all fingers proximal to the middle of the proximal phalanx and an unaffected thumb or a thumb amputated distal to the interphalangeal joint. This type is further detailed and treatment recommendations are given in Table 1. Type II hands are characterized by the amputation of all fingers proximal to the middle of the proximal phalanx and thumb amputation proximal to the interphalangeal joint (Table 2).

Conclusions.—Metacarpal hands may be classified into 2 basic types: those requiring reconstruction of the fingers and those requiring reconstruction of the fingers and thumb. Further subclassification is based on amputation level and the functional status of the remaining thumb, including the adequacy of thenar musculature and the integrity of the first carpometacarpal joint. The choice of type and technique of toe transfer should be based on this classification.

▶ The authors use their wealth of experience to classify proximal finger and thumb amputations. They recommend different modifications of toe-to-hand transfers for different types of amputations (see Tables 1 and 2). They report details of 4 cases. Although the authors give lots of advice, they do not provide objective proof of enhanced function after the procedures they advocate. In 1 case of bilateral metacarpal hand, they borrowed 5 toes, causing considerable foot deformities. Still, their classification and guidelines make sense and provide us with a useful framework for treating patients with these devastating injuries.

M.A. James, M.D.

Results of Functioning Free Muscle Transplantation for Elbow Flexion

Chuang DC-C, Carver N, Wei F-C (Chang Gung Med College, Taipei, Taiwan)

J Hand Surg (Am) 21A:1071–1077, 1996 15–5

Introduction.—Functioning free muscle transfer (FFMT) may be used for muscle reconstruction when no musculotendinous donor units are available locally. Patients with brachial plexus injury need reconstruction of elbow flexion. There have been few reports of the use of FFMT for this purpose. A 6-year experience with FFMT for restoration of elbow flexion, using various nerves for reinnervation, was reported.

Methods.—The experience included 38 patients undergoing FFMT for reconstruction of elbow flexion, most because of brachial plexus injury in motorcycle accidents. Thirty-two patients had had paralysis for more than 1 year, and 26 had not been operated on previously. The gracilis muscle was transferred in 34 patients and the rectus femoris in 4. Reinnvervation was accomplished using the musculocutaneous nerve in 3 patients (who had traumatic biceps loss; group 1), the intercostal nerves in 31 patients (group 2), and the spinal accessory nerve in 4 patients (group 3). The Medical Research Council grading system was used to evaluate the results. Muscle strength of M4 was considered a successful result.

Results.—All 3 patients in group 1 had successful results within 1 year. In group 2, the success rate was 78% when 3 intercostal nerves were transferred. Complete rehabilitation took an average of 2 years. When 2 intercostal nerves were used, rehabilitation took 3 years, and the final muscle strength and range of motion were not as good. Muscle strength was no better than M2–M3 for the 4 patients in group 3, even after 3 years of rehabilitation (Table 1).

Conclusion.—For patients with traumatic biceps loss, a nerve-reinnervated FFMT provides better results than regional latissimus dorsi transfer. When the intercostal nerves are used for reconstruction after brachial plexus injury, it is best to use 3 nerves for reinnervation. The results are not as good when the spinal accessory nerve is used, probably because of the need for interposition grafts.

▶ Chuang et al. report on the outcome of reconstruction of elbow flexion in a large series of patients. There is a lot of practical information in this report, including several different reconstructive schemes, depending on the interval between plexus injury and injury. The idea of using intercostal nerve grafts to the musculocutaneous nerve and adding a free muscle graft, also innervated by other branches of the intercostal nerve, is a novel one.

The concept is that the free muscle transfer becomes innervated and begins working early, but that, as time goes by, the biceps-brachialis muscles also begin to function, providing ultimately greater elbow flexion power. Chuang believes that in more delayed cases, 3 intercostal nerve transfers are better than 2, with the third nerve undergoing direct implantation into the muscle. Krakauer and Wood,[1] in a smaller series of patients,

TABLE 1.—Reinnervating Nerve, Technique of Reconstruction With Functioning Free Muscle Transplantation to Restore Elbow Flexion, and Results

Group	*Reinnervating Nerve and Reconstructive Technique*	*No. of Patients (n = 38)*	*No. of Patients Achieving Muscle Strength of M4*
1. Traumatic biceps loss	Original MC nerve to FFMT for biceps replacement	3	3
2. Brachial plexus injury	3 IC nerves to FFMT for biceps replacement	19	14
	3 IC nerves to FFMT for biceps and FDP replacement	4	4
	2 IC nerves to FFMT for biceps replacement	5	4*
	2 IC nerves to FFMT for biceps enhancement plus 2 IC nerves to MC nerve	3	3
3. Brachial plexus injury	XI nerve to FFMT for biceps replacement	4	0†

*Muscle strength M4 but weaker than other techniques.
†Muscle strength M2+.
Abbreviations: FFMT, functioning free muscle transfer; *MC*, musculocutaneous; *IC*, intercostal; *XI*, spinal accessory; *FDP*, flexor digitorum profundus.
(Courtesy of Chuang DC-C, Carver N, Wei F-C: Results of functioning free muscle transplantation for elbow flexion. *J Hand Surg [Am]* 21A:1071–1077, 1996.)

found no difference between 2 and 3 intercostal nerves, but in their cases, only nerve-to-nerve repair was carried out.

V.R. Hentz, M.D.

Reference

1. Krakauer JD, Wood MB: Intercostal nerve transfer for brachial plexopathy. *J Hand Surg (Am)* 19:829–835, 1994.

The Quadrifoliate Flap: A Combination of Scapular, Parascapular, Latissimus Dorsi and Scapula Bone Flaps

Bakhach J, Peres JM, Scalise A, et al (Hópital du Tondu, Bordeaux, France)

Br J Plast Surg 49:477–481, 1996 15–6

Background.—The scapular area has become a popular donor site for flap acquisition. The use of a composite pedicled flap with 4 different units nourished by the same pedicle was described.

Case Report.—Man, 25, sustained a complete amputation of the left arm as a result of a motor vehicle accident. The limb root was crushed, with muscle and nerve tearing. After the arm wounds were healed, the patient was referred for stump lengthening. There was almost no stump, and at least 10 cm was needed to fit a prosthesis. Stump lengthening required vascularized bone, muscle padding, and a large area of skin cover for the arm circumference. The scapular area was the only possible donor site. A pedicled flap could be obtained because of the proximity of the stump to the donor site. The parascapular flap (30 × 13 cm), scapular flap (20 × 12 cm), lateral border of the scapula, and lateral border of the latissimus dorsi muscle were outlined. The multiple tissue flap was transferred to the arm stump, with the proximal edge of the bone flap inserted into the humerus diaphysis. The latissimus dorsi muscle, left attached to the humerus proximally, was rolled up to pad the end of the bone flap. The skin flaps were turned at least 180 degrees. The parascapular flap was wound around the arm, and the scapular flap was placed on the end of the stump. At the donor site, the teres major and minor muscles were re-inserted onto the scapula. The skin was sutured, and a central area was covered with a thin skin graft. After 2 weeks of immobilization, passive physiotherapy was begun. Active physiotherapy was initiated 6 weeks later. At 4 months, the bone was healed. A Z-plasty was then done to free the posterior axillary fold so that a definitive prosthesis could be used.

Conclusions.—The quadrifoliate flap used in this patient appears to be the only possible solution for a multiple tissue reconstruction of a short limb stump. This flap provides a bony framework, muscle padding, and 2 cutaneous flaps as covering.

► This case illustrates the application of anatomy to flap design for treatment of a multicomponent defect. The subscapular pedicle can be used to support a tissue complex including skin (scapular, parascapular), muscle (latissimus, serratus), and bone (scapula, rib), and these tissue combinations can be used regionally (as in this article) or as microvascular flap transplants.

W.L. Lineaweaver, M.D.

Free Flap Cover of Acute Burns and Post-burn Deformity

Barisoni D, Bortolani A, Sanna A, et al (Istituti Ospitalieri di Verona, Italy)

Eur J Plast Surg 19:257–261, 1996 15–7

Background.—Microsurgery in the treatment of acute burns and secondary deformities allows single-stage reconstruction with minimal patient discomfort. In postburn hand deformities, free tissue transfer provides an effective method of reconstruction. The outcomes of free tissue transfer in 1 series of patients with acute burns or postburn sequelae were described.

Methods and Findings.—Twenty-three patients underwent microsurgical procedures. Ten were treated for acute burns. In the hand and upper limb, the recipient vessels were the radial artery and nearby vein. Outcomes were satisfactory in 22 patients. Flap failure was caused by venous thrombosis in 1 patient with acute electrical burn of the left wrist. In the other 10 patients treated for postburn deformity, contracture release, functional recovery, and cosmetic outcomes were satisfactory at 1 year.

Conclusions.—The results achieved with a variety of microsurgical repairs of burn and postburn injuries are good. However, before using a free flap, surgeons must consider the techniques available, the patient's general health, the condition of the local wound, and the availability of a well-trained surgical staff.

► The authors present a series of burn wounds treated with microsurgical flap transplants. Their 96% success rate establishes the reliability of these procedures in these patients, and their application of this technique to hand injuries (11 cases) exemplifies the potential of aggressive salvage attempts of severe burns of the hand.

W.L. Lineaweaver, M.D.

The Clinical Reliability of Vein Grafts in Free-Flap Transfer

Germann G, Steinau H-U (BG-Trauma Hosp, Ludwigshafen, Germany; BG-Univ Hosp, Bochum, Germany)

J Reconstr Microsurg 12:11–17, 1996 15–8

Introduction.—The use of interposition vein grafts in microsurgery has been criticized for high complication and flap failure rates. One research group has recommended using vein grafts or arteriovenous (A-V) loops instead of microsurgical anastomoses in "high-risk" patients with posttraumatic vascular disease or radiation exposure. The results of venous micrografting in such high-risk patients were evaluated.

Methods.—The retrospective/prospective study included all vein grafts used in free-flap transfers over a 4-year period. Ninety-three vein grafts in 55 patients (mean age, 43 years) were evaluated. Thirty-seven patients had severe trauma to the extremities, 18 had had resection of soft-tissue cancer, and 7 had received regional cytostatic limb perfusion or irradiation. The grafts consisted of 52 arterioarterial and 41 venovenous grafts; 27 patients with critical vascular situations had an A-V loop created before free-flap transfer. Twenty patients underwent a 1-stage procedure in which the A-V loop was created immediately after débridement or tumor resection but before the flap was raised. End-to-end anastomoses were performed only in small arteries; the larger vessels, except for the greater saphenous vein, underwent end-to-side anastomoses.

Results.—The flap survival rate in this series was 96%. Eight patients required revision of the vein grafts. Five patients had arterial thrombosis and 4 had venous occlusion; 4 of these cases involved A-V loops. The results were similar in the retrospectively and prospectively studied patients. The limb salvage rate was 75%. The success rate, revision rate, and salvage rate were comparable to those of a series of flaps performed without vein grafting during the same period.

Conclusion.—Contrary to conventional thinking, vein grafts can be performed in free-flap transfers with no increase in the flap failure rate. Although the complication rate is somewhat higher, vein grafting can give good results with careful planning, meticulous monitoring, early revision, and knowledge of the technical dangers of the procedure. Vein grafts are particularly advantageous in vessels affected by posttraumatic vascular disease.

► In this series of 55 flap cases, use of vein grafts was associated with a higher rate of pedicle thrombosis when compared with flap cases without vein grafts (14% vs. 8.7%). Flap survival was ultimately the same in flaps with grafts as in flaps without grafts. The flap survival rate in this series is encouraging when compared with other series that have reported increased failure rates in flaps with vein grafts. The high thrombosis rate, however, still indicates that use of vein grafts is associated with significant complications.

W.L. Lineaweaver, M.D.

Antithrombotic Potencies of Enoxaparin in Microvascular Surgery: Influence of Dose and Adminstration Methods on Patency Rate of Crushed Arterial Anastomoses

Korompilias AV, Chen L-E, Seaber AV, et al (Duke Univ, Durham, NC)

J Hand Surg (Am) 22A:540–546, 1997 15–9

Introduction.—Anastomotic thrombosis remains a major problem among patients undergoing microvascular surgery, particularly when crush and avulsion injuries are involved. A number of experimental studies have used anticoagulants to prevent thrombus formation in this setting, but results are inconclusive. Investigators used a rat model of microvascular thrombosis to evaluate the influence of dose and administration methods of enoxaparin on patency at the anastomosis site in crushed femoral arteries.

Methods.—After anastomosis of the crushed vessels using a standard microsurgical technique, the rats were allowed to recover from the anesthesia. The arteries were divided into 5 groups of 20 vessels each according to the dosage and administration method of enoxaparin, a low–molecular-weight heparin. Group 1 received systemic enoxaparin alone (45 IU) twice a day for 3 days. Groups 2 and 3 received topical irrigation with a lower (15 IU/mL) and a higher (45 IU/mL) concentration of enoxaparin, respectively. Group 4 animals were treated with systemic and topical application at a dose of 15 IU and a concentration of 15 IU/mL. Group 5 received both systemic and topical treatment at the higher dose (45 IU) and concentration (45 IU/mL).

Results.—Two animals from group 4 died for unknown reasons at day 4. All vessels were patent immediately after anastomosis. Day 1 patency rates for groups 1 through 5 were 5%, 35%, 60%, 60%, and 70%, respectively. Day 7 patency rates were similar: 5%, 35%, 60%, 62.5%, and 75%, respectively. When compared with group 1, the patency rates in groups 2 through 5 were significantly higher at both day 1 and day 7.

Discussion.—The systemic administration of enoxaparin did not prevent thrombus formation after anastomosis in this rat model of crushed femoral arteries. Topical application of the agent was effective, however, in preventing thrombus formation. No additional advantages were gained when systemic enoxaparin was added to topical irrigation. The concentration of 45 IU/mL (3 times the dose recommended for clinical systemic use adjusted by body weight) was most effective.

► I enjoyed reading and studying this research article from the orthopedic research laboratories at Duke University. The authors concluded that in a rat femoral artery crush model, topical administration of enoxaparin at 45 IU/mL within and about the vessel during anastomosis results in effective antithrombotic action. Enoxaparin is a heparin salt derivative. The study provides excellent histologic follow-up of the damaged vessels. Statistical significance was achieved at 3 times the recommended topical dose in preventing thrombosis.

I am not sure how this experimental model can be helpful to the practicing clinician. First of all, no one in microsurgery would consider doing an anastomosis within the field of injury of a crushed vessel. I believe everyone agrees that we would not use damaged vessels and would go instead to vein graft techniques. Secondly, it would have been very beneficial to have compared this heparin derivative topically with topical heparin in the usual dose of irrigation, which, in our practice, is 10 units of heparin/mL of normal saline.

We will continue in our microsurgery practice to use topical heparin irrigation without systemic anticoagulation in elective and urgent microsurgical procedures. Enoxaparin (Lovenox) is approximately 8 times the cost of heparin when dose potencies are equilibrated. In this day of cost-effective medical practice, I am not convinced by this article that this product is any better than topical irrigation with heparin. The article will not change my current practice.

N.B. Meland, M.D.

Heat-induced Tissue Fusion for Microvascular Anastomosis

Cooley BC (Med College of Wisconsin, Milwaukee)

Microsurgery 17:198–208, 1996 15–10

Introduction.—Use of the carbon dioxide laser has been advocated as a means of creating a faster anastomosis during the welding of small vessels. Because heat appears to be the final pathway for effecting the weld, another form of heat delivery might also be successful in creating functional microvascular welds. This hypothesis was tested in a comparison of laser tissue welding and bipolar coagulator-generated heat application.

Methods.—The 2 methods of heat-induced welding were examined in rat microarterial anastomoses. Femoral arteries were anastomosed with 3 triangulated stay sutures, then treated with either carbon dioxide laser welding or bipolar coagulator welding. In control anastomoses, 9 stitches were placed around the circumference of the repair, and there was no treatment with either laser or bipolar coagulation. Vessels were evaluated with a standard empty-and-refill patency test at periods ranging from 10 minutes to 84 days postoperatively.

Results.—The control anastomoses that received no heat treatment had a patency rate of 100% when evaluated at 1 or more days postoperatively. For vessels treated with 0.1-second laser pulses, the patency rate at 1 or more days postoperatively was 90%. The patency rate for laser-welded vessels did not differ significantly from that of controls or of coagulator-welded anastomoses (88%). Both laser- and coagulator-treated vessels had higher rates of pseudoaneurysm than control vessels (9% and 14% vs. 0%, respectively), but the difference was not significant. A large percentage of laser-assisted anastomoses required extra laser application when the initial weld ruptured upon reflow. The pattern of healing was similar among control, laser-treated, and coagulator-treated anastomoses.

Discussion.—Laser-assisted microvascular anastomosis is, at best, equal to standard microvascular repair and is not superior to the crude weld formation from heat generated by a bipolar coagulator. A critical factor in the success of microvascular laser welding is precision in laser energy delivery, but the precision achieved with a carbon dioxide laser demonstrated no advantage in microvascular tissue welding.

▶ Dr. Cooley has proven what I have thought all along, i.e., that carbon dioxide laser microvascular coaptation is not applicable to the practice of clinical microvascular surgery. In his article, he concludes, and I agree wholeheartedly, that it is not time saving, it is not cost effective, and that the coaptation between the vessel and the skin leads to thrombosis and microaneurysm difficulties. It is a nicely planned study, I enjoyed reading it, and I agree wholeheartedly with his conclusions.

N.B. Meland, M.D.

Use of Distal Arteries for Microvascular Reconstruction in Forearm and Hand Surgery

Ge X-Z, Huang G-K (Lianyungang First People's Hosp, China; Shanghai First People's Hosp, China)

Microsurgery 17:180–183, 1996 15–11

Introduction.—To correct an arterial deficiency in hand surgery, the most common method is use of vein or arterial grafts. For revascularization of an extremity or for replantation or as a recipient site artery for a free tissue transfer, a method has been recently used that involves division of one of the forearm arteries and use of distal vessels. This technique was used on 3 vascularized bone grafts, 3 toe-to-hand transfers, 1 free cutaneous flap, 1 brachial artery reconstruction, and 1 replantation of an amputated palm.

Methods.—Nine patients had one of 3 techniques used with distal arteries for microsurgical reconstruction in forearm and hand surgery. There were 3 women and 6 men ranging in age from 20 to 30 years. The 3 techniques involved distal-based supply from the deep branch of the radial artery; proximal reversal of the radial artery; and distal-based supply from the ulnar artery.

Cases.—There were 2 pathologic metacarpal fractures from enchondromas, 2 patients with amputations of the thumb resulting from electric saw injuries, 2 with a 4-digit amputation, 1 with a loss of forearm skin and underlying flexor tendons in an explosion, 1 open humerus fracture, 1 pathologic fracture of the humeral shaft from metastatic thyroid cancer, and 1 avulsion amputation of the palm. The distal-based supply from the deep branch of the radial artery was used for toe-to-hand transfer for reconstruction of the thumb or index finger and for vascularized iliac crest bone graft to a metacarpal bone defect. The proximal reversal of the radial artery was used for a reconstruction of a cutaneous defect of the forearm with an anterolateral thoracic flap, a reconstruction of the brachial artery, and a vascularized fibular free tissue transfer.

Conclusion.—A number of advantages are reported with this technique, including the elimination of the need for vein grafts, the requirement of a single arterial microvascular anastomoses, minimization of microvascular size discrepancies, preparation of the distal artery in the same operative field as the rest of the reconstruction, and enablement of an undamaged artery to be brought into a zone of trauma and used as a recipient vessel. The disadvantage of this technique is that it sacrifices some of the collateral circulation to the hand. The blood supply to the hand must be checked before surgery.

▶ The authors have presented a short article on ideas to avoid vein grafting in hand surgery for microsurgical reconstruction by dividing major arteries to the hand and to the forearm, dissecting these arteries, and reversing them to provide access for microvascular reconstruction. This resulted in division of the radial artery at the wrist, and transposing it distally for an index finger revascularization and transposing an entire radial artery to replace a pulse to the brachial artery. I believe that this article should be included in the YEAR BOOK OF HAND SURGERY simply because I totally disagree with the author's presumption and technique in doing this. I do not feel that it has been shown that vein grafts are a hinderance in traumatic hand surgery, and I think the sacrifice in a traumatized extremity of an artery to facilitate microvascular access, instead of using a vein graft, is not warranted and could lead to further problems of ischemia. I, therefore, respectfully disagree with the authors' ideas and feel that the hand surgeon would have better results using vein grafts instead of transposed intact arteries.

N.B. Meland, M.D.

Suggested Reading

Becker HJ, Lassner F, Dagtekin FZ, et al: Morphometric changes in free neurovascular latissimus dorsi flaps: An experimental study. *Microsurgery* 16:786–792, 1995.

▶ In spite of the fact that in the introduction the authors speak of the necessity to have a similarity of muscle fiber typology between the transferred muscle and the muscle to be replaced in case of free neurovascular muscle transfer, they have not chosen an experimental model to explore this subject.

The observation of the fiber type grouping in the histologic analysis of the reinnervated latissimus dorsi muscle is not a new phenomenon. Fiber type grouping is nearly always observed during the early period after muscle reinnervation.

Some other studies of interest, not cited in this article, have already been published.[1–4]

M. Chammas, M.D., Ph.D.

References

1. Donovan CM, Faulkner JA: Plasticity of skeletal muscle: Regenerating fibers adapt more rapidly than surviving fibers. *J Appl Physiol* 62:2507–2511, 1987.

2. Guelinckx PJ, Carlson BM, Faulkner JA: Morphologic characteristics of muscles grafted in rabbits with neurovascular repair. *J Reconstr Microsurg* 8:481–489, 1992.
3. Kuzon WM, Rosenblatt JR, Pynn BR, et al: Fiber type morphometry and capillary geometry in free, vascularised muscle transfer. *Microsurgery* 12:352–360, 1991.
4. Terzis JK, Sweet RC, Dykes RW, et al: Recovery of function in free muscle transplants using microneurovascular anastomoses. *J Hand Surg (Am)* 3A:37–59, 1978.

Chang LD, Buncke G, Slezak S, et al: Cigarette smoking, plastic surgery, and microsurgery. *J Reconstr Microsurgery* 12:467–474, 1996.

▶ This is a very comprehensive review article about the effects of smoking, adverse or otherwise, on the outcome of microvascular and non-microvascular reconstructive procedures. The take-home message is that cutaneous flaps fare poorly in smokers and replants fail but microvascular free tissue transfers, especially muscle flaps, can be successful.

V.R. Hentz, M.D.

Chu N-S: Recovery of finger sensibility and somatosensory evoked potentials following digit-to-digit replantation in man. *Scand J Rehab Med* 28:125–131, 1996.

▶ This is the first study of changes in somatosensory evoked potentials using a replanted finger as the model. Replantation avoids problems such as crossover from other non-injured nerve territories. The authors equate the absence of specific corticol responses to alterations of function such as reduced vibratory sense. This is an interesting approach to analyzing outcome following nerve injury.

V.R. Hentz, M.D.

Kind GM, Buncke GM, Buncke HJ: Foreign-body sensation following 3M coupler use in the hand. *Ann Plast Surg* 37:418–421, 1996.

▶ The authors report on having to remove the 3M anastomotic coupler device in 2 patients who experienced discomfort because the device was palpable in the dorsum of the hand. Could not these rings be made of biodegradable materials?

V.R. Hentz, M.D.

Yilmaz M, Menderes A, Karataş Ö, et al: Free arterialised venous forearm flaps for limb reconstruction. *Br J Plast Surg* 49:396–400, 1996.

▶ This paper describes the use of large arterial venous flaps based on the forearm venous system. Four of the 5 flaps survived completely and the other resulted in a 30% loss of the flap. No anti-coagulation was used and the thin flaps that were produced were excellent reconstructive options for the particular problems that were addressed. The discussion offers a brief theoretical basis for the success of these flaps. The utility of these flaps seems somewhat limited as the thickness is not that different from that of a radial forearm flap. However, there do appear to be instances where these would be useful solutions for specific wound healing problems. Overall, this is a technical article with a small series of patients who did relatively well following the use of arterialized venous flap reconstruction for problem wounds. However, nothing really new is presented and no anatomic studies have been done to validate the concept as superior to standard arterial free flaps.

S.M. Shenaq, M.D.

16 Vascular and Dystrophic Disorders and Infection

Reflex Sympathetic Dystrophy Treated With Gabapentin

Mellick GA, Mellick LB (Loma Linda Univ, Calif; American Pain Specialists, Inc, Elyria, Ohio)

Arch Phys Med Rehabil 78:98–105, 1997 16–1

Objective.—Reflex sympathetic dystrophy (RSD), characterized by severe burning pain, hyperpathia, allodynia, vasomotor and sudomotor changes, edema, stiffness, and discoloration, usually begins about 3 months after injury and progresses to atrophy about 6 months after injury. Six case reports of improvement of RDS after using gabapentin, an anticonvulsant, were presented.

Case 1.—Woman, 52, with right arm RSD after falling, had pain that was untreatable with nerve blocks, electrical nerve stimulation, physical and occupational therapy, and various analgesics and nonsteroidal anti-inflammatory drugs (NSAIDs). After 1 month of gabapentin therapy, color and texture of her skin had normalized, she had regained the use of her middle finger, and her grasp was stronger and pain free.

Case 2.—Woman, 43, with left arm RSD after falling and dislocating her elbow, had severe RSD pain, swelling, and sensation problems even after nerve blocks. Treatment with gabapentin reduced her pain and normalized her skin temperature.

Case 3.—Woman, 57, had posterior tibial nerve entrapment causing unrelieved RSD pain in her right foot, leg, and back. Gabapentin therapy provided good pain relief.

Case 4.—Woman, 45, had bilateral RSD leg pain, swelling, stiffness, and discoloration after a fall. She began having burning back spasms. After 1 week on gabapentin, her pain was reduced by 75%.

Case 5.—Woman with right arm RSD after a fall had severe arm pain that also involved her shoulder, rib cage, and neck, and later, her left hand. She lost some sensation in her left hand. Gabapentin provided pain relief. She has mild pain after exercise.

Case 6.—Woman, 68, had pain and stiffness in her fingers and thumb from RSD after right thumb basal joint arthroplasty. She had decreased pain and temperature sensation in her thumb and index finger. Nerve blocks were unsuccessful at relieving her pain. After using high doses of gabapentin for her late acute or early dystrophic stage disease, she regained mobility in her fingers, her pain was reduced, and hypersensitivity and swelling decreased.

Conclusions.—Gabapentin therapy relieved RSD pain that was untreatable by other methods. Common side effects including headache, euphoria, disorientation, dizziness, drowsiness, leg cramps, and diarrhea gradually diminished with use of the drug. Randomized, double-blind studies are needed to confirm these results.

▶ Gabapentin (Neurontin) has been reported to relieve somatic neuropathic pain,[1] but this is the first report of its use for RSD. Currently, this is a first-line medication for neuropathic pain at our institution. We use it before tricyclic antidepressants (TCAs) and carbamazepine (Tegretol) because of its efficacy and minimal side effects. At times TCAs may be preferable to gabapentin because of cost.

Mellick and Mellick report 6 cases of RSD with remarkable response to gabapentin. They also state that they have never seen a treatment failure with gabapentin for RSD. I must admit that my experience is less dramatic. I have only used this drug for RSD with elements of causalgia (complex regional pain syndrome type 2), and have seen only mild-to-moderate pain relief. Nonetheless, any pain relief is appreciated with this difficult problem. The discussion section provides an excellent review of sympathetic pain mechanisms and plausible explanations for the action of gabapentin. Certainly, 6 case studies are not conclusive evidence of efficacy. However, gabapentin is worth considering in intractable cases of RSD.

K.A. Bengtson, M.D.

Reference

1. Rosner H, Rubin L, Kestenbaum A: Gabapentin adjunctive therapy in neuropathic pain states. *Clin J Pain* 12:56–58, 1996.

Reflex Sympathetic Dystrophy: Treatment With Long-acting Intramuscular Corticosteroids

Grundberg AB (Des Moines Orthopaedic Surgeons, Iowa)

J Hand Surg (Am) 21A:667–670, 1996 16–2

Purpose.—Patients with reflex sympathetic dystrophy (RSD) have pain, swelling, and limited motion of the hand. In many patients, chronic pain and limited motion develop, with or without treatment. The usual recommended treatment is exercise and sympathetic interruption with a stellate ganglion block. However, the results of stellate ganglion blocks do not last long. Results of long-acting corticosteroid treatment were studied in patients with RSD.

Patients.—Sixty-nine patients with RSD, defined as pain, swelling, limited motion, and discoloration of the hand after an injury or operation, were included. The status of all patients was followed for at least 1 year. Patients who did not improve with active exercises were given IM injections of long-acting methylprednisolone (Depo-Medrol), 80 mg. Twenty-two patients had compression syndromes in addition to RSD and required surgical treatment.

The other 47 patients were treated with Depo-Medrol and active exercises. There were 31 women and 16 men; average age, 54 years. They started RSD treatment a mean of 15 weeks after the inciting cause, most commonly an injury. Depo-Medrol injections were given no more frequently than every 2 weeks, although as many as 4 injections were given at 2-week intervals. The average number of injections per patient was 2.3, or 184 mg of Depo-Medrol.

Outcomes.—The treatment relieved night and rest pain for all patients. Motion of the proximal interphalangeal joint increased from 39 degrees before surgery to 75 degrees afterward. Grip strength improved from 7 to 29 lb. Twenty-two of 26 employed patients were able to return to work, and 3 went to lighter duties. There were some mild, transient corticosteroid side effects, none of which required cessation of Depo-Medrol treatment.

Conclusions.—Intramuscular injection of long-acting methylprednisolone gives good results in the treatment of RSD. Through their anti-inflammatory action, corticosteroids improve the compression syndrome and inflammation of RSD by reducing carpal tunnel swelling. The IM route of administration avoids problems with compliance and gastrointestinal symptoms.

▶ The author provides his rationale for treating patients who have pain, swelling, or stiffness that lasts too long or is out of the ordinary. Intramuscular Depo-Medrol injection is preferred because it obviates problems associated with oral routes of administration, such as compliance or gastric upset. No patient had avascular necrosis, and few had other corticoid-associated side effects.

Many of the patients who did not respond to this regimen were determined to have nerve compression pathology, which, in theory, perpetuates symptoms of RSD. Release of compression improved the clinical picture of RSD in these patients.

I am a strong believer in early steroid use in these patients but have used orally given agents, turning quickly to stellate blocks if the patient did not respond promptly. I will try the IM route.

V.R. Hentz, M.D.

Technical Considerations in Endoscopic Cervicothoracic Sympathectomy

Josephs LG, Menzoian JO (Boston Univ)

Arch Surg 131:355–359, 1996 16–3

Introduction.—The use of videoendoscopic equipment has rekindled interest in cervicothoracic sympathectomies. A technique using standard equipment was perfect for the performance of videoendoscopic cervicothoracic sympathectomy. This technique and the experience with 10 transthoracic cervicothoracic sympathectomies performed for hyperhidrosis or reflex sympathetic dystrophy were reviewed.

Methods.—Ten videoendoscopic transthoracic sympathectomies were performed in 9 patients using standard endoscopic equipment. The procedure encompassed the lower third of the stellate ganglion to the fourth thoracic ganglion and was performed with general anesthesia using 3 incisions, each 1-cm long, for instrument placement. Intraoperatively, bilateral hand temperature probes were taken. Four of the procedures were in the right hemithorax, and 6 were in the left. There was a mean postoperative follow-up of 14 months, and the main outcome measure was relief of the symptoms for which the patient was referred.

Results.—Partial or complete relief of symptoms occurred in 9 of 10 patients. Complete relief of symptoms occurred in the 3 patients with sympathectomies performed for hyperhidrosis. Increased range of motion and decreased pain resulted in 6 of 7 procedures performed for reflex sympathetic dystrophy. Nail and hair regrowth occurred in 2 patients with severe atrophic reflex sympathetic dystrophy. There was an average operating time of 91 minutes, an average length of hospital stay of 3.5 days, and a mean increase in skin temperature of 2.4°C. Symptoms persisted in 1 patient with severe dystrophic reflex sympathetic dystrophy. No patient had Horner's syndrome, but pneumothorax developed in 1 patient for 48 hours.

Conclusion.—For reflex sympathetic dystrophy and hyperhidrosis of the upper extremity, endoscopic cervicothoracic sympathectomy is an effective, minimally invasive therapy.

► Endoscopic cervicothoracic sympathectomy is gaining popularity because of a perception that it is less invasive, shortens hospital stay, and returns the patient to normal activities in a short time. However, the results of this particular study are comparable to a surgical sympathectomy performed through a small incision in the second to third intercostal space. The length of hospital stay and the results are similar to a small thoracic or supraclavicular incision, and the current endoscopic technique takes approximately 30 minutes longer than surgery. Consequently, endoscopic cervicothoracic sympathectomy may be considered an excellent alternative to patients with reflex sympathetic dystrophy or hyperhidrosis of the upper extremity, but its benefits may not be significantly different from a surgical approach through a small thoracotomy or cervical incision. The choice of technique should depend upon the surgeon's experience and the patient's body habitus.

J.W. Hallet, Jr., M.D.

Upper Dorsal Thoracoscopic Sympathectomy for Palmar Hyperhidrosis: Improved Intermediate-term Results

Kopelman D, Hashmonai M, Ehrenreich M, et al (Rambam Med Ctr, Haifa, Israel; Technion-Israel Inst of Technology, Haifa, Israel)

J Vasc Surg 24:194–199, 1996 16–4

Background.—Patients with primary palmar hyperhidrosis have excessive perspiration of unknown cause, resulting in severe occupational, emotional, and social problems. Surgical thoracoscopic sympathectomy is the treatment of choice. A previous randomized comparison of open supraclavicular surgery to 3-port thoracoscopic access found no obvious advantage of the thoracoscopic approach. The technique was, therefore, modified by use of a single-lumen endotracheal tube without total intraoperative lung collapse and only two 5-mm thoracoscopic ports. The immediate and mid-term results of this modified approach to upper dorsal thoracoscopic sympathectomy were reported.

Methods.—The experience included 106 sympathectomies in 53 patients with palmar hyperhidrosis. There were 34 women and 19 men (mean age, 23 years). All patients underwent general anesthesia with a single-lumen endotracheal tube. A 5-mm incision was made in the midclavicular line in the second intercostal space for insufflation of carbon dioxide and subsequent endoscopic trocar placement. A second port was placed in the anterior axillary line in the fourth intercostal space, through which an endoscopic diathermy hook was placed. The T2-T3 sympathetic ganglia were resected with the hook and removed for histologic examination. Both sides were operated on at the same procedure. The status of 104 limbs in 52 patients was followed for a mean of 19 months.

Results.—All procedures were successfully carried out by the thoracoscopic approach. All hands were completely dry immediately after surgery. Throughout follow-up, there were no cases of recurrent palmar hyperhidrosis. The short-term postoperative complication rate—mainly atelectasis, pneumonia, pneumothorax, and hemothorax—was 11%. Eighty-one percent of patients had some type of long-term sequela, including compensatory hyperhidrosis in 67%, unilateral Horner's syndrome in 17%, and neuralgia in 14%. These sequelae varied in severity and were not always permanent. Six patients expressed dissatisfaction with their results, primarily because of compensatory sweating. Three regretted having the operation.

Conclusion.—The authors' modified technique of upper dorsal thoracoscopic sympathectomy for palmar hyperhidrosis provides mainly satisfactory results. Although most patients have some type of long-term sequela, dry hands were obtained immediately and on mid-term follow-up. Although some drawbacks remain, thoracoscopic sympathectomy is still the surgical treatment of choice for severe primary palmar hyperhidrosis.

▶ The hand surgeon, along with the dermatologist, sees patients with palmar hyperhydrosis. This report indicates that less than 20% of patients undergoing this procedure will persist in experiencing Horner's syndrome. The introduction of the thorascope, together with carbon dioxide insufflation to collapse the lung, has made this a very benign procedure (no chest tube).

V.R. Hentz, M.D.

Reflex Sympathetic Dystrophy: Skin Blood Flow, Sympathetic Vasoconstrictor Reflexes and Pain Before and After Surgical Sympathectomy

Baron R, Maier C (Christian-Albrechts-Universität Kiel, Germany)

Pain 67:317–326, 1996 16–5

Introduction.—Reflex sympathetic dystrophy (RSD) may develop after trauma affecting the limbs. Although clinical signs and symptoms vary considerably, 3 major components have been distinguished: sensory abnormalities, vascular and sweating abnormalities, and motor abnormalities. Some studies suggest that patients with RSD are characterized by sympathetic overactivity in the affected limb. To better understand the mechanisms of vascular disturbances in RSD and the role of the sympathetic nervous system, 12 patients were studied with laser Doppler flowmetry.

Methods.—Study participants were 12 consecutive patients referred for evaluation of RSD of the hand. Eleven recalled a previous trauma to the affected limb. Controls were 12 healthy volunteers. Cutaneous blood flow, skin resistance, and skin temperature were measured at the affected and contralateral hands. To measure the function of sympathetic vasoconstrictor fibers, autonomic reflexes were examined after deep inspiration. Eleven patients were treated with local anesthetic stellate ganglion blocks and/or regional guanethidine blocks. One experienced long-term relief, 5 had temporary relief, and 4 did not respond to sympathetic blocks. Four of those who had temporary relief underwent surgical sympathectomy.

Results.—In 10 patients, both blood flow and skin temperature were considerably lower after acclimatization in a cold environment (18°C or less), indicating vasoconstriction of cutaneous vessels. No additonal vasoconstrictor reflexes were elicited ipsilaterally under these conditions. In a warm environment (22°C to 24°C), blood flow and skin temperature exhibited no significant side differences. Sympathetic vasoconstrictor responses to deep inspiration were also quantitatively the same on both sides in a warm environment. Vasoconstrictor reflexes were absent after sympathectomy, and skin resistance was considerably higher on the affected hand. For 4 weeks after the procedure, the affected hand was warmer and blood flow higher compared with the unaffected hand. There was a subsequent slow decrease in skin temperature and perfusion, and the affected hand turned from warm to cold. The 2 patients who experienced long-term pain relief had postsympathectomy skin temperature and blood flow values that were only slightly less in the affected hand than in the normal hand.

Conclusion.—Side differences in patients with RSD must be interpreted with care because skin temperature and blood flow vary according to changes in environmental temperature. Vascular disturbances do not result from constant overactivity of sympathetic vasoconstrictor neurons. Some patients experience a relapse of pain after sympathectomy, perhaps because of denervation supersensitivity of blood vessels and vasomotion.

▶ Reflex sympathetic dystrophy, as defined by the criteria for complex regional pain syndrome, remains a clinical entity without pathonemonic physiologic findings. This article presents 4 important concepts: (1) hand temperature(s) without environmental control(s) and/or stress is an unreliable measurement; (2) side-to-side differential temperature is neither diagnostic nor consistent in RSD; (3) proximal irreversible cervicothoracic sympathectomy produces delayed receptor hypersensitivity and should be used with caution in RSD; and (4) RSD is a dynamic process.

L.A. Koman, M.D.

Hand Infections in Patients With Diabetes

Kour AK, Looi KP, Phone MH, et al (Natl Univ of Singapore)

Clin Orthop 331:238–244, 1996 16–6

Background.—Diabetic patients have a known predisposition to sepsis that can result in significant morbidity. One group of diabetic patients hospitalized for hand infections was reviewed.

Methods and Findings.—Twenty-five adults with hand infections were studied. Eighty percent were younger than 60 years and had had diabetes mellitus for less than 5 years. Twenty percent of the patients had secondary neurologic, vascular, or cutaneous changes in the hands. Sixteen percent had a documented instance of trauma. None of the infections was nosocomial. Ninety-six percent of the patients needed surgery. Débridement alone was done in 21 patients, and amputation of 1 or more digits of the hand was performed in 3 patients, either as a primary procedure or after débridement. Fifty-five percent of the positive cultures grew multiple organisms. In 73% of the positive cultures, gram-negative organisms were documented. The entire spectrum of causative organisms was covered by an antibiotic combination of gentamicin, penicillin G, and cloxacillin. At a 2-year follow-up, there were no repeat episodes of the hand infections.

Conclusions.—Effective management of sepsis, reduction of morbidity, and hand salvage were accomplished by using an aggressive treatment protocol consisting of hospitalization, IV combination antibiotics, surgical débridement, appropriate diabetic control, and strict elevation of the hand. No recurrences of the hand infections occurred.

► Twenty-five patients with diabetes had upper-extremity infections, predominantly of gram-negative origin. All except 1 patient required surgical débridement, and, in fact, amputation of digits in 2 patients and amputation of the forearm in 1 patient was required to manage the infection. Of importance is that the majority of patients in this study were in their fifth decade and were not necessarily old and debilitated. Only 4 patients had open injuries, whereas the remaining patients were believed to have inadvertent minor trauma to the skin, unrecognized by the patient. In 80% of the patients, diabetes mellitus was present for 5 years or less, and 3 patients had diabetes diagnosed after their presentation with sepsis.

P. Dell, M.D.

Necrotizing Fasciitis of the Upper Extremity

Gonzalez MH, Kay T, Weinzweig N, et al (Univ of Illinois, Chicago; Cook County Hosp, Chicago)

J Hand Surg (Am) 21A:689–692, 1996 16–7

Background.—Necrotizing fasciitis, a severe, insidious infection, spreads rapidly along soft-tissue planes. Initially, its true severity is often not appreciated. The pathology, natural history, and treatment of necrotizing fasciitis of the upper extremity were retrospectively studied.

Methods and Findings.—A retrospective review identified 12 patients with necrotizing fasciitis. In all patients, the infection was associated with a history of substance abuse by injection or with diabetes. Eleven infections were β-hemolytic *Streptococcus*, mixed anaerobic-aerobic, or both (Table 1). Testing for HIV infection was positive in 3 of 5 patients. Necrotic fascia were débrided using a wide extensile approach. One to 6 débridements were needed. Uncontrollable infection resulted in shoulder disarticulation in 2 patients.

Conclusions.—Necrotizing fasciitis is a rapid, destructive disease. Early recognition, aggressive débridement, and antibiotic treatment are needed to minimize morbidity.

► Nectrotizing fasciitis has gained increased significance in recent years because of its apparent increased incidence among immunocompromised patients. This excellent article by Gonzales et al. summarizes the experience

TABLE 1.—Bacteriology of Cases of Necrotizing Fasciitis

Causative Agent	No. Cases
Beta-hemolytic *Streptococcus*	7
Alpha-hemolytic *Streptococcus*	6
Bacteroides species	6
Peptostreptococcus	3
Eikenella corrodens	2
Enterococcus	2
Staphylococcus aureus	2 (1 methicillin resistant)
Bacillus species	1
Staphylococcus hemolyticus	1
Pseudomonas	1
Fusobacterium	1
Prevotella melaninogenica	1
Prevotella buccae	1
Escherichia coli	1

(Courtesy of Gonzalez MH, Key T, Weinzweig N, et al: Necrotizing fasciitis of the upper extremity. *J Hand Surg [Am]* 21A:689–692, 1996.)

with a large group of patients (12) with a diverse bacteriology. The case example shows the extensive nature of dissection involved and alerts the reader to the aggressive nature of the wound and the aggressive nature of surgical management that permits recovery.

Our experience is similar to that of Gonzales et al. with the insidious onset of rapidly progressive infection in patients who initially appear less predisposed to infection. Surgical exploration with extensive attention to fasciotomy, drainage, exposure, débridement, and aggressive antibiotic treatment is important, along with consultating specialists from infectious disease, general medicine, and surgery to discover comorbidities which predispose to the rapid progression of this infection. This is an important article for contemporary managers with responsibility for hand infections.

M. Keith, M.D.

Suggested Reading

Bruehl S, Lubenow TR, Nath H, et al: Validation of thermography in the diagnosis of reflex sympathetic dystrophy. *Clin J Pain* 12:316–325, 1996.

► Thermography is useful when documentation of asymmetrical or abnormal skin temperature is needed. Strict attention to baseline acclimatization in a climate-controlled room is essential if the results are to be valid and reproducible.

P.C. Amadio, M.D.

Field J, Atkins RM: Algodystrophy is an early complication of Colles' fracture: What are the implications? *J Hand Surg (Br)* 22B:178–182, 1997.

► Tenderness of the fingers to palpation and decreased range of motion of finger joints were found to be excellent predictors of later development of reflex sympathetic dystrophy/algodystrophy/complex regional pain syndrome—take your choice. When both were present at 1-week follow-up, the sensitivity was 96% and the specificity 73%. Patients who had neither tenderness nor decreased range of motion of uninjured joints had a less than 5% chance of later being diagnosed with RSD/algo/CRPS. The latter group may well have a better prognosis than the former.

P.C. Amadio, M.D.

Hudson DA, Duminy F: Microembolectomy in the treatment of arterial occlusion of the hand: Report of two cases. *J Hand Surg (Am)* 21A:884–887, 1996.

▶ The authors have described a useful technical tip. They construct a microembolectomy out of a nylon suture chosen so that its diameter is about half that of the vessel to be embolectomized. The tip of the suture is blunted and rounded by melting the end with an ophthamalogic cautery. The blunted end acts like a ladle that scoops the clot out of the vessel. I will surely try this.

V.R. Hentz, M.D.

Nancarrow JD, Rai SA, Sterne GD, et al: The natural history of cold intolerance of the hand. *Injury* 27:607–611, 1996.

17 Research

Long-Segment Nerve Allograft Regeneration in the Sheep Model: Experimental Study and Review of the Literature

Strasberg SR, Mackinnon SE, Genden EM, et al (Washington Univ, St Louis; Univ of McMaster, Hamilton, Ont; Univ of Toronto)

J Reconstr Microsurg 12:529–537, 1996 17–1

Introduction.—Nerve autografts have been used to treat peripheral nerve injuries. However, reconstruction of severe injuries is difficult because of the limited number of nerves available for grafting. The use of nerve allografts in the reconstruction of peripheral nerve injuries offers several advantages, including a larger supply of donor nerves and decreased donor-site morbidity. Long-segment nerve-allograft reconstruction and the effects of cold temperatures on nerve regeneration were studied.

Methods.—Twenty outbred ewes received 8-cm nerve autografts for a surgically created defect in the median nerve in the right forelimb and a nerve allograft in the contralateral forelimb. One group received fresh grafts, and the second group received grafts that had been cold-preserved for 7 days before use. In vivo nerve conduction studies were performed, after which the animals were killed at either 6 or 10 months. The nerve grafts were removed and examined by microscopy and morphometric analyses.

Results.—Histologic examination found no difference between the fresh and cold-preserved autografts at 6 or 10 months; both types showed normal-appearing architecture. A dense population of well-myelinated fibers was present, suggesting regeneration. The distal host nerve was also densely populated with normally myelinated nerve fibers. However, both the fresh and cold-preserved allografts showed evidence of poor regeneration. Few regenerated fibers were present at 6 or 10 months, and fiber concentration of the distal host segments was markedly reduced. In the allograft group, both the graft and the distal median nerve showed significantly worse nerve fiber width, density, and number compared with the autograft group. Morphometric indices examined were similar between the fresh and cold-preserved autografts and between the fresh and cold-preserved allografts. No nerve conduction velocity could be obtained from any allografts at 6 or 10 months. Similar nerve conduction velocities were obtained across the fresh and cold-preserved autografts (27.9 m/s at 10 months for both groups).

Conclusion.—Evidence of nerve regeneration was found when either a fresh or cold-preserved long-nerve autografts were used for repair of a nerve defect. In contrast, use of a nerve allograft resulted in poor nerve regeneration. Cold preservation of the nerve before grafting did not appear to enhance nerve regeneration.

▶ The authors are to be congratulated for introducing an animal model that can permit experiments with long grafts. The sheep model avoids the ethical concerns of using primates, and the sheep nerve is relatively similar to the human nerve in its histologic morphology, especially in terms of connective tissue content. The literature review is very extensive and helpful.

V.R. Hentz, M.D.

Peripheral-Nerve Allotransplantation in Rats Immunosuppressed With Transient or Long-term FK-506

Weinzweig N, Grindel S, Gonzalez M, et al (Univ of Illinois, Chicago)

J Reconstr Microsurg 12:451–459, 1996 17–2

Background.—Significant peripheral nerve gaps can be treated with autogenous nerve grafting, but expendable donor sites are limited and result in secondary neurologic defects. Use of peripheral nerve allografting (PNA) would increase the supply of grafting material and eliminate donor-site morbidity. To increase the chances of success with PNA, immune suppression is necessary. The 2 most promising agents for immune suppression are cyclosporine (Cs) and FK-506. Immunosuppression may not have to be continued indefinitely, as the PNA functions as a scaffolding to permit functional host nerve regeneration. Regeneration across PNA was evaluated in rats receiving transient or long-term immunosuppression with Cs or FK-506.

Methods.—Lewis rats served as recipients of sciatic nerve isografts (LEW) or allografts (ACI), a major histoincompatable mismatch. There were 7 groups with 8 rats in each group: group 1, LEW/LEW isograft control; group 2, Lew/ACI allograft control; group 3, allograft + Cs subcutaneously for 2 weeks; group 4, allograft + Cs daily for 2 weeks and then subcutaneously biweekly; group 5, allograft + FK-506 by single injection; group 6, allograft + FK-506 daily for 2 weeks; and group 7, allograft + FK-506 daily for 2 weeks and then biweekly. After 7 months, conduction velocities were evaluated.

Results.—Neural regeneration with good results was detected in the isograft group, the allograft groups with long-term immunosuppression, and in the transient FK-506 group. The transient Cs group, allograft control group, and the single-dose FK-506 group had significantly worse results.

Conclusions.—Transient immunosuppression with FK-506 permitted excellent regeneration across peripheral nerve allografts in inbred rats.

FK-506 has demonstrated promise in this animal model and should be investigated as an agent to assist in peripheral nerve allotransplantation.

► The authors have demonstrated successful regeneration across short nerve allografts in a rodent model using FK-506 as the immunosuppressive agent. Their conclusion that transient immunosuppression allows for the restoration of anatomical and physiologic function of a PNA is in keeping with experimental[1] and preliminary clinical results.[2] It provides optimism for the cautious introduction of nerve allotransplantation in the clinical situation of an otherwise irreparable nerve injury.

S.E. Mackinnon, M.D.

References

1. Evans PJ, Midha R, Mackinnon SE: The peripheral nerve allograft: A comprehensive review of regeneration and neuroimmunology. *Prog Neurol* 43:187–233, 1994.
2. Mackinnon SE: Nerve allotransplantation following severe tibial nerve injury. *J Neurosurg* 84:671–676, 1996.

Nerve Coaptation Studies With and Without a Gap in Rabbits

Hasegawa J, Shibata M, Takahashi H (Niigata Univ, Japan)

J Hand Surg (Am) 21A:259–265, 1996 17–3

Background.—There are several methods of achieving appropriate matching of proximal and distal nerve fibers during nerve repair. However, there is evidence that neurotropic factors affect motor–sensory specificity and thus the functional outcome. This suggests that it might be better to leave a gap between the 2 nerve ends. The outcomes of cut nerve ends that were directly coapted and those in which a gap was left—with or without sensory and motor alignment—were compared in rabbits.

Methods.—Rabbit radial nerves were cut and treated in 1 of 4 ways. Two groups of cut nerve ends were directly coapted inside a 5-mm collagen tube, 1 with and 1 without appropriate motor and sensory alignment. In the other 2 groups, the cut ends were placed in a 10-mm collagen tube with a 5-mm gap, also with and without motor and sensory alignment. After 24 weeks, the rabbits were killed for electrophysiologic, histologic, and muscle contraction studies.

Results.—There were no significant differences in nerve conduction velocity, dry muscle, weight, or motor axon count between the 4 groups. Sensory nerve regeneration was better and muscle contraction was less for nerves that were left malaligned without a gap than in the other 3 groups. Muscle contraction force was equal in the group that was left malaligned with a gap and in the group that was aligned with a gap.

Conclusions.—In cut rabbit radial nerves, leaving a short gap between the nerve ends reduces misdirection of motor fibers after coaptation of the nerve ends. Using a conduit will make nerve regeneration more specific, whereas leaving a short gap will decrease mismatching of motor and sensory fibers.

▶ The results of this study suggest that nerve repair using a tubulization technique with a short nerve gap is not superior to the ideal microneurosurgical nerve repair. However, in a situation in which the topography is unknown and an inappropriate anatomical alignment is likely, reconstruction using a short nerve gap with a conduit appears superior to an inappropriate microsurgical repair in which sensory and motor topography is misaligned. The results of this study are similar to those of Evans et al.[1] and suggest that should a readily absorbable biodegradable nerve conduit be available in a situation in which the surgeon is uncertain as to the motor sensory alignment, consideration could be given to using a nerve conduit with a short gap.

S.E. Mackinnon, M.D.

Reference

1. Evans PJ, Bain JR, Mackinnon SE, et al: Selective reinnervation: A comparison of recovery following microsuture and conduit nerve repair. *Brain Res* 559:315–321, 1991.

A Primate Model for Studying Focal Dystonia and Repetitive Strain Injury: Effects on the Primary Somatosensory Cortex

Byl NN, Merzenich MM, Cheung S, et al (Univ of California at San Francisco)
Phys Ther 77:269–284, 1997 17–4

Introduction.—Discomfort in arms, wrists, and hands can occur among workers doing automated tasks under highly demanding conditions. Excessive and repetitive end-range motions, recessive force, stretching, and awkward postures can lead to repetitive strain injuries with symptoms of chronic soft-tissue inflammation, scarring, pain, fatigue, muscle spasm, and postural imbalance. Another complication is reflex sympathetic dystrophy and occupational hand cramps or focal dystonia of the hand. There is an increase in job-related repetitive strain injuries, and few treatment strategies have been successful in helping the injured workers return to work. The behaviorally induced cortical plasticity effects of repetitive strain injuries and focal dystonia symptomatology in 2 owl monkeys were evaluated.

Methods.—Training for 20 weeks occurred with 2 owl monkeys who repetitively closed a handpiece against an 80-g force. One monkey performed active, repetitive hand opening and closing using a highly articulated hand-squeezing strategy. The other monkey used a proximal arm-pulling strategy performing this task. Recordings were taken of changes in motor performance. Comparisons were made of the electrophysiologic maps of the hand representation on the trained primary sensor cortex with those of untrained control animals and untrained sides of the trained monkeys.

Results.—More motor deterioration and dedifferentiation of the normally sharply segregated areas of the hand representation of the primary somatosensory cortex occurred in the monkey using the articulated hand-squeezing strategy. The monkey using the proximal arm-pulling strategy had mild degradation of the hand, but no motor dysfunction.

Conclusion.—Hand degradation and motor control interferences occur with attended, highly articulated, repetitive finger squeezing. The sensory degradation was minimized and motor control was preserved with a proximal, more variable repetitive strategy. For patients with chronic repetitive strain injuries, restoring the hand representation may be a critical part of treatment.

▶ This is excellent and creative work that provides evidence that the strategy used in accomplishing a repetitive movement determines the likelihood of changes in cortical sensory representations and presumably occupational dystonia or repetitive strain injury. This is a unique model of acquired dystonia that holds great promise in aiding our understanding of these disorders.

J.R. Daube, M.D.

Influence of the Delay of Denervation on Slow Striated Muscle Resistance to Slow-to-Fast Conversion Following Cross-Innervation

Chammas M, Coulet B, Micallef JP, et al (Lapeyronie Hosp, Montpellier, France; NIH and Med Research, Montpellier, France; Arnaud de Villeneuve Hosp, Montpellier, France)

Microsurgery 16:779–785, 1995 17–5

Background.—Cross-reinnervation refers to a situation common after conventional microsurgical repair or nerve transfer, when a slow or fast twitch muscle is innervated by the opposite type of nerve. The nerve of a slow muscle is able to convert a fast muscle to a functional slow type, whereas a fast muscle nerve has only incomplete control over the functioning of a slow muscle. To determine whether timing of reinnervation might affect the expression of fast motoneuron properties in slow cross-reinnervated muscle, a rat model of cross-reinnervation was employed.

Methods.—Eight adult male rats were assigned to a control group for the determination of normal soleus muscle fiber type composition. In the remaining rats, the medial gastrocnemius nerve (MG) and the combined lateral gastrocnemius and soleus nerve (LG-soleus) were severed, and the ends electrocoagulated, ligated, and fixed to prevent muscle reinnervation and nerve retraction. Other leg muscles were denervated to prevent reinnervation from neighboring muscles. Branches of the sciatic nerve were sectioned and muscle cross-reinnervation was performed in 24 rats. In the remaining 24 rats, the nerves were resutured to themselves (self-reinnervation). These procedures were performed immediately (T0), 6 weeks (T6), or 12 weeks (T12) after the severance of the nerve, with 8 rats in each group.

Results.—Normal soleus muscle contained over 80% type I slow fibers, normal medial gastrocnemius muscle contained over 89% type II fibers, and normal lateral gastrocnemius muscle contained over 90% type II fibers. In the T0 group, after cross-reinnervation, type I fibers were significantly reduced in the soleus, whereas type II fibers were significantly increased. In the self-reinnervation T0 group, type I fibers were also decreased. In the T6 group, type I fibers significantly decreased, whereas type II fibers increased to become predominant. In the self-reinnervation group, these changes were less marked. In the T12 group, the inversion in the proportion of type I and type II fibers was detected only in the cross-reinnervated group.

Conclusions.—The results of these studies using an adult rat model of cross-reinnervation indicate that a significant slow-to-fast transformation of the soleus muscle was obtained when nerve repair was delayed. Maximal benefit was detected when repair was performed 6 weeks after nerve section in the adult rat. An initial phase of muscle denervation appears to be adaptive and to permit better muscle-nerve interaction in cases of cross-reinnervation.

▶ This experimental work explores the morphological consequences in reinnervated muscle of the changes in the type of motor innervation after conventional microsurgical nerve repair. The situation in which the type of motor innervation can be changed is called cross-innervation. Cross-innervation, as was emphasized by the authors, is frequently present in cases of conventional microsurgical nerve suture because of misdirection of nerve regeneration and also in case of nerve transfer. Muscle fibers of the slow twitch type have shown strong resistance for their conversion to the fast twitch type if they are reinnervated by motoneurons of the fast type in case of cross-reinnervation. This fact has functional consequences as was previously shown experimentally.

This work suggests that the negative consequences on nerve and muscle relationship caused by cross-reinnervation in the case of wrong connections between slow and fast motorneurons after conventional nerve suture or in the case of nerve transfer could be minimized by imposing a delay before nerve repair. The initial phase of muscle denervation should no longer be considered only as a period of muscle degeneration but also as a period of improved muscle plasticity. This denervation time allows the reinnervated muscle to adapt to changes in the pattern of innervation and to improve muscle-nerve interaction on muscle properties.

M. Chammas, M.D., Ph.D.

Biomechanical and Histologic Characteristics of Canine Flexor Tendon Repair Using Early Postoperative Mobilization

Aoki M, Kubota H, Pruitt DL, et al (Washington Univ, St Louis)

J Hand Surg (Am) 22A:107–114, 1997 17–6

Background.—Flexor tendon repair with traditional suture techniques, such as that of Kessler, is usually followed by postoperative rehabilitation through passive mobilization. Recently, postoperative active flexion protocols have been advocated, but the traditional 2-strand suture methods may not have the strength to withstand this stress. New suture techniques with increased tensile strength, such as the 6-strand Savage suture, have been developed. The tendon healing process was analyzed in a canine model of flexor tendon repair, followed by immediate postoperative active motion. The modified 2-strand Kessler, modified 6-strand Savage, and dorsal splint repair techniques were compared.

Methods.—A group of 25 mongrel dogs weighing from 20 to 25 kg were used for this study. Each dog was anesthetized and the flexor profundus (FP) tendons exposed in zone II. A transverse laceration was made in the FP tendons of the fourth and fifth digits. The 47 tendons were repaired using either modified Kessler, modified Savage, or dorsal tendon splint techniques (Fig 1). Postoperatively, the operated upper extremity was immobilized in a wrist extension block shoulder-elbow-forearm spica cast that permitted active wrist and digit flexion and extension but did not permit weight bearing. The intensity of active movement was not fully controlled in this experimental model system. The controls for these procedures consisted of 21 fresh canine cadaver FP tendons from 6 mongrel dogs. Tendon repairs were inspected and failure was defined as rupture or adhesions that prevented tendon gliding. Biomechanical testing was performed on controls and on 5-, 10-, and 21-day specimens. Five Savage and 2 dorsal tendon splint specimens were subjected to macroscopic and histologic evaluation.

Results.—Of the 9 Kessler repairs, 8 were ruptured by day 10. None of the 19 Savage repairs or the 19 dorsal tendon splint repairs ruptured. Three of the dorsal tendon splint repairs failed as the result of adhesions. The gap strength values for the Savage and dorsal tendon splint repairs were significantly improved on day 21 compared with day 5 and day 10. Ultimate tensile strength was not decreased during the 3-week healing period. Histologically, there was evidence of progressive healing without adhesions in successful repairs.

Conclusion.—Using a canine model of flexor tendon repair has shown that those tendon repair techniques, such as Savage and dorsal tendon splint which have increased ultimate tensile strength, have the potential to withstand the stress of active postoperative digital motion protocols and promote successful tendon healing. The tensile properties of tendons repaired with these techniques did not decrease throughout the 21-day healing period of this study. The study also demonstrated that the canine

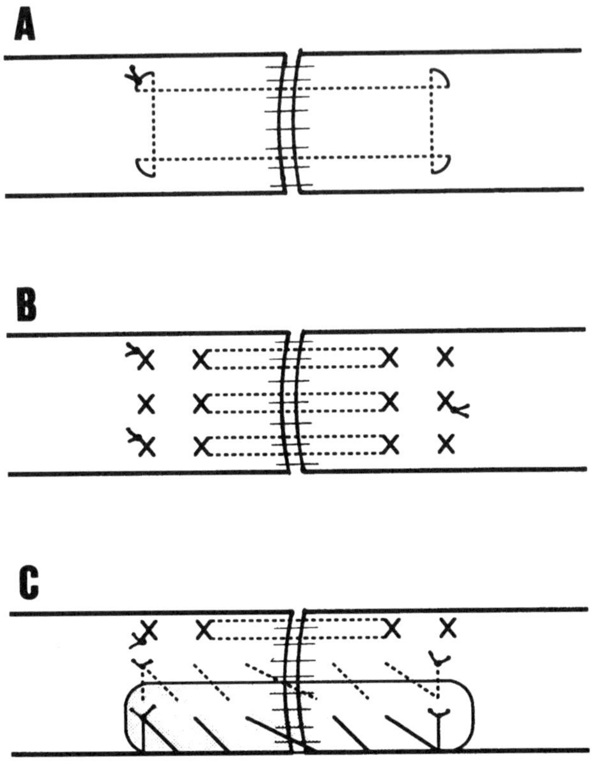

FIGURE 1.—Flexor tendon repair techniques: **A**, modified Kessler; **B**, modified Savage; and **C**, dorsal tendon splint. (Courtesy of Aoki M, Kubota H, Pruitt DL, et al: Biomechanical and histologic characteristics of canine flexor tendon repair using early postoperative mobilization. *J Hand Surg [Am]* 22A:107–114, 1997.)

model is useful in the analysis of the response of the healing tendon to active postoperative rehabilitation protocols.

► Here is in vivo evidence that the Savage repair provides better results in dogs than the standard 2-strand Kessler repair when early active motion is allowed. Unfortunately, the authors did not have an early passive motion control arm in their study, so it is not clear whether the final results of an active motion protocol are any better than that of a passive one. This is relevant, as Gelberman showed an 11% increase in ultimate tensile strength after 21 days of a passive protocol,[1] whereas this study showed a 2% to 3% decrease at 21 days. I believe that the essential element of tendon rehabilitation is the fact that the tendon moves; whether this is done by active or passive exercise is more a matter of technique than anything else. There is a risk of overdoing things with active protocols; they need to be approached cautiously.

P.C. Amadio, M.D.

Reference

1. Gelberman RH, Woo SL-Y, Lothringer K, et al: Effects of early intermittent passive mobilization on healing canine flexor tendons. *J Hand Surg (Am)* 7A:170–175, 1982.

Mechanical Characteristics of Cross-Stitch Epitenon Suture in Association With Various Two-Strand Core Sutures: A Biochemical Study Using Canine Cadaver Tendons

Aoki M, Ito K, Wada T, et al (Sapporo Med Univ, Japan)

Injury 27:703–707, 1996 17–7

Background.—With the introduction of early mobilization after flexor tendon repair, the mechanical properties of sutures have assumed increasing importance. The recently introduced cross-stitch epitenon suture technique provides the greatest tensile strength without interference with tendon gliding. It is possible to combine this suture technique with one of the many core suture techniques used in tendon repair to increase tendon stabilization. This biomechanical study examined the properties of several 2-strand core sutures in association with the cross-stitch epitenon suture in a canine cadaver model of tendon repair.

Methods.—The study was performed on 24 flexor profundus tendons from 3 adult mongrel dogs. The flexor profundus tendons in the second to fifth digits were lacerated and then repaired as follows: group 1, cross-stitch; group 2, modified Kessler plus cross-stitch; group 3, Tsuge plus cross-stitch; and group 4, 2-strand Savage plus cross-stitch (Fig 1). Each group was composed of 6 tendons. Ultimate tensile strength was evaluated with a tensile testing machine, and stiffness was recorded by a video dimension analyzer system.

Results.—The ultimate tensile strength of group 2 was significantly greater than that of all other groups (group 4, group 3, and group 1 followed in that order). The stiffness of group 2 was significantly greater than that of all other groups (group 4, group 3, and group 1 followed in that order).

Conclusion.—The results of this canine cadaver model study of the mechanical characteristics of the cross-stitch epitenon suture technique in association with several 2-strand core sutures for tendon repair suggests that the modified Kessler technique was the best 2-strand core suture technique and should be used in association with the cross-stitch epitenon suture. These results may be useful to surgeons in determining which core suture technique to use in conjunction with the cross-stitch epitenon suture for tendon repair.

► As Lin first pointed out,[1] the epitenon stitch does more than tidy up the repair. If it is designed as a grasping or locking stitch, it provides considerable strength as well. This paper uses a cross-stitch variation to confirm

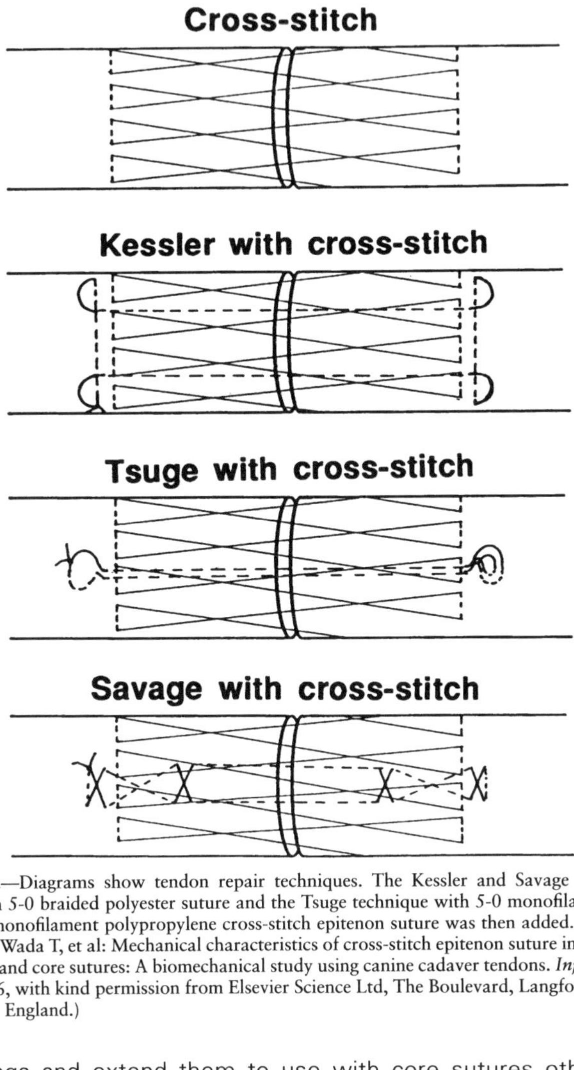

FIGURE 1.—Diagrams show tendon repair techniques. The Kessler and Savage techniques were performed with 5-0 braided polyester suture and the Tsuge technique with 5-0 monofilament loop nylon suture. A 6-0 monofilament polypropylene cross-stitch epitenon suture was then added. (Reprinted from Aoki M, Ito K, Wada T, et al: Mechanical characteristics of cross-stitch epitenon suture in association with various two-strand core sutures: A biomechanical study using canine cadaver tendons. *Injury* 10:703–707. Copyright 1996, with kind permission from Elsevier Science Ltd, The Boulevard, Langford Lane, Kidlington OX5 1GB, England.)

Lin's findings and extend them to use with core sutures other than the standard Kessler one.

P.C. Amadio, M.D.

Reference

1. Lin GT, Cooney WP, An KN, et al: Biomechanical study of running suture for flexor tendon repair. *J Hand Surg (Am)* 13A:553–538, 1988.

Single Exposures to 5-Fluorouracil: A Possible Mode of Targeted Therapy to Reduce Contractile Scarring in the Injured Tendon

Khan U, Occleston NL, Khaw PT, et al (Univ College, London; Univ of Florida)
Plast Reconstr Surg 99:465–471, 1997 17–8

Objective.—After injury, tendon adhesions may develop that prevent tendon excursion. Because fibroblasts are the primary cells involved in scar formation, fibroblasts were isolated from the parietal synovial sheath and from the endotenon to characterize the relative rates of collagen lattice contraction and to investigate the effect of single 5-minute exposures to the antimetabolite 5-fluorouracil on lattice contracture.

Methods.—Fibroblasts isolated from New Zealand White rabbits were cultured, suspended in 1-mL collagen lattices, and exposed in triplicate to a single 5-minute treatment with 0.25, 0.5, 2.0, and 25 mg/mL of 5-fluorouracil or buffered saline. Each lattice was then washed, incubated, and photographed for 7 days. Fibroblast-populated collagen lattice contracture was quantified, and differences were analyzed statistically.

Results.—Synovial fibroblasts produced significantly more contracture than did endotenon fibroblasts. All concentrations of 5-fluorouracil reduced the contracture of the lattice for both cell populations. Treatment with 5-fluorouracil did not significantly affect cell viability or actin organization in either cell population.

Conclusion.—These findings suggest that a single local treatment with 5-fluorouracil can prevent adhesion formation and contractile scarring in injured tendons without causing cell death. Synovial fibroblasts produced significantly more contracture than did endotenon fibroblasts.

► This interesting article suggests that a single topical application of 5-fluorouracil may decrease adhesion formation after tendon injury. It may, of course, also retard healing. An in vivo experiment is needed to see which effect occurs (but, based on studies in the past to block collagen crosslinking with other agents, I would bet on the latter).

P.C. Amadio, M.D.

Comparative Biomechanical Analysis of a New Circumferential Flexor Tendon Repair and a Modified Kessler Repair

Ion LE, Sykes PJ, Cassell OCS, et al (Morriston Hosp, Swansea, Wales; Univ of Wales, Cardiff)
Br J Plast Surg 50:236–241, 1997 17–9

Introduction.—A 2-part study was designed to test the biomechanical behavior of a new circumferential repair for flexor tendons in zone II. Repair of these tendons must meet particularly stringent requirements to provide good recovery of motion in the injured tendon.

Methods.—The first part of the study compared the mechanical properties of the new circumferential suture with a modified Kessler suture. In the second part of the study, the effects of the suture material on the behavior of the new circumferential suture were examined. Both investigations used fresh human cadaver flexor tendons. A Kessler-Tajima core suture with the Strickland modification was used for repair of the first group of 12 tendons. The second group of 12 tendons was repaired with the new technique which uses a single, continuous, inverting and locking suture of the periphery of the tendon. In the second investigation, 8 tendons were repaired with 5/0 multifilament steel by the new circumferential technique. Repaired tendons were tested at longitudinal stress to failure.

Results.—The first 2 groups of tendons were tested at 2 crosshead speeds (20 and 70 mm/min). Because crosshead speed had no statistically significant effect on ultimate tensile strength, data were pooled for comparison of the 2 types of repair. The third group of 8 tendons was tested at 70 mm/min crosshead speed. The 5/0 polypropylene circumferential repair was significantly stronger than the Kessler repair (median, 32.29 N vs. 24.03 N), and the circumferential repair was significantly stronger when 5/0 multifilament steel was used (median, 56.04 N) than when 5/0 polypropylene was used (median, 32.39 N).

Conclusion.—The new circumferential repair appears to have a number of biomechanical advantages over the modified Kessler suture and may be preferable for tendon repairs in zone II. Video recordings showed the new circumferential repair to have a higher breaking strength without gap formation, suggesting that its rigidity is at least as good as, if not better than, that of the Kessler repair.

▶ We know from the work of Lin et al.[1] that a running, locking peripheral stitch adds to the strength of a tendon repair. This paper goes the next step and shows that using 5/0 rather than 6/0 suture improves the strength even further. A four-strand core and a 5/0 circumferential repair may be what we need to start early active motion after zone II flexor tendon repair.

P.C. Amadio, M.D.

Reference

1. Lin GT, An KN, Cooney WP III, et al: Biomechanical studies of running suture for flexor tendon repair in dogs. *J Hand Surg (Am)* 13A:553–558, 1988.

Tensile Properties of Canine Intrasynovial and Extrasynovial Flexor Tendon Autografts

Noguchi M, Seiler JG III, Boardman ND III, et al (Univ of Pittsburgh, Pa; Emory Univ, Atlanta, Ga; Washington Univ, St Louis)

J Hand Surg (Am) 22A:457–463, 1997 17–10

Background.—Previous research has shown that grafted intrasynovial tendons heal with minimal adhesions and normal cellularity and collagen organization up to 6 weeks after surgery, whereas extrasynovial tendons heal by early ingrowth of peripheral adhesions and increased cellularity. However, the functional and structural features of these donor tendons after grafting to the synovial space are not known. The biomechanical properties of intrasynovial and extrasynovial flexor tendon autografts were studied in a canine model.

Methods.—In each dog, flexor digitorum profundus tissue from the fifth toe of the hindpaw was harvested and transplanted as an intrasynovial graft to the second toe of the left forepaw. Peroneus longus tendon from the lateral compartment of the hind leg was used for the extrasynovial graft that was transplanted to the fifth toe in each dog's left forepaw. The right forepaw served as a control. After surgery, the dogs underwent a regimen of daily controlled passive mobilization. Six dogs were killed 3 and 6 weeks after grafting, and their grafts were evaluated for gliding function and tensile properties.

Findings.—Angular rotation of the proximal interphalangeal joint was significantly greater in the digits receiving intrasynovial grafts, compared with those receiving transplanted extrasynovial tendon, at 3 and 6 weeks. Tendons receiving extrasynovial grafts had significantly greater linear stiffness than did those of the intrasynovial group. These findings were consistent with histologic findings of postoperative adhesions in specimens with an extrasynovial graft. The extrasynovial tendon graft complex had significantly higher ultimate loads than the intrasynovial tendon graft complex at 6 weeks.

Conclusion.—These data suggest a donor tissue–specific healing process after flexor tendon grafting with autogenous grafts. Intrasynovial tendon grafts enhance inherent cellularity with less need for tissue ingrowth, whereas extrasynovial tendon grafts depend on the ingrowth of tissue from extrinsic sources. Thus, the latter are associated with greater postoperative adhesion formation and result in decreased tendon gliding function.

▶ Noguchi and colleagues have published a series of papers confirming the fact that tendons which have a synovial sheath are different, in many ways, from those that do not. Sheathed, or intrasynovial, tendons glide with less friction; heal with fewer adhesions; and now apparently, also heal more slowly than their extrasynovial brethren. Most of the time, the latter drawback will be outweighed by the obvious advantages of better motion.

Unfortunately, intrasynovial tendon *grafts* are hard to come by. Most expendable tendon sources are extrasynovial, such as the palmaris and plantaris tendons. It is possible that the extensor indicis, which has an intrasynovial component at the wrist, may serve if the intrasynovial part is placed in the sheath to be grafted. Otherwise, we will probably have to make do with extrasynovial grafts as we always have; only now, we will know *why* they don't work so well.

P.C. Amadio, M.D.

Effect of Immobilization, Immediate Mobilization, and Delayed Mobilization on the Resistance to Digital Flexion Using a Tendon Injury Model

Halikis MN, Manske PR, Kubota H, et al (Washington Univ, St Louis)

J Hand Surg (Am) 22A:464–472, 1997 17–11

Background.—Instituting passive or active motion after flexor tendon repair can ameliorate the negative effects of tendon immobilization, the limiting factor being the strength of the repair site. Determinations of the minimum strength of repair allowing mobilization rehabilitation without repair rupture have been based on previous research. However, current values do not account for the effect of adhesions on resisting flexion nor compensate for the potential effects of surgical trauma and early motion on the properties of the digit. Such factors may increase the force or work necessary for flexing the digit.

Methods and Findings.—A tendon injury model in chickens was used to determine the effect of immobilization, immediate mobilization, and delayed mobilization on the energy needed to fully flex the digit after surgical trauma to the tendon, as determined by measurement of the work of flexion (WOF). No increased WOF was observed in the immobilized group at 3 days, compared with the zero time control values. However, at 1, 2, and 3 weeks, WOF was increased significantly by 36%, 41%, and 63%, respectively. The tendons immobilized immediately had an initial 36% increase in WOF at 3 days, increasing to 40% at 1 week, and declining to baseline values by 3 weeks. Delaying mobilization until 5 days did not significantly decrease the peak WOF value at 1 week. However, delaying it until 3 days reduced that peak WOF value to 13%. In both the 3- and 5-day delayed-mobilization groups there was a return to baseline WOF values by 3 weeks (Fig 5).

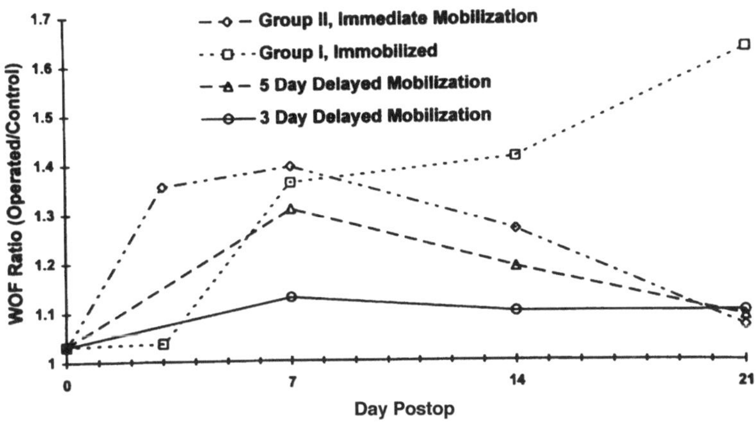

FIGURE 5.—Results for day 0 and groups 1, 2, and 3 to show comparison of work of flexion (*WOF*) ratios at 7, 14, and 21 days. The 3-day delayed-mobilization subgroup of group 3 has a much lower WOF ratio at 7 days than the other groups. (Courtesy of Halikis MN, Manske PR, Kubota H, et al: Effect of immobilization, immediate mobilization, and delayed mobilization on the resistance to digital flexion using a tendon injury model. *J Hand Surg [Am]* 22A:464–472, 1997.)

Conclusion.—There is an early increase in the work needed for flexion of the injured operated digit and tendon that is present in the immediately mobilized tendons at 3 days, persisting to 1 week. This increase does not appear in immobilized tendons until 1 week. The rise in WOF may be ameliorated by delaying the institution of mobilization.

► It is generally believed that early mobilization of flexor tendon repairs improves outcome, at least as far as final motion is concerned. But how early? Some surgeons initiate motion a day or 2 after surgery; others wait a few days for hemostasis and for edema to subside. It appears that patience is a virtue. Waiting 3 days (in chickens; in humans probably about the same time) seems to reduce gliding resistance. This should translate into better clinical results.

P.C. Amadio, M.D.

Sarcomere Length Changes After Flexor Carpi Ulnaris to Extensor Digitorum Communis Tendon Transfer

Lieber RL, Pontén E, Burkholder TJ, et al (Univ of California, San Diego; Univ of Umeå, Sweden; Gothenburg Univ, Sweden)

J Hand Surg (Am) 21A:612–618, 1996 17–12

Background.—Tendon transfers are commonly performed to restore function in the upper extremity after trauma, peripheral nerve injury, spinal cord injury, brain injury, and neuromuscular disease. However, neither the specific functional and structural characteristics of the donor muscles nor the specific length at which the muscles should be attached has been investigated thoroughly. Sarcomere length in the flexor carpi ulnaris (FCU) muscle before and after transfer into the tendons of the extensor digitorum communis muscle (EDC) was measured.

Methods and Findings.—Five patients who were undergoing tendon transfer of the FCU to the EDC for radial nerve palsy were included. The absolute sarcomere length and sarcomere length operating range of the FCU increased after transfer into the EDC. Before surgery, the mean FCU sarcomere length was 4.22 μm with the wrist fully extended and fingers flexed and 3.19 μm with the wrist fully flexed. Thus, the overall sarcomere length range was 1.03 μm. All sarcomere lengths increased significantly after tendon transfer using standard recommended techniques. At the increased sarcomere lengths, the FCU muscle was predicted to develop relatively high force only during movement involving synergistic wrist flexion and finger extension. The transferred FCU muscle was predicted to produce maximum force over approximately 30 degrees of wrist flexion and 0 degrees of finger flexion to 90 degrees of wrist extension and 90 degrees of finger flexion. Transferring the muscle at a longer length would be more desirable.

Conclusion.—The shorter-fibered FCU acting on a larger moment arm at the wrist and digits results in longer sarcomere lengths and concomitantly lower muscle forces than normally observed for the FCU. Overstretch of the FCU has profound consequences in tendon transfer, as it is the shortest-fibered muscle acting at the wrist. In addition, transferring the FCU at a longer sarcomere length dramatically increases muscle force in the position of functional grasp, which may result in significant functional advantages. The disadvantage of this is that less force is produced by the muscle when the wrist is in the more flexed position. It is unknown whether this would represent a functional loss.

▶ The sarcomere length of the donor muscle is the muscle architectural parameter that can be surgically adjusted to produce greater muscle force in specific wrist and finger positions. Making accurate intraoperative sarcomere length adjustments by setting the resting length of the donor tendon, however, has remained a challenge. The authors combine fundamental muscle architecture principles, optimum sarcomere length data for the FCU, and laser diffraction techniques to show that intraoperative manipulation of muscle architecture is possible. They propose that transferring the FCU to the EDC at a longer sarcomere resting length (i.e., more stretched) than is currently done may improve FCU force production for functional finger and wrist positions. However, the authors acknowledge that their small sample size and the ability of some musculotendons to add sarcomeres postoperatively may preclude generalization of their results.

Optimizing the sarcomere resting length of the transferred FCU may be desirable because adequate index finger extensor tendon force is essential to maintain finger position while producing high key and tip pinch forces.[1, 2] Lastly, the authors emphasize that force production of the transferred FCU will be compromised at other positions because the increased tendon excursion will place its sarcomeres further into the descending limb of the force-length curve. Although these techniques may not yet be applicable in the typical operating room, this paper's application of fundamental principles of muscle architecture and new techniques is worth noting.

F.J. Valero-Cuevas, Ph.D.

References

1. Valero-Cuevas FJ: Muscle coordination of the human index finger (thesis). Stanford University, Stanford, California, 1997.
2. Valero-Cuevas FJ, Zajoc F, Burger C, et al: Musculoskeletal interactions which limit finger tip forces. Presented at the 5th International Conference of Surgical Rehabilitation of the Upper Limb in Tetraplegia, Melbourne, Australia, 1995.

Ultrasound Velocity Measurement in Long Bones: Measurement Method and Simulation of Ultrasound Wave Propagation

Lowet G, Van der Perre G (KU Leuven, Belgium)

J Biomech 29:1255–1262, 1996 17–13

Introduction.—There is increasing interest in quantitative measurement of the mechanical properties of bone for clinical purposes, for example, monitoring of fracture healing. Several techniques have been suggested for measuring the stiffness of long bones, such as vibration methods and the use of strain gauges on external fixators. Ultrasound velocity determination is 1 proposed method for evaluating the elastic properties of bone, although its in vivo application has been limited by several problems. A new approach to the measurement of ultrasound velocity in bone was presented.

Methods and Findings.—The new technique, based on the principle of pulse transmission, uses a high-voltage pulse transmitted through the bone to a receiver at a known distance (Fig 1). Propagation times are recorded as the 2 transducers are moved farther apart, and a graph is made showing the linear relationship between the distance and propagation time (Fig 2). The method includes automatic correction for the influence of soft tissue. A series of simulations, using intact bars and bars with gaps of variable width and depth, was performed to test hypotheses regarding the ultra-

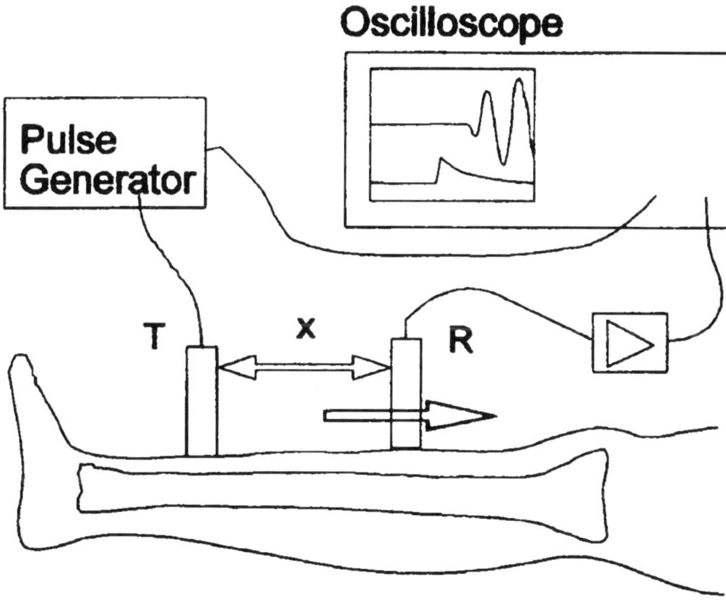

FIGURE 1.—Measurement principle. (Reprinted from Lowet G, Van der Perre G: Ultrasound velocity measurement in long bones: Measurement method and simulation of ultrasound wave propagation. *J Biomech* 29:1255–1262. Copyright 1996, with kind permission from Elsevier Science Ltd, The Boulevard, Langford Lane, Kidlington OX5 16B UK.)

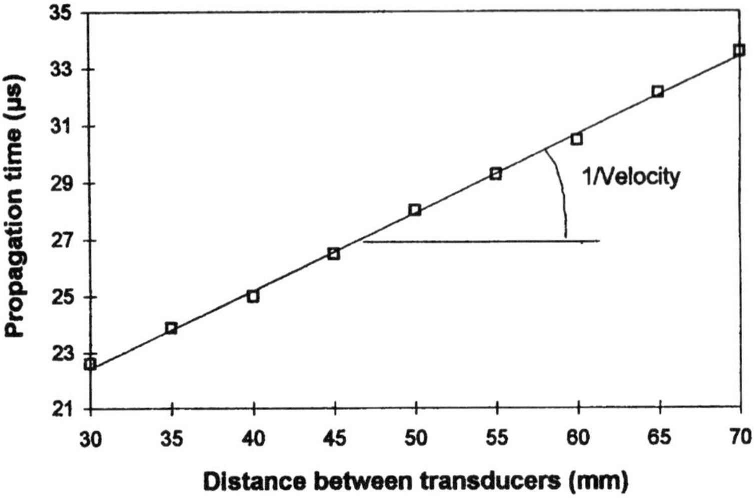

FIGURE 2.—Measurement graph. (Reprinted from Lowet G, Van der Perre G: Ultrasound velocity measurement in long bones: Measurement method and simulation of ultrasound wave propagation. *J Biomech* 29:1255–1262. Copyright 1996, with kind permission from Elsevier Science Ltd, The Boulevard, Langford Lane, Kidlington OX5 16B UK.)

sound wave path through the bone. There was good agreement between the predicted wave path and the measurements obtained in the experimental setup. When the setup included a fracture gap of sufficient size, even the local velocity of the material in the gap was measurable.

Conclusions.—This new technique of measuring ultrasound velocity through bone may be useful in assessing fracture healing, such as monitoring callus formation, and in studying bone metabolic disorders, such as osteoporosis. If the ultrasound wave path is not straight, this will have to be considered in the data interpretation.

▶ This article focuses on the problem of soft-tissue interference in measurement of the speed of sound through bone tissue, and it offers—at least for long bones and, in particular, the tibia—an interesting effective mathematical approach. The study is relevant for a recently introduced measurement technique for the ultrasound diagnosis of osteoporosis at the tibia. The method investigates the transmission of ultrasound on the longitudinal axis of the tibial anterior surface.[1] Although the article contains several formulas, the clear exposition allows even a reader not familiar with mathematics to follow the text easily.

Actually, different assumptions are undertaken concerning the homogeneity of the materials, and only in vivo studies will demonstrate how the dishomogeneity, both of the bone tissue and the thickness variation of the soft tissue, will affect the measurements. This method also seems to be able to find out the effect of the presence of a gap in the homogeneity of the "bone tissue" and to quantify its characteristics. It would be important if these observations have significant clinical correspondences.

Certainly this is a new approach for evaluation by ultrasound of the progression of bone healing. The method appears to be much easier, more reproducible, and more practicable than what has been described previously in literature. References to the use of ultrasound for the evaluation of bone tissue are not sufficiently updated.[2]

R. Cadossi, M.D.

References

1. Orgee JM, Foster H, McCloskey EV, et al: A precise method for the assessment of tibial ultrasound velocity. *Osteoporosis Int* 6:1–7, 1996.
2. Cadossi R, Cane V: Pathways of transmission of ultrasound energy through the distal metaphysis of the second phalanx of pigs. *Osteoporos Int* 6:196–209, 1996.

A Dynamic Model for Simulating Movements of the Elbow, Forearm, and Wrist

Lemay MA, Crago PE (Case Western Reserve Univ, Cleveland, Ohio)

J Biomech 29:1319–1330, 1996 17–14

Introduction.—Various models of the upper extremity have been developed to study the static effects of muscle actions and joint forces. However, they have not been useful in studying the motions of the limbs, as moved by muscles with time-varying activation. Such models are much more useful if they include motion dynamics. A dynamic upper extremity model was developed to simulate the movements of the forearm and wrist.

Methods.—The skeletal model includes the elbow, forearm, and wrist. The skeletal structure is dynamically controlled using a Hill-type model of muscles and is capable of elbow flexion/extension, forearm pronosupination, wrist flexion/extension, and radial/ulnar deviation. The passive moments providing limits on joint motion are modeled after experimental studies. The model was used to study muscle output force sensitivity, together with wrist flexion/extension motion sensitivity to variations in the parameters.

Results.—The sensitivity analysis demonstrated the importance of muscle fiber-length, force, and moment arm on the joint movement–generating capacity of a muscle, providing important insights into the planning of tendon transfer operations. The factors with the greatest influence on muscle output and flexion/extension of the wrist were tendon slack length and muscle fiber length. Tendon stiffness had little influence on muscle force output at ratios of tendon slack length to muscle length of less than 2. The model accurately reflected the moment vectors at the wrist. However, the moments predicted by the model were much higher than those measured by stimulation of the paralyzed muscles of 1 patient with tetraplegia.

Conclusion.—A dynamic model of the elbow, forearm, and wrist confirms the important contributions of muscle length, force, and moment arm on the ability of muscles to produce motion. The model's dynamic capabilities are more fully explored in a companion article. The authors hope that their model will improve evaluation of tendon transfer and functional neuromuscular stimulation in tetraplegics.

▶ It is understandable that a given upper-extremity function (e.g., lifting force of the arm) is dependent on some anatomical factors (e.g., the strength of the biceps muscle, its moment arm at the elbow) more than others. Identifying the critical factors from the many biomechanical elements of the upper limb is difficult. The functional outcome of upper-extremity reconstructions stands to benefit greatly from the identification of these factors, specially if they are surgically alterable.

This paper presents a sophisticated model of the upper limb in which biomechanical (e.g., moment arms) and muscle architectural parameters (e.g., resting tendon length) are individually specified. This allows the calculation of the sensitivity of arm function to each factor. Tendon resting length and muscle fiber length were found to influence muscle forces and wrist motion most. Tendon resting length is surgically alterable. Therefore, this work shows that detailed biomechanical models hold great promise for the optimization of current surgical techniques and the development of innovative surgical techniques for restoring upper-extremity function.

F.J. Valero-Cuevas, Ph.D.

Isolation and Quantitation of Debris Particles Around Failed Silicone Orthopedic Implants

Hirakawa K, Bauer TW, Culver JE, et al (Cleveland Clinic Found, Ohio; Cleveland Ctr for Joint Reconstruction, Ohio)

J Hand Surg (Am) 21A:819–827, 1996 17–15

Introduction.—Silicone elastomer arthroplasty of the finger, wrist, and elbow has become more popular since the 1960s, and the implants have had a low rate of complications; however, there have been reports of inflammatory reactions related to wear debris. The composition, number, size, and shape of debris appears to have an effect on the tissue reaction, but the size and dose of debris adjacent to the failed silicone implants are not clear. A recently developed assay was used to characterize the debris associated with silicone-induced granulomas in 10 patients.

Methods.—Ten patients, ranging in age from 33 to 70 years, with silicone elastomer implants in the wrist, elbow, or finger, had their debris particles in the periarticular tissues isolated and quantified. The indications for implant insertion where rheumatoid arthritis and avascular necrosis of the lunate after injury. At the time of removal of fragmented silicone elbow, wrist, or metacarpophalangeal joint implants, the 10 specimens were obtained. As controls, 5 rheumatoid synovia without implants were used. Studies included morphologic and chemical characterization of particles, the effect of digestion on debris materials, and light microscopic analysis.

Results.—All patients had particles of foreign material in the connective and synovial tissue. Nearly all particles were silicone, according to x-ray spectroscopy; the number of particles ranged from 0.99 to 24.8 × 10^{-9} g (dry weight) of tissue, and they were small with a mode particle diameter of 0.59 ± 0.057 µm. For the 5 wrist implants, the number of particles correlated with duration in vivo, and the implantation duration for all ranged from 3.2 to 10.6 years.

Conclusion.—Adjacent to failed silicone implants are billions of particles, most of which are smaller than 1 µm, and may be associated with bone resorption and inflammation. The mechanisms of osteolysis and local tissue injury induced by silicone particles require further study.

► The authors have performed an extremely thorough and careful investigation to characterize the size and number of silicone debris particles present in the periarticular tissues of 10 patients with failed wrist, elbow, or finger implants.

This study points out that high doses of very small particles (0.5 µm) are released into tissues adjacent to failed implants. The study further suggests that the high doses present may be even greater because of instrument limitations on the detection of even smaller particles. It is interesting that the authors report a wide variability of particles/g × 10^9 in tissue, even within the same patient, e.g., in 1 patient, 8.99 particles/g x 10^9 and 24.8 particles/g × 10^9 were present in periarticular wrist tissues. It is not known whether tissues were taken from bilateral wrists in this patient. An interesting finding was the uniform infiltrate of lymphocyte and plasma cells associated with silicone debris particles suggesting the possibility of an immune mediated response. It is very difficult in rheumatoid patients to determine whether this inflammatory response is the result of the disease or is caused by the silicone. However, the authors did observe this inflammation in nonrheumatoid patients who received implants for posttraumatic ischemic necrosis of the lunate.

The authors have performed an excellent study, which denotes that billions of silicone particles may be released from failed implants into periarticular tissues. Further study should help to clarify the consequences of this regarding osteolysis and the mechanisms of implant failure itself.

M.A. Badalamente, Ph.D.

Suggested Reading

Amadio PC, Higgs P, Keith M: Prospective comparative clinical trials in *The Journal of Hand Surgery (American)*. *J Hand Surg (Am)* 21A:925–929, 1996.

► The authors reviewed volumes 1–19 of the American *Journal of Hand Surgery* and identified 25 articles with methodology satisfying the criteria of a "controlled clinical trial" and 8 articles satisfying criteria for a "randomized controlled trial." The survey included over 3,000 articles, case reports, etc. The actual number of "gold standard" type studies is unimpressive. This is probably a reflection of the difficulty in planning and conducting rigorous clinical research.

V.R. Hentz, M.D.

Hermann RP, Novak CB, Mackinnon SE: Establishing normal values of moving two-point discrimination in children and adolescents. *Dev Med Child Neurol* 38:255–261, 1996.

▶ This study of 313 subjects evenly divided between males and females concluded that normal values of moving 2-point discrimination for individuals ages 4–18 years old is 2–4 mm. Since this study has confirmed others' work, a more interesting finding was that for children aged 5 years and younger, this test is of little practical value given the high likelihood of an unreliable response.

R.M. Szabo, M.D., M.P.H.

Jensen CH, Jensen CM: Biodegradable pins versus Kirschner wires in hand surgery. *J Hand Surg (Br)* 21B:507–510, 1996.

▶ This small but well-done prospective randomized study shows that the latest generation of biodegradable pins made of poly-p-dioxanone may not have the bone lysis properties of the earlier polyglycolic acid pins. However, there are still problems with insertion technique as the pins require predrilling. Also, adequate mechanical strength needs to be demonstrated as the pins degrade.

L.K. Ruby, M.D.

Tang JB, Shi D, Zhang QG, et al: Biomechanical and histologic evaluation of tendon sheath management. *J Hand Surg (Am)* 21A:900–908, 1996.

▶ Using a relatively standard chicken tendon/tendon sheath model, the investigators analyzed the effects on tendon gliding of enlarging, narrowing, and closing the sheath after tendon repair. Sheath closure remains controversial. This study clearly shows that if sheath closure results in narrowing of the sheath, the results are compromised. From a practical standpoint, it is very difficult to simply reapproximate the sheath once it is incised, even in an uninjured digit. The study suggests that if one believes that a closed sheath promotes better results, closure should include interposing some additional autogenous tissue to avoid sheath narrowing.

V.R. Hentz, M.D.

Subject Index*

A

* *All entries refer to the year and page number(s) for data appearing in this and previous editions of the* Year Book.

B

D

E

G

I

J

L

M

N

O

P

S

T

U

V

W

X

Z

Author Index

A

B

C

D

E

F

G

H

I

J

K

L

M

N

O

P

R

S

T

U

V

W

Y

Z